NEURAL PLASTICITY AND COGNITIVE DEVELOPMENT

Neural Plasticity and Cognitive Development

INSIGHTS FROM CHILDREN WITH PERINATAL BRAIN INJURY

Joan Stiles, PhD
EMERITUS PROFESSOR OF COGNITIVE SCIENCE
UNIVERSITY OF CALIFORNIA, SAN DIEGO
LA JOLLA, CA

Judy S. Reilly, PhD
EMERITUS PROFESSOR OF PSYCHOLOGY
SAN DIEGO STATE UNIVERSITY
SAN DIEGO, CA; AND
UNIVERSITÉ DE POITIERS-CNRS, FRANCE

Susan C. Levine, PhD
STELLA M. ROWLEY PROFESSOR
DEPARTMENTS OF PSYCHOLOGY, COMPARATIVE HUMAN DEVELOPMENT, AND COMMITTEE ON EDUCATION; AND
CHAIR, DEPARTMENT OF PSYCHOLOGY
UNIVERSITY OF CHICAGO
CHICAGO, IL

Doris A. Trauner, MD
PROFESSOR OF NEUROSCIENCES AND PEDIATRICS
UNIVERSITY OF CALIFORNIA, SAN DIEGO SCHOOL OF MEDICINE
LA JOLLA, CA; AND
CHIEF, PEDIATRIC NEUROLOGY
UNIVERSITY OF CALIFORNIA, SAN DIEGO SCHOOL OF MEDICINE AND RADY CHILDREN'S HOSPITAL SAN DIEGO
SAN DIEGO, CA

Ruth Nass, MD
PROFESSOR OF CHILD NEUROLOGY, CHILD AND ADOLESCENT PSYCHIATRY, AND PEDIATRICS
NEW YORK UNIVERSITY SCHOOL OF MEDICINE
NEW YORK, NY

OXFORD
UNIVERSITY PRESS

OXFORD
UNIVERSITY PRESS

Oxford University Press, Inc., publishes works that further
Oxford University's objective of excellence
in research, scholarship, and education.

Oxford New York
Auckland Cape Town Dar es Salaam Hong Kong Karachi
Kuala Lumpur Madrid Melbourne Mexico City Nairobi
New Delhi Shanghai Taipei Toronto

With offices in
Argentina Austria Brazil Chile Czech Republic France Greece
Guatemala Hungary Italy Japan Poland Portugal Singapore
South Korea Switzerland Thailand Turkey Ukraine Vietnam

Published by Oxford University Press, Inc.
198 Madison Avenue, New York, New York 10016
www.oup.com

Library of Congress Cataloging-in-Publication Data

Neural plasticity and cognitive development : insights from children
with perinatal brain injury/Joan Stiles . . . [et al.].
p.; cm.
Includes bibliographical references and index.
ISBN 978-0-19-538994-4 (hardcover)
I. Stiles, Joan.
[DNLM: 1. Brain Injuries—complications. 2. Infant, Newborn. 3. Brain—growth & development.
4. Child Development. 5. Child. 6. Developmental Disabilities—etiology. 7. Infant. 8. Neuronal
Plasticity—physiology. WS 340]
617.4'81044—dc23 2011043998

"Language is a new machine built out of old parts emerging from a nexus of skills in attention, perception, imitation, and symbolic processing that transcend the boundaries of language proper."

—Elizabeth A. Bates

We dedicate this volume to our friend and colleague Liz Bates. The core questions addressed in this book were central to her scientific quest. She pursued these ideas with great dedication, verve, and infectious enthusiasm. Our only regret is that she could not be here to help with the integration and synthesis of the theory and data from this project that has been such a big part of all of our scientific lives.

Preface

THIS BOOK ORIGINATED with a collaboration that began more than 30 years ago. In the ensuing years, the changes in developmental cognitive neuroscience have been both exciting and dramatic. Thirty years ago collaborations between brain and cognitive scientists were more the exception than the rule. The disciplinary boundaries were high and the conversations limited, but threads of what would become cognitive neuroscience were beginning to emerge. One venue for this new discipline was an initiative begun by George Miller at Princeton University and Mike Gazzaniga at the Cornell Medical School in New York City, aimed at bridging the disciplinary divide and initiating the crucial conversations between cognitive psychologists and neuropsychologists. The initiative took the form of colloquia and pilot research projects among scientists at George's cognitive psychology laboratory and Mike's brain sciences laboratory. One of those conversations had an important impact on the work presented in this book and the direction of the careers of several of its authors. In 1980, Joan Stiles (JS) was a graduate student in cognitive psychology at Princeton and Ruth Nass (RN), who had studied with Rita Rudel during her residency, was a pediatric neurologist at Cornell Medical Center. A colloquium on cognitive development given at Cornell prompted RN to explore the possibility of a collaboration focused on an interesting but understudied population, children with focal perinatal brain lesions (PL). That collaboration was the basis of JS's Ph.D. thesis, the subject of 30 years of collaborative research, and the impetus for this book. In the ensuing years, the research initiative grew. JS moved to UCSD and in 1985 helped to found what later became the Project in Cognitive and Neural Development, which was a focal point for studying the PL population in San Diego. Our multidisciplinary collaborative group also grew to include Doris Trauner (pediatric neurologist) who had trained with Peter Huttenlocher at the University of Chicago, Judy Reilly (linguist), and our late colleague Elizabeth Bates (psycholinguist). Our collaboration with

Susan Levine, a developmental psychologist who had studied with Hans-Lucas Teuber as a graduate student and later worked with Peter Huttenlocher, began more recently when the group at the University of Chicago initiated a parallel study of language development in the PL population.

The changes we have observed in both theory and methods over these 30 years have been dramatic. When we began, the dominant neuropsychological views were based on strongly localizationist models derived from studies of adult lesion patients. These models were derived from the available data at the time. Neuroimaging data were extremely limited; thus, diagnosis of lesion location was based upon behavioral assessment. This approach promoted a modular view of brain organization that involved strongly localized structure–function mappings. Nonetheless developmental models diverged from this strong localizationist view. Several prescient studies hinted that the developing brain did not share this modular organization, and this was particularly evident in cases of early neuropathology. Language was a central focus of many early studies, and a number of early investigators noted that language function was spared in children with right hemiplegia or left early hemidecortication, relative to adults with lesions to mature language regions. This finding led to the suggestion that the brain may organize differently in the wake of early injury. However, there were no direct measures of brain function to support these hypotheses. Indeed, an important impetus for RN's proposed collaboration was newly available imaging technology that would allow for direct assessment of the lesion size and site, which could then be mapped to behavioral profiles.

This book is the story of how our knowledge and perspective concerning neurobehavioral development has changed in the intervening 30 years, and how advances in theory and technology have fundamentally altered our ways of thinking about the development of brain-behavior relations. As can be seen in the range of expertise in our collaborative group, the study of brain–behavior relations has become an increasingly multidisciplinary endeavor. Advances in our understanding of neurobiological development, improvement of brain imaging technologies, and refinement of behavioral methodologies have all contributed to our changing view of neurobehavioral development. This book is intended to capture the extent of progress in each of these areas. The book ends with an attempt to provide a framework for understanding neurobehavioral development that captures the breadth and scope of the multidisciplinary advances that we have both participated in and observed over these many years.

Over the years a great many people have contributed to the work reported here. Indeed, the list is much too long to include here, but we would like to express our appreciation and gratitude to all of our many colleagues and collaborators from around the world who have contributed to this important enterprise. We would also like to express our thanks to a number of colleagues who have provided thoughtful input and helpful critiques of various chapters in this volume. These include Natacha Akshoomoff, Tim Brown, Jason Carmel, Frank Haist, and Annette Karmiloff-Smith. We are grateful for all of their insights. We would also like to thank the children and families who have worked with us for so many years. Their enthusiasm and dedication makes this work possible. Finally, we would like to acknowledge the institutions that over many years have provided funding for this work. These include: The March of Dimes, United Cerebral Palsy, the Kavli Institute for Brain and

Mind, and the many institutes and agencies of the United States National Institutes of Health, including the National Institute of Neurological Disorders and Stroke, the Eunice Kennedy Schriver National Institute of Child Health and Human Development, the National Institute on Deafness and Other Communicative Disorders, and the National Institute of Mental Health.

Joan Stiles
Judy Reilly
Susan Levine
Doris Trauner
Ruth Nass
(October 2011)

Contents

PART ONE

Neurobiology

1

Neuroplasticity and the Developing Brain

OVER THE PAST several decades, developmental neurobiologists have made tremendous progress in defining basic principles of mammalian brain development. This work has fundamentally changed the way we think about how the brain develops. Forty years ago, the dominant model was strongly deterministic (Gottlieb, 1976, 1998; Johnson, 2001; Oyama, 2000), reflecting the influences of maturational models of embryological development and simplified views of gene expression. The relationship between brain and behavioral development was viewed as unidirectional; that is, brain maturation enables behavioral development. The advent of modern neurobiological methods has provided a very different view of how brains develop. There is now overwhelming evidence that it is the *interaction* of genetic factors and the experience of the individual that underlies brain development (Stiles, 2008). Brains do not develop normally in the absence of critical genetic signaling, *and* they do not develop normally in the absence of essential environmental input. Together genetic signaling and environmental cues work in concert to support the progressive development of the mammalian brain.

Because brain development is a dynamic process, it is also adaptive and capable of adjusting to various contingencies that may arise from either the biological system or the environment. The term "neural plasticity" has been used to capture this adaptive aspect of development (Stiles, 2000). Neural plasticity is a ubiquitous term that has been applied to virtually all levels of the neurocognitive system from molecules to behavior (Collignon, Voss, Lassonde, & Lepore, 2009; Green & Bavelier, 2008; Kuczewski, Porcher, Lessmann, Medina, & Gaiarsa, 2009; Mehler, 2008; Morita, 2009; Tropea, Van Wart, & Sur, 2009). It thus encompasses a vast array of potential mechanisms and functional effects. Indeed, its usage is so wide-ranging that the utility of the term may be questioned (Berlucchi & Buchtel, 2009). However, there is a common conceptual thread that unites the different levels of description and defines a fundamental principal of brain development—specifically, the principle of neural adaptation. In the broadest sense and at all levels of the neurocognitive system, neural plasticity refers to the capacity of the developing brain to adapt to current demands and circumstances, whether that involves epigenetic modulation of gene expression, the responsiveness of axons to guidance molecules, neuronal competition for trophic factors at synaptic junctions, adjustments of neural networks to variations in input, or the reorganization of neural systems in the wake of injury or insult. At every point in development and at every level of the neural system, the capacity to adapt is essential to the functional viability of the organism; indeed, failure to adapt can have catastrophic consequences (Kalia, 2008). As such, neural plasticity is a central feature of brain development (Pascual-Leone, Amedi, Fregni, & Merabet, 2005).

Much of what is known about the plasticity of the developing mammalian brain has come from studies of animal species as diverse as mouse, ferret, cat, and rhesus macaque. These studies have provided critical information about the range and limits of plasticity in the developing brain. The early studies of Kennard (1936, 1938a, 1938b) demonstrated the resilience of young animals to early neural insult. The seminal studies of Hubel and Wiesel (Hubel & Freeman, 1977; Hubel & Wiesel, 1963a, 1963b, 1977; Hubel, Wiesel, & LeVay, 1977; Wiesel & Hubel, 1963a, 1963b, 1963c, 1965a, 1965b) were among the first to show that primary sensory cortices organize differently in response to altered input. The now-extensive body of work examining the effects of rearing conditions on brain development has documented the dramatic effects that impoverished environments can have on all aspects of the neural system, from the elaboration of dendritic arbors to enhancement of the cerebral vascular system (Denenberg, 1981; Greenough, 1993; Greenough, Black, & Wallace, 1987; Greenough, Hwang, & Gorman, 1985; Nithianantharajah & Hannan, 2006; Rosenzweig & Bennett, 1972; Rosenzweig, Krech, Bennett, & Diamond, 1962; Rosenzweig, Krech, Bennett, & Zolman, 1962; Rosenzweig, Love, & Bennett, 1968). Experimental lesion studies have documented the capacity of the complex neural systems to organize differently in the wake of early injury (Bachevalier & Mishkin, 1994; Goldman-Rakic, 1981, 1988; Goldman-Rakic & Leung, 2002; Kolb, 1987, 1995; Kolb, Cioe, & Muirhead, 1998; Kolb & Elliott, 1987; Kolb, Holmes, & Whishaw, 1987; Kolb & Tomie, 1988; Kolb & Whishaw, 2000; Sur, Angelucci, & Sharma, 1999; Sur, Garraghty, & Roe, 1988; Sur & Leamey, 2001; Sur, Pallas, & Roe, 1990; Sur & Rubenstein, 2005). More recently, studies of synaptic plasticity have begun to elucidate the complex molecular factors that underlie learning and memory at the cellular level (Alberini, 2009; Barker, 2009; Kuczewski et al., 2009; Mattson, 2008).

While all of the animal work has been critically important to our understanding of the role and mechanisms of plasticity in mammalian brain development, its applicability to our understanding of human brain development is indirect and its contribution to our understanding of the effects of early injury on higher cognitive functions, such as language or problem solving, is limited. The invasive nature of the animal methodologies precludes comparable experimental studies of humans; however, the unfortunate occurrence of "natural experiments" presents a means for exploring questions that cannot be studied by traditional experiment approaches. One such natural experiment involves a rare population of children who suffered localized, unilateral brain lesions in the perinatal period. The study of children with perinatal brain injury provides the opportunity to examine the effects of very early-occurring lesions on brain and cognitive development in humans, and offers a way of exploring the role of neural plasticity in human brain development.

The remaining sections of this chapter will examine the larger sets of issues that serve to frame the essential questions about neurocognitive development following perinatal brain injury. The first section of the chapter reviews in greater detail the evidence from animal studies on developmental neural plasticity in the mammalian brain. It focuses primarily either on the effects of altering the early experience of the organism, or on the effects of explicit experimental manipulation of the developing neural substrate. The purpose of this section is to establish the case for neural plasticity in the developing mammalian brain. The next section addresses the question of limitations on plasticity. While animal studies have been the source of considerable evidence supporting the construct of neural plasticity, they also provide insight into the limits of plasticity. This section examines factors such as location and extent of injury, timing of insult, and variation in effects of injury on different neural subsystems. The section also examines the construct of the critical or sensitive period as a constraining factor on neural plasticity. The final two sections of this chapter return to questions concerning the effects of perinatal injury on neurocognitive functioning in human children. The discussion begins by considering the historical role of the "lesion method" as a general approach to studying neural organization in adult populations. It then focuses on the differences in the logic of the lesion method when applied to child populations. It argues that while studies of adult lesion patients are designed to elucidate basic structure–function mapping within the neurocognitive system, studies of children provide a window on questions of neurocognitive plasticity and developmental adaptation (Moses & Stiles, 2002). Finally, taking as background the studies of neural plasticity in other species, the last section of this chapter asks fundamental questions about the nature and extent of neural plasticity in the developing human brain. It argues that longitudinal studies of children with discrete, early occurring neural injury can make significant contributions to our understanding of fundamental mechanisms of neural plasticity, and will extend our understanding to the relationship between neural plasticity and higher cognitive processes, including language. It thus sets the stage for the remainder of this book.

NEURAL PLASTICITY: EVIDENCE FROM ANIMAL STUDIES

The idea that the developing brain may exhibit resilience not observed among adults is not new. Clinical observations and experimental studies documenting mitigation of functional loss following early injury date from at least the 19th century (Broca, 1865; Brown, 1915; Kennard, 1936, 1938a, 1938b; Kennard & Fulton, 1942; Langworthy, 1924; Weed & Kennard, 1917). By the 1940s Hebb (Hebb, 1949) had begun to explore the idea that experience alone could alter neural development. This section reviews evidence for neural plasticity from animal studies. Three primary categories of experiments are considered. These include studies on the effects of (1) experimental alteration of the neural substrate; (2) alteration of sensory input; and (3) experimental variation in environmental complexity.

The Effects of Experimentally Altering the Neural Substrate

By mid-gestation, most neocortical neurons have been produced (Clancy, Darlington, & Finlay, 2001), and within weeks they will have completed their migration to the neocortex. A number of studies have explored questions about the extent to which the fate of neurons in different cortical regions is fixed at the time they are produced or whether it can be altered by changes in the local environment. Put simply, can, for example, the function of neurons initially fated to become part of visual or somatosensory cortex be altered by exposure to a different set of signaling cues? These questions have been addressed experimentally in two types of studies. Cortical explant studies involve the experimental transplantation of tissue from a typical cortical region in a donor animal to an atypical region in a host animal, and ask whether the neurons retain their original characteristics or take on those of the atypical region in the host. Experimental lesion studies ask what happens to cortical organization when particular brain regions or pathways are removed or disconnected.

Cortical Explant Studies

In an early series of cortical explant studies, O'Leary and Stanfield (1989) moved sections of somatosensory tissue (tissue explants) from the brain of a fetal donor animal to the occipital region of a newborn host animal (Fig. 1.1). They also did the converse, moving donor occipital tissue to the host's sensorimotor region. The experiment was designed to test the fundamental question of whether the tissue explants would adapt to the host environment or whether they would retain the characteristics of the donor. For both of these procedures, the transplanted cells survived and began to take on characteristics of cells in the host environment. Visual neurons transplanted to the somatosensory areas extended permanent axonal connections to the spinal cord, a subcortical target for sensorimotor neurons. Sensorimotor neurons transplanted into visual cortex extended axons to the superior colliculus, a subcortical visual target. Transplanted tissue in both areas established callosal and thalamic projections typical of their host environment. In addition, the transplanted cells developed intra-regional patterns of organization typical of the host cortical area. For example, somatosensory regions of rat cortex normally form well-demarcated anatomical features, called "barrel fields." Each component barrel within a cortical barrel field reflects input from one whisker on the animal's face. The two dimensional spatial layout of whiskers on the animal's face is maintained at the level of cortex and that organization defines the cortical barrel field. Within somatosensory cortex, transplanted visual tissue not only formed connections appropriate for somatosensory cortex, it also developed the characteristic barrel field patterning, further supporting the capacity of tissue to adapt to the local signaling cues (Schlaggar & O'Leary, 1991). The cortical explant studies suggest that the early functional specificity of neurons is not fixed. Rather, exposure to cues arising from different brain areas can alter the developmental trajectory of the young neurons and induce the cells to adapt to the signaling cues and patterns of connectivity appropriate to the experimentally re-specified brain region.

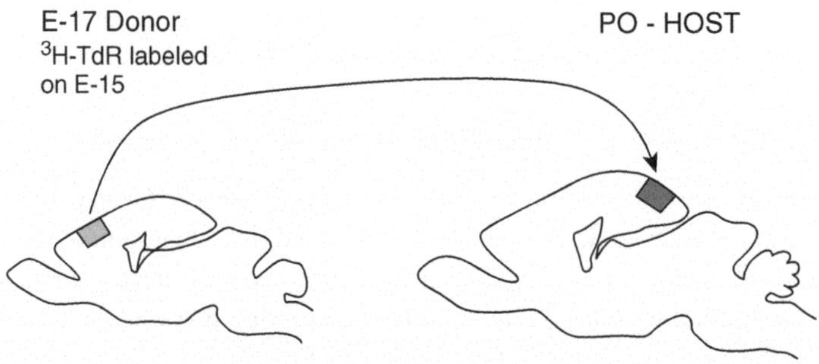

FIGURE 1.1 In the cortical explant experiments a section of tissue is removed from a donor animal and implanted in an atypical location in a host animal. In this example a section of somatosensory cortex is removed from the donor fetus and implanted in primary visual cortex of the host fetus. (Figure adapted with permission from O'Leary and Stanfield, 1989.)

Experimental Lesion Studies

The experimental lesion studies are designed to examine the plasticity of the developing brain by examining behavioral resilience following specifically targeted injury to the brain. Many of these studies explore the extent to which function can be maintained when brain areas that are critical to normal functioning in adult animals are injured early in life. Other studies examine the effects of altering neural input to a developing cortical region and ask whether the function of a cortical area could be changed by variation in the input it receives; for example, is it possible to transform auditory cortex into a visual area by altering its input early in development? These later studies introduce the construct of cross-modal plasticity as an extreme form of neural plasticity.

Dorsolateral prefrontal cortex plays an important role in spatial working memory. Lesions to these regions in adult monkeys impairs performance on spatial working memory tasks (Goldman, 1971; Goldman, Rosvold, & Mishkin, 1970). Goldman-Rakic used both a delayed response task and a delayed alternation task to assess the effects of early and late lesions on performance, and showed that the timing of cortical lesions has markedly different effects on performance (Fig. 1.2). In the delayed response task, bait is hidden under an object and the monkey is required to wait before retrieving it. In the delayed alternation task, the animal watches as the bait is hidden under Object A, and after a delay, the original Object A and a novel Object B are presented. The monkey must learn that the bait is always hidden under the novel object. Goldman-Rakic compared the performance of monkeys lesioned as neonates with that of monkeys lesioned at 1 year. On both tasks the monkeys with neonatal cortical lesions performed better than monkeys lesioned later. Further, compared to nonlesioned

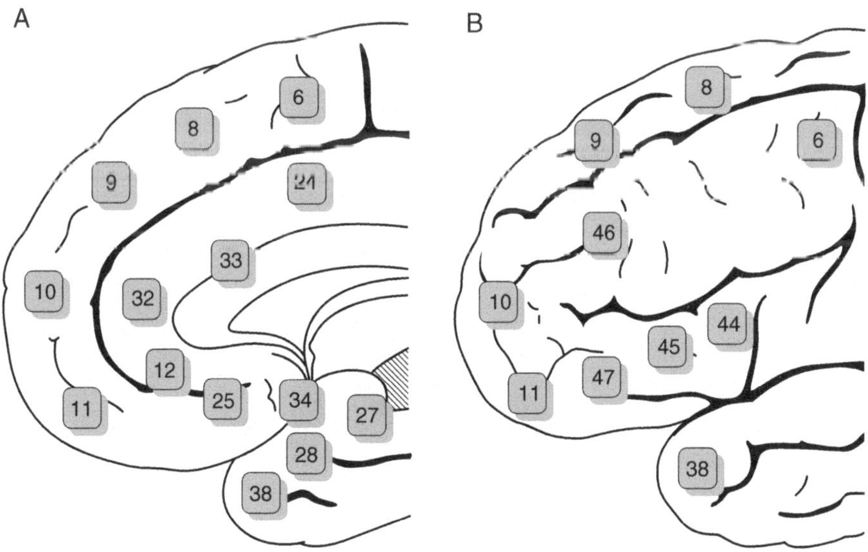

FIGURE 1.2 Dorsolateral prefrontal cortex encompasses BA 9 and BA 46 on the lateral (A) and medial (B) surface of the brain. (Images adapted from Gray's Anatomy of the Human Body, originally published in 1918 and the public domain.)

controls, the performance of monkeys with neonatal lesions was comparable on the delayed response task and only slightly worse on the delayed alternation task. However, in a longitudinal follow-up study a year later, monkeys with neonatal lesions had lost ground relative to normally developing monkeys on the delayed alternation task. Rather than showing the normal profile of developmental improvement with age, no change in performance was observed. These studies suggest that the developing neocortical system is capable of adapting to the effects of lesions more effectively than the mature neocortical system in that the performance of animals lesioned early in life is largely preserved. However, subtle differences, at least on more challenging tasks, are observed, and the typical pattern of developmental improvement observed in nonlesioned animals is attenuated in animals with early lesions.

Bachavelier, Miskin, and colleagues studied the effects of experimental lesions to another important cortical memory system within the inferior temporal lobe (Mishkin, 1982; Webster, Bachevalier, & Ungerleider, 1995; Webster, Ungerleider, & Bachevalier, 1991a, 1991b). Visual recognition memory relies in part on the neural pathway involved in processing information about objects (Fig. 1.3). This pathway begins in primary visual cortex, projects to multiple prestriate areas in occipital cortex, to area TEO in the posterior inferior temporal lobe, to area TE in anterior inferior temporal lobe, and then to limbic structures in the medial temporal lobe (amygdala, hippocampus, rhinal cortex). In adult animals, interaction of area TE with the limbic system structures is critical for visual recognition memory. Lesions to area TE impair performance on a delayed non-match to sample (DNMS) task, a novel object recognition task very similar to the delayed alternation task used by Goldman-Rakic. As with dorsolateral prefrontal lesions, the timing of TE lesions affects performance on the DNMS task (Bachevalier & Mishkin, 1994). When the performance of normal infant and adult monkeys was compared to that of monkeys with neonatal or adult-onset lesions to area TE, performance differences were marked. Accuracy of normal infant

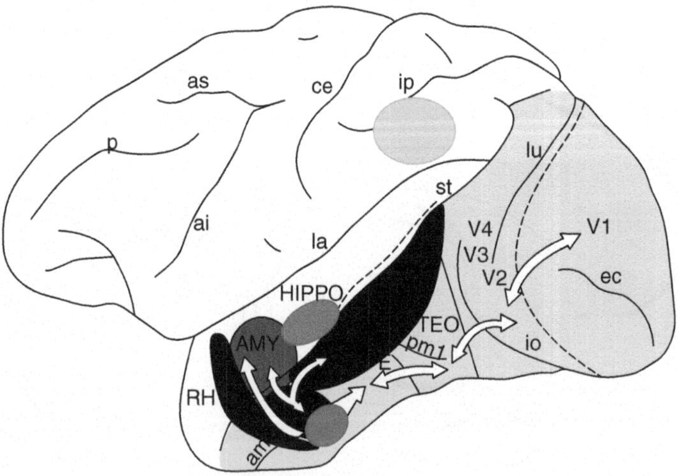

FIGURE 1.3 The regions involved in the serial lesion studies of Bachevalier et al (Webster, Bachevalier, & Ungerleider, 1995). The initial lesions involved area TE; subsequent lesions included TEO and visual association areas, including STP (red), PG (green), and TF (blue). (See color insert.)

and adult monkeys was above 90%, while that of adult TE lesioned monkeys was only 71%. Monkeys with neonatal lesions performed at 84%, suggesting mild impairment with neonatal as compared to adult lesions to area TE. Further, when the infant-lesioned monkeys were tested 4 years later as adults, they retained their high level of performance (Malkova, Mishkin, & Bachevalier, 1995). Consistent with the data on lesions to dorsolateral prefrontal cortex, these studies suggest that neural substrate may be capable of compensatory reorganization.

Additional studies with this same group of monkeys provided insight into the nature of reorganization following neonatal TE lesions. In these studies, a second surgical procedure was performed on the monkeys with neonatal TE lesions after they reached adulthood. The second surgery targeted brain regions believed to be part of a more exuberant cortical network that is typical in young animals. Specifically, in the normal course of early brain development both areas TE and TEO make connections with limbic system structures. As development proceeds, TEO–limbic system connections are withdrawn, while TE–limbic system connections strengthen and stabilize, becoming principal components of the mature neural pathway for visual recognition memory. In addition, a number of visual association areas, including the superior temporal polysensory area (STP), area PG in inferior parietal cortex and TF in the posterior parahippocampal gyrus, which are not typically part of the mature visual recognition memory system, are part of the early cortical network (Webster et al., 1991a). The second surgery targeted one or more of these exuberantly connected brain regions. In one group of neonatal TE-lesioned monkeys, the second lesion involved area TEO only. In a second group, only visual association areas STP, PS, and TF were involved, and in a third group areas TEO plus STP, PG, and TF were all lesioned. Only the third group of monkeys showed evidence of impairment on the DNMS task. Removal of only TEO or the visual association areas was not sufficient to impair performance on this task; impaired visual recognition performance was observed only when both TEO and the visual association areas were lesioned (Webster, Bachevalier, & Ungerleider, 1995). These findings demonstrated that when area TE is lesioned early in development, the normally transient connections between TEO and limbic structures, as well as connections involving STP, PS, and TF, are retained, thus providing a possible alternative pathway for visual memory processing. These findings suggest that there is considerable capacity for neural plasticity within the developing temporal lobe system.

Studies of early cross-modal plasticity used what have come to be known as "cortical rewiring" procedures to experimentally alter input into cortical sensory areas. In these studies, normal connection pathways or brain regions are systematically eliminated, thus altering the typical competition for neural resources in targeted brain regions. The central question in these studies is whether systematic alteration in competitive inputs will modify the patterns of connectivity in cortex and affect the basic anatomical organization and functioning of the targeted cortical area. The first study to demonstrate that lesions of subcortical structures could alter the projection patterns of major sensory pathways came from Schneider's work with hamsters (Schneider, 1973). Subsequent studies have elaborated upon that early work. In an important series of studies with neonatal ferrets, Sur et al. (Pallas, Roe, & Sur, 1990; Sur et al., 1988) manipulated inputs to primary auditory cortex (PAC) by severing the connection between the cochlea and PAC and between the inferior colliculus and the auditory nucleus of the thalamus, thus leaving PAC without its principal auditory sensory input pathways (Fig. 1.4). They also ablated primary visual cortex and the superior colliculus, thus

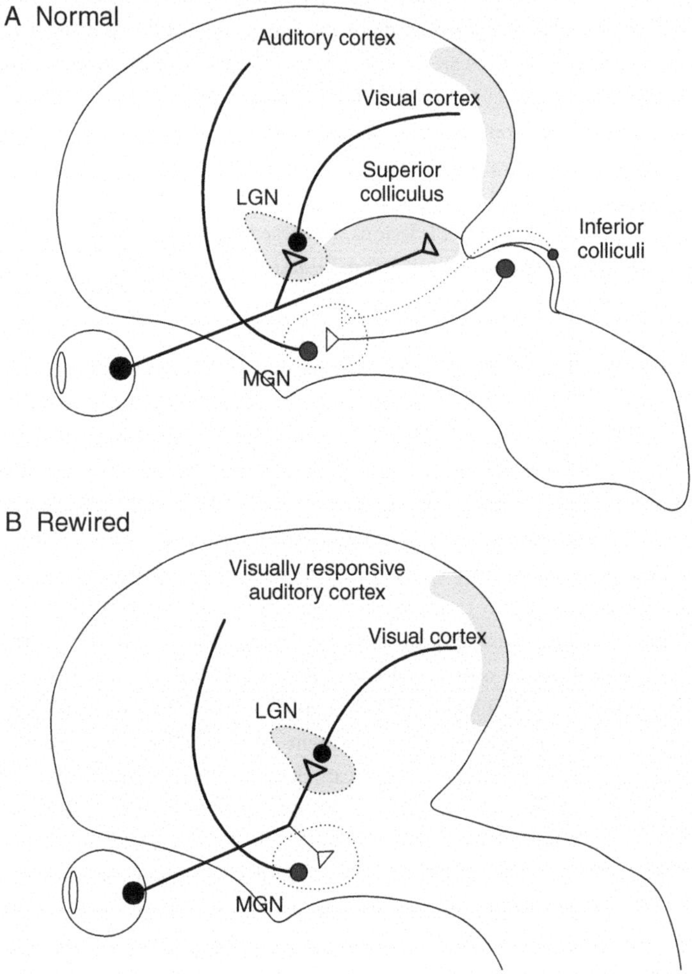

FIGURE 1.4 (A) The normal patterns of visual and auditory input. The auditory system projects from the cochlea in the ear to the inferior colliculus to the medial geniculate nucleus (MGN) of the thalamus to primary auditory cortex. The visual system projects from the retina to the superior colliculus and to the lateral geniculate nucleus (LGN) of the thalamus, and then from the LGN to primary visual cortex. (B) Pattern of visual input in the rewired ferret. The visual system projects from the retina to both the LGN and MGN. LGN then projects to primary visual cortex, and MGN projects to visually responsive auditory cortex. (Note: In the early experiments primary visual cortex was removed and in later experiments it was left in place. Retinal inputs project to auditory cortex in either case.) (Figure adapted with permission from Sur, Angelluci, & Sharma, 1999.)

eliminating the major cortical target of the primary visual pathway. The neonatal lesions fundamentally changed both the anatomical organization and function of PAC. Specifically, fibers of the visual pathway projected to the auditory nucleus of the thalamus and then to PAC, thus creating a visual input pathway to PAC. Further, the organization of the "rewired" PAC took on the characteristics of primary visual cortex (PVC). In typical development, PVC is organized into a two-dimensional "retinotopic" map of space, while PAC is organized into a one-dimensional map of auditory frequencies. Two-dimensional, retinotopic organization was reported for the rewired PAC. In addition, other features of typical PVC organization, including orientation and direction-specific mapping, also emerged in the rewired PAC. However, the visual maps in PAC were less well defined than those observed in PVC (Sur & Leamey, 2001). Finally, in addition to the anatomical similarities to PVC, rewired PAC has been shown to function as a visual area in that animals can be trained to effectively respond to visual cues. However, measures of visual acuity suggest somewhat reduced function (von Melchner, Pallas, & Sur, 2000).

The cortical rewiring studies provide a dramatic cross-modal demonstration of the capacity of the developing neural system to adapt to unconventional input and establish alternative patterns of connectivity and functionality. As in the earlier studies, while the rewired system may be functional, it is not optimal or as efficient in mediating the acquired function.

The Effects of Altered Sensory Input on Brain Development

Alteration of cortical organization does not require the invasive procedures used in the experimental lesion studies. Changes in cortical organization and function can be induced by simply altering the input to the neural system. The effects of altered sensory input on the development of brain organization have been studied across a range of sensory modalities. Data suggest that alteration of input can affect the internal organization of a cortical sensory area. Interestingly, complete deprivation beginning in the neonatal period can result in the functional reassignment of a sensory area. We have seen examples of this kind of cross-modal plasticity in the cortical lesions studies. The sensory deprivation studies suggest that similar functional changes can be induced by altered experience alone.

The seminal work by Hubel and Wiesel (Hubel & Wiesel, 1964 Hubel, Wiesel, & LeVay, 1976; 1977; LeVay, Wiesel, Hubel, 1980; Wiesel & Hubel, 1963a, 1963b, 1963c; 1965a; 1965b) provided one of the first demonstrations that alteration of sensory input can have a dramatic effect on the organization within a cortical sensory area. Their work highlighted the importance of both specific input and timing of experience on the development of conventional patterns of cortical organization. One important organizational feature of the input layer of PVC is the ocular dominance columns (ODC). Neurons within an ODC are preferentially driven by inputs from one eye. The segregation of eye-specific inputs begins at the retina and continues along the extent of the primary visual pathway. Within layer 4 of PVC, the inputs from each eye cluster into the distinct bands that make up the ODCs.

Hubel and Wiesel experimentally manipulated the early visual experience of kittens and newborn rhesus macaque monkeys by suturing closed one eye, thus altering the balance of visual input to PVC. Following a period of monocular deprivation, vision in the deprived eye was initially profoundly impaired and there was no hint of any ability to perceive form. Within PVC, the great majority of cortical cells were driven exclusively by input from the nondeprived eye. In other experiments, Hubel and Wiesel manipulated the timing of deprivation and found that disruption of cortical organization was most severe when deprivation began prior to 10 weeks of age. Some change was detectable with onset at 1 year, and no changes were observed when adult animals were monocularly deprived. The effects of duration of deprivation co-varied with time of onset; with earlier onset, less time was required to induce substantial change. Recovery from early deprivation depended on both time of onset and duration.

A human analog to visual deprivation experiments comes from studies of children with congenital cataracts. Cataracts are a clouding or opacity of the lens of the eye (Levin, 2003), which, when dense, can block patterned vision (Maurer, Lewis, & Mondloch, 2005). Maurer et al. have studied a large group of children with binocular or monocular congenital cataracts and compared their visual development to typical controls. The evaluation of the initial effects of deprivation on visual development (Maurer, Lewis, Brent, & Levin, 1999) were based on a study of infants with congenital cataracts who received surgery within the first year of life. During surgery the cataracts were removed and corrective lenses implanted, thus providing the children with their first exposure to patterned visual input. The children were tested three times: within 10 minutes of their surgery, 1 hour after surgery, and 1 year after surgery. Immediately after fitting with the corrective lens, vision in the deprived eye(s) was poor, but improvement began within an hour and continued through the end of the first year of life in both binocular and monocular cases. However, although considerable improvement was observed, specific deficits persisted. Among children with early binocular cataracts, subtle but permanent deficits in contrast sensitivity, visual acuity, and peripheral vision were evident (Lewis & Maurer, 2005). Although the initial effects of monocular and binocular deprivation followed a similar pattern of recovery, competitive effects resulting from early monocular deprivation became more apparent after the first year of life. Without treatment, outcomes across a range of measures of visual function for the monocularly deprived eye were worse than for cases of binocular deprivation. Early intensive intervention involving patching of the unaffected eye resulted in good final acuity and contrast sensitivity, with outcomes comparable to or better than binocular cases. For children who did not receive intensive early treatment or who did not comply with the treatment protocols, outcomes for the deprived eye were much worse than for children with bilateral cataracts on measures of visual acuity, contrast sensitivity, and peripheral vision. Thus, both the early experience of deprivation and the intervention to restore a competitive balance of activity from the two eyes can have dramatic effects on functional vision. Both reflect the underlying plasticity of the developing neural system for vision.

Cross-modal plasticity has also been examined using animal models in which visual input is eliminated either by very early enucleation (removal of the eyes) or by congenital disorders that disrupt eye formation. These studies examine the functional reassignment of brain areas as a consequence of early sensory deprivation. Krubitzer et al. (Kahn & Krubitzer, 2002; Karlen, Kahn, & Krubitzer, 2006) examined change in cortical cytoarchitecture and in patterns of neural connectivity in opossums enucleated prior to the normal formation of the thalamocortical pathway. Two principal findings emerged from these studies. First, even in the absence of all visual input, a cortical area cytoarchitectonically similar to visual area 17 (i.e., PVC) could be identified in the enucleated animals, and neurons within this cortical area made connections with major visual association areas within cortex as well as with the major visual nuclei of the thalamus. Thus, fundamental features of typical visual system organization were maintained without visual experience. However, the studies also revealed significant differences in cortical organization and function that reflect the cross-modal plasticity of the developing neural system (Fig. 1.5). The size of area 17 was greatly reduced in enucleated animals. In addition, a novel cortical area, referred to as area X, was reported

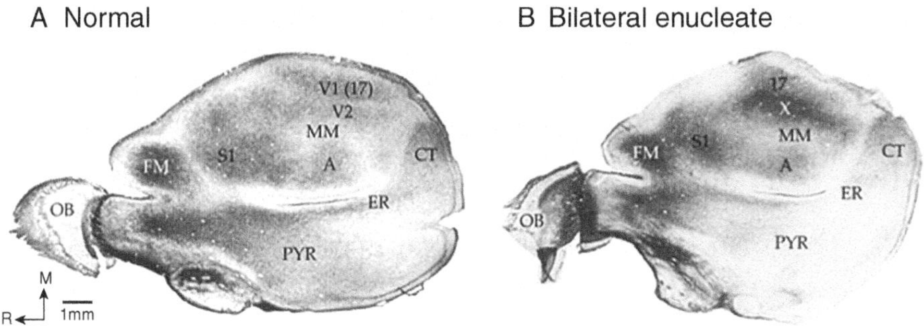

FIGURE 1.5 Flattened cortical sections of a normal (A) and bilaterally enucleated (B) opossum. In normal animals primary sensory areas (V1/17, S1, A) are darkly myelinated. Most cortical areas are normal in the bilateral enucleate animals; however, Area 17 is much smaller, and there is a novel area, area X, adjacent to Area 17. (Figure adapted with permission from Karlen, Kahn, & Krubitzer, 2006.)

lateral to area 17, in the region typically occupied by visual area 18. This area was architectonically distinct from area 18 in normal animals and appears to represent a newly emergent cortical structure. Functionally, neurons within both area 17 and area X were responsive to auditory and somatosensory stimulus input. In some animals the neurons responded in a multimodal fashion, while in others discrete populations of auditory- or somatosensory-specific neurons were reported. Cortico–cortico connectivity also differed. In addition to the typical connections with visual association areas, connections with primary auditory and somatosensory cortices, as well as with multimodal association areas, were found. Thalamocortical connections also exhibited this increased diversity. In addition to input from the typical visual thalamic nuclei, area 17 in the enucleated animals also received input from nuclei associated with somatosensory, auditory, motor, and limbic/hippocampal functions. Finally, the effects of early enucleation extended beyond the visual system. A large proportion of neurons in primary auditory and primary somatosensory cortices exhibited bimodal responsivity in that they fired to both auditory and somatosensory input. Studies of congenitally blind mice reported similar findings. Neurons in PVC respond to auditory input in these animals (Chabot et al., 2008; Izraeli et al., 2002; Laemle, Strominger, & Carpenter, 2006; Piche et al., 2007; Piche, Robert, Miceli, & Bronchti, 2004), although the range and level of responsiveness appear to be reduced compared to auditory cortex (Izraeli et al., 2002; Piche et al., 2007). Reorganization of subcortical input pathways appears to be implicated in the altered patterns of responsivity in these animals.

A growing body of neuroimaging data suggests that analogous patterns of cross-modal plasticity may be operating in humans with congenital sensory abnormalities. A large number of studies have reported activation of visual cortex to auditory and somatosensory stimuli in congenitally blind individuals (Bavelier & Neville, 2002; Noppeney, 2007; Pascual-Leone et al., 2005). Recent work has also documented changes in neural anatomy that involve volumetric loss throughout visual areas, including BA17, BA18/19, MT (Ptito, Schneider, Paulson, & Kupers, 2008; Shimony et al., 2006), and the right hippocampus

(Chebat et al., 2007), as well as attenuation of the visual thalamocortical pathways as measured with diffusion-weighted imagining techniques (Shimony et al., 2006). Analogous behavioral (Bavelier, Dye, & Hauser, 2006; Bavelier & Neville, 2002) and anatomical (Emmorey, Allen, Bruss, Schenker, & Damasio, 2003; Emmorey, Grabowski, et al., 2003) changes have been reported for congenitally deaf individuals.

THE EFFECTS OF ENVIRONMENTAL COMPLEXITY ON BRAIN DEVELOPMENT

The most general case for the impact of the environment on brain development comes from studies that examine the effects of the rearing conditions on major indices of brain development. These studies provide the most unambiguous evidence for the role of experience in neural development, because the only factor that is manipulated is the complexity of the local environment. One of the first reports of the effects of environmental complexity on development was a study by Donald Hebb (Hebb, 1949). Hebb compared a group of rats reared as pets in his home with a group reared in standard laboratory cages. He attributed the superior maze learning in home-reared groups to the effects of rearing environment. The first systematic series of studies on the role of environment on brain development were conducted by Rosenzweig et al. (Bennett, Rosenzweig, & Diamond, 1969; Rosenzweig & Bennett, 1972; Rosenzweig, Krech, Bennett, & Zolman, 1962; Rosenzweig, Love, & Bennett, 1968). These were among the first studies to demonstrate explicit effects of environmental enrichment on brain anatomy and chemistry.

The most comprehensive body of work examining the effect of environment on brain development comes from Greenough et al. (Greenough & Chang, 1988; Grossman, Churchill, Bates, Kleim, & Greenough, 2002; Markham & Greenough, 2004). In an extensive series of studies with rats, they demonstrated that variation in environmental conditions can affect both neural and non-neural elements of the developing brain. In the standard experimental protocol, identical strains of rats are reared from birth to adolescence under three conditions: individual cage (IC), social cage (SC), and environmental complexity (EC). In the IC and SC condition, animals are housed either individually or on small groups in standard laboratory cages containing only food and water. In the EC condition, groups of 12 or more animals are free to explore in large enclosures filled with a variety of objects that are regularly changed.

Rearing condition has dramatic effects on many aspects of brain development. Measures of brain morphometry showed that animals reared in the EC condition have 20% to 25% more dendrites per neuron than animals reared in the other two conditions. These effects were not associated with any specific feature of the enriched environment condition, nor were they accounted for by general metabolic differences in animals reared in the enriched condition. For example, animals fitted with a monocular visual occluder and reared in the EC environment showed evidence of *unilateral* exuberance of dendrites in visual areas (Chang & Greenough, 1982). Similar effects of EC exposure are observed for the number and complexity of astrocytes, the brain's support cells (Jones & Greenough, 1996), as well as for the myelin-producing oligodendrocytes (Sirevaag & Greenough, 1987; Szeligo & Leblond, 1977). Experience also induces change in the cerebral vascular system, as evidenced by findings that animals reared in EC environments have larger and more complex capillary systems (Black, Sirevaag, & Greenough, 1987). Finally, enhancement effects appear to vary in terms of persistence. Changes in synapse morphology and in the oligodendrocytes appear to persist beyond the period of exposure. Animals returned to the IC after 30 days of exposure to EC showed no loss of dendritic spines or myelination (Briones, Klintsova, & Greenough, 2004; Markham & Greenough, 2004). Effects for astrocytes and the vasculature appear to be more transient (Markham & Greenough, 2004).

LIMITATIONS ON NEURAL PLASTICITY

The data from the animal lesion and altered sensory input studies make an impressive case for plasticity in the developing brain. Early experimental manipulations can induce reorganization of cortical areas that is adapted to the demands imposed by the experimental procedures. Some manipulations induce reorganization within a cortical area (e.g., monocular deprivation and ODC change), while others can promote more extensive changes in cortical function (e.g., cross-modal plasticity). However, as suggested throughout the last section of this chapter, while functional outcomes for early lesioned animals are often good relative to adults, performance rarely matches that of normal control animals, and subtle but persistent performance decrements are often reported. These data suggest that while the developing neural system has the capacity for considerable adaptation and exhibits substantial plasticity, deprivation or lesioning procedures also come with a cost that results in a functional but suboptimal neurobehavioral system. Such findings raise the more general issue of constraints or limits on neural plasticity in the developing brain.

The capacity for plastic adaptation is a property of the developing neural system, but it always operates within a context that reflects the current developmental state and history of the organism. As such, plasticity is limited by the process of development itself, and thus by the particular constraints on the capacity for plastic adaptation that differ at different points in development. At one extreme, specific gene anomalies or toxic insults that interrupt early embryonic patterning can introduce catastrophic defects that preclude adaptive compensation (Kalia, 2008; Stiles, 2008) and can result in serious, permanent disability or even death. Other effects can have more variable effects on outcome. For example, teratogens such as radiation or cocaine introduced during the critical period of neuronal migration can affect corticogenesis, but the degree of disruption varies depending on the timing and duration of exposure to the teratogen. The effects of more specifically targeted factors such as localized brain lesions differ depending on timing and the specific site of insult. The last section reviewed some of the large literature documenting neural plasticity following early localized brain injury. This section first examines data that point to limits on plasticity following early brain lesions, and then considers the more general issue of critical periods in neural development

Neural Plasticity and the Timing of Brain Injury

As discussed earlier, neonatal cortical lesions involving dorsolateral prefrontal or inferior temporal regions have minimal effects on the development of visual working memory task performance (Goldman, 1971; Goldman et al., 1970; Webster et al., 1995). However, neonatal lesions to selectively targeted subcortical structures within these same neural systems can produce severe deficits that are comparable to those observed with adult-onset lesions.

Goldman-Rakic examined the effects of neonatal and adult lesions to the caudate nucleus, a critical subcortical structure with extensive connections to dorsolateral prefrontal cortex. In contrast to the findings from the study of neocortical lesions, she reported that caudate nucleus lesions produced severe and comparable deficits on the delayed response tasks in both neonatal and adult lesion groups (Goldman, 1974). Further, the effects of the early subcortical lesions did not resolve with development.

A similar but somewhat more complex pattern is observed within the temporal lobe. As discussed earlier, neonatal TE lesions induce extensive reorganization of the inferior temporal pathway that supports high levels of performance on visual working memory tasks (Bachevalier & Mishkin, 1994; Malkova et al., 1995; Webster et al., 1995). By contrast, lesions to either the hippocampal complex (which includes the hippocampus, dentate gyrus, subicular complex, and underlying areas of TH and TF of the parahippocampal gyrus) or the amygdaloid complex (which includes the amygdaloid nucleus, piriform cortex, and the anterior portion of the entorhinal cortex) within the medial temporal lobe result in serious but task-specific deficits (Alvarado & Bachevalier, 2000; Alvarado, Wright, & Bachevalier, 2002; Bachevalier, Beauregard, & Alvarado, 1999). The studies documenting these dissociated patterns of impairment examined the effects of neonatal lesions on two visual working memory tasks. The first was the *object-based* delayed non-match to sample task (ODNMS) used in the studies of the inferior temporal lobe. The second was a *spatial* delayed non-match to sample task (SDNMS) that is similar in structure to ODMNS except that during the test phase two identical objects are presented in the original location and a novel location, and the task is to find the reward at the novel location. ODNMS thus places demands on visual object memory, while SDNMS taxes memory for spatial relations. The neonatal hippocampal lesions produced severe and permanent deficits in spatial but not object memory, while lesions to the amygdaloid complex produced moderate deficits in object but not spatial memory.

Neonatal amygdala lesions also affect the development of emotional and social behaviors in monkeys, but with outcomes that differ from those observed among animals lesioned as adults. Amygdala lesions in adults monkeys result in reduced fear responses to novel inanimate objects and enhanced affiliative behavior in social interactions (Prather et al., 2001). Both behaviors suggest that damage to the amygdala affects the animal's ability to discern danger, and thus results in reduced caution in interactions with both objects and other animals. Early amygdala lesions produce both similarities and differences to the adult pattern. Specifically, like amygdala-lesioned adults, monkeys with neonatal lesions exhibit reduced fear of inanimate objects (Prather et al., 2001); however, unlike the adults they show enhanced fear reactions in social interactions (Bauman, Lavenex, Mason, Capitanio, & Amaral, 2004; Prather et al., 2001). These findings suggest a complex dissociation of fear responses associated with early lesions of the amygdala.

More general questions about the location and timing of lesions were examined by Kolb et al. (Kolb & Whishaw, 1989) in their studies of the effects of unilateral versus bilateral lesions introduced in rats at different postnatal ages. In this series of studies, lesions involved either hemispherectomy or removal of either the frontal or parietal lobes bilaterally. Lesions were introduced on postnatal day 1 (D1), D5, or D10 or as adults (DA). Spatial problem-solving was tested using the Morris Water Maze task, in which rats are placed in a tank filled with opaque liquid and trained to find a submerged platform (Morris, 1984). Kolb et al.

found that bilateral lesions, whether to the frontal (Kolb & Elliott, 1987) or parietal (Kolb et al., 1987) lobes, resulted in much greater impairment than hemidecortication. In addition, the effects of lesion timing differed in the two cases (Kolb & Tomie, 1988). Specifically, regardless of the exact timing of the early lesion, hemidecorticated young animals performed better than animals unilaterally lesioned as adults, and they performed better than animals with either early or late bilateral lesions. Further, not only did bilateral lesions, in general, produce the most serious overall level of impairments, but the effects were greatest for animals with the earliest lesions. Performance of D1 animals was worse than that of DA, while performance of D10 was better than DA. This study suggests that unilateral lesions allow for greater neural compensation than bilateral lesions, and that the earlier the onset of a unilateral lesion, the greater capacity for reorganization. By contrast, bilateral lesions appear to limit the capacity for reorganization, and thus the more immature the neural system at time of injury, the more debilitating the impact of the lesion. These findings, like those reporting differences in outcome with subcortical versus cortical prefrontal and temporal lobe lesions, raise important questions about the limits on the capacity of the developing brain to respond to early injury. An important construct related to these questions about the effects of timing, location, and extent of injury is the old and well-established idea in developmental neuropsychology of critical or sensitive periods in neurocognitive development.

Critical or Sensitive Periods in Brain Development

Studies reporting greater capacity for neural plasticity in the developing brain imply that there must be windows of time when sensitivity to input and capacity to adapt to altered early experiences are enhanced. The term "critical period" has been used to describe the temporally circumscribed periods of postnatal development when specific input is required to establish a particular behavior, presumably because the input is necessary to support the establishment of the neural system (Knudsen, 2004). These periods of sensitivity also appear to be related to capacity for neural adaptation. The early definitions of the critical period (e.g., Bowlby, 1969; Lenneberg, 1967; Lorenz, 1937/57) made very strong claims about intrinsic control of the time window during which experience could affect development. However, subsequent work provided substantial evidence for greater flexibility in both the onset and termination of the critical period for many behaviors, and for the idea that critical period effects could be modified, or in some cases even reversed, by variations in experimental conditions (Michel & Tyler, 2005). These kinds of findings led to a revision of the initial concept and the introduction of the term "sensitive period" as a more moderate alternative (Johnson, 2005; Knudsen, 2004; Michel & Tyler, 2005).

The sensitive period terminology endorses the concept that experience has a greater impact on emerging neural organization and associated behavior during specific developmental windows, but does not subscribe to a simple maturational account of these important time periods. Studies of sensitive period events focus on identifying the underlying mechanism for a particular event as well as the complement of factors that might affect its development. Johnson (2001, 2005) has offered three competing accounts of sensitive period effects: maturational, skill learning, and interactive specialization. The maturational view is similar to the critical period view in that sensitive periods are defined by the physical development of the brain. The skill learning view suggests that the apparent insensitivity to new learning after the close of the "sensitive period" actually reflects the stabilization of a particular neural system as specific expertise in a skill area is acquired. Thus, stabilization of neural pathways constrains plasticity indirectly by limiting sensitivity to novel input. Interactive specialization suggests that the response properties of a given region are dependent on its connections with other brain regions. As learning proceeds, patterns of connectivity sharpen and functions within a region become more specifically defined. Thus, the end of the sensitive period is associated with the learning process itself. For both skill learning and interactive specialization, the sensitive period appears to be an epiphenomenon of the underlying developmental processes associated with learning, rather than a product of physical maturation. As learning-associated input shapes the patterns of connectivity and refines the neural systems, the sensitive period gradually declines.

The construct of a sensitive period, thus, introduces a number of important ideas. First, it postulates specific periods during which input is critical for establishing neurocognitive systems. The timing of these periods differs for different neural systems. In that sense, sensitive periods capture what Greenough has termed experience-expectant learning processes (Black & Greenough, 1986; Greenough, Black, & Wallace, 1987). Second, the periods of dependency on input for establishing specific pathways coincide with periods of enhanced neural plasticity; thus, an essential feature of a sensitive period is the capacity for plastic adaptation. Such adaptation most typically involves the "expected" inputs to the system (e.g., patterned visual input, the spectral range of auditory frequencies, sensorimotor exploratory behaviors in the world) and results in "typical" patterns of development. But this same capacity for adaptation is available when circumstances vary and organism internal (e.g., brain lesions) or external (e.g., deprivation) factors intervene. Under such conditions, alternative patterns of neural organization can emerge. Finally, the very properties that make sensitive periods critically important for development must be constrained as the neurocognitive system stabilizes and matures. It is not adaptive for well-functioning sensory or cognitive systems to be highly susceptible to fluctuation and change. Thus, while the capacity for learning and adaptation to environmental circumstance is never completely lost, the mature system is stable and less receptive to the effects of variation input.

THE LESION METHOD IN ADULT AND CHILD POPULATIONS

Historically, the study of individuals with localized brain injury has provided an important approach to understanding the relationship between human behavior and the mature brain. The logic of the lesion method is one of subtraction. In other words, by associating specific functional loss with injury to a particular brain area, it is possible to infer the original function of the area, or more precisely to infer that the region plays a role in the support of the function. The idea of associating functional and neural loss is an ancient one. The oldest known record of such speculations, the Sir Edwin Smith Surgical Papyrus, dates to the Egyptians in approximately 3000 BC (Finger, 1994). The first modern case to establish the efficacy of the lesion method was reported by the French neurologist Paul Broca in 1861 (Broca, 1861). The case of Tan, as Broca's patient was known, provided evidence of an association between injury to left inferior frontal regions and loss of productive language functioning. In 1876, Wernicke reported the case of a patient with a stroke in the region of temporal-parietal junction and profound impairment of language comprehension.

Following on these early reports, the lesion method became a mainstay of neuropsychological research for the next century (Damasio, 2000; Damasio, Adolphs, & Damasio, 2003; Damasio & Damasio, 2000; Rorden & Karnath, 2004).

The logic of the lesion method is not without controversy. Throughout much of the past two centuries debates persisted among proponents of strongly localizationist view of structure–function mapping and those advocating an aggregate field view in which function is widely distributed among many brain areas. Ultimately the study of adult neuropsychology pursued what might be called a modified localizationist framework in which parallel, distributed neural networks act in concert to support function. Recent advances in brain imaging techniques such as positron emission tomography (PET), functional magnetic resonance imaging (fMRI), and event-related electrophysiology (ERP) have made it possible to study localization in healthy brains. With the advent of these new technologies, the convergence of patient lesion data and systems neuroscience has been possible (Damasio et al., 2003; Fellows et al., 2005; Rorden & Karnath, 2004; Schuren, 1997).

While the lesion method has served as a critical source of data in the debate over functional localization in the mature brain, it has been used to inform a somewhat different set of issues about the developing brain. Beginning with the earliest experimental (e.g., Brown, 1915; Kennard, 1936, 1938a, 1938b; Kennard & Fulton, 1942; Langworthy, 1924; Weed & Kennard, 1917) and clinical (e.g., Broca, 1865; Brown-Sequard, 1877; Osler, 1987) studies on the effects of early brain lesions, the focus of discussion has been on the resilience of the young organism to the effects of early neurological insults and the level of plasticity exhibited by the developing brain. While the question of functional localization has been a part of the clinical and experimental inquiry, the central question concerns the multiple, alternative patterns of brain organization that can arise following early injury to the developing brain.

Clinical observations of the resilience of the developing human brain date back to at least the 19th century. Broca (1865) reported the case of a woman who at autopsy was found to have a large congenital lesion of the left third frontal convolution, but during her life this woman exhibited no signs of "aphemia" (aphasia). Broca concluded that a lesion that can "produce lasting aphemia in an adult, will not prevent a small child from learning to talk" (see Finger & Almli, 1988; Schiller, 1979, chapter 10). Brown-Séquard (1877) noted that children with injury to brain regions associated with speech show recovery not usually seen in adults.

Subsequent experimental studies examining the outcome of development following early unilateral brain injury reported mixed results. Some studies emphasized the "resilience" of young children to the effects of early injury and argued that the early capacity for neuroplastic change allowed children to develop normal or near-normal cognitive functioning following injuries to the brain that would have left an adult permanently impaired (Alajouanine & Lhermitte, 1965; Brown, 1975; Carlson, Netley, Hendrick, & Prichard, 1968; Gott, 1973; Hammill & Irwin, 1966; Krashen,1973; Lenneberg, 1967; Reed & Reitan, 1969). However, other investigators argued that a more fine-grained analysis of behavior showed evidence of persistent cognitive deficit (Day & Ulatowska, 1979; Dennis, 1980; Dennis & Kohn, 1975; Dennis & Whitaker, 1976; Kohn, 1980; Kohn & Dennis, 1974; McFie, 1961; Rudel & Teuber, 1971; Vargha-Khadem & O'Gorman, 1983; Vargha-Khadem, O'Gorman, & Watters, 1985; Woods, 1980; Woods & Carey, 1979). These apparent contradictions suggested a complex interplay between plasticity and specialization of function in the developing brain, but the nature and course of that interaction remained unclear. Systematic, longitudinal investigation of children with localized perinatal brain injury can elucidate these complex sets of issues.

PERINATAL BRAIN INJURY AS A WINDOW ON NEURAL PLASTICITY AND DEVELOPMENT

As suggested by the studies reviewed in this chapter, animal studies of neurobehavioral development have redefined ideas about the role of plasticity in early neurobehavioral development. This work has important implications for the study of human brain development in both typical populations and in populations of children with brain disorders. Older ideas from the pediatric clinical literature portrayed early brain plasticity as a secondary system that is recruited in the wake of early injury (Stiles, 2000; Teuber, 1974; Witelson, 1985). However, the emerging view of the developing brain as dynamic and constantly adapting to internal biological signals and input from the outside world provide a very different perspective on the nature of plasticity, and thus on the development of children with early brain injury. By this view, the early brain injury, itself, becomes a factor in the developmental trajectory of the individual child, and as such it becomes integrated into the ongoing, dynamic, and adaptive processes of brain development, which are inherently plastic. Early pathology is never optimal or beneficial to the child, but its consequences and effects are best understood as the product of a dynamic set of processes that reflect fundamental properties of neurobehavioral development. The study of children with localized perinatal brain injury can provide a window on these important and dynamic processes.

The remainder of this volume explores the available data on cognitive, linguistic, and affective development in children with unilateral perinatal brain injury. Much of the focus is a comprehensive review of the small number of mostly longitudinal studies that identified children during infancy and followed their development through childhood to document the trajectories of change in essential functions as they unfold. These studies are important because they allow us to examine prospectively the emergence of important aspects of cognitive functioning, and to compare developmental trajectories across cognitive domains. Four questions are central to the study of neurocognitive development in children with perinatal brain injury:

1. Is there evidence of cognitive deficit early in development?
2. Is the association between pattern of behavioral deficit and site of brain injury among children comparable to the patterns of association observed among adults?
3. Do behavioral deficits persist over time?
4. What is the nature of the change and how does this change occur?

As will be evident, the answers to the four questions differ depending on the behavioral domains under examination, suggesting that the developmental trajectories and capacity for plastic adaptation may vary by behavioral function. These contrasting profiles have important implications for understanding the development of brain–behavior relations.

THE PLAN OF THIS BOOK

This book is about the neurobehavioral consequences of perinatal brain injury, and what the study of this important population of children can tell us about the fundamental nature of human brain development. The book is divided into three parts. Part 1 provides background and context for the central questions about the effects of early brain injury. Part 2 constitutes the heart of the book, presenting an in-depth account of what is known about the effects of perinatal brain injury on neurobehavioral development. Part 3 provides both a summary and reflection on what we have learned from this population, as well as a chapter on what can be done to clinically assist children afflicted by this disorder.

Part 1 of this book provides an overview of the basics of brain development (Chapter 2) and the specific effects of perinatal lesions (PL) on the developing brain (Chapter 3). Chapter 2 reviews the major milestones of prenatal brain development and presents a model of typical brain development as a dynamic and adaptive process that relies upon both molecular and experiential factors. As discussed in the chapter, plasticity is a fundamental property of brain development that reflects the dynamic interactions of intrinsic and extrinsic factors that define the developmental process as it unfolds over time. Critically, the state of the organism at a given point in development imparts specific susceptibilities and vulnerabilities. The specific developmental state of the neural system determines which factors can, as well as which factors cannot, affect its subsequent development. Such a model of brain development provides a critical context for understanding development in the wake of perinatal injury.

Chapter 3 considers the nature of the brain injury, itself. The major focus of this chapter is on perinatal stroke, which accounts for the great majority of cases of children with unilateral perinatal brain lesions. The chapter discusses the timing, etiology, and mechanisms of perinatal stroke, focusing on both neuroanatomy and vascular organization, and differences that may be associated with prenatal versus postnatal onset. The chapter provides an overview of the clinical presentation and diagnostic indicators and considers maternal, neonatal, and genetic factors that may contribute to or complicate the clinical presentation.

Part 2 (Chapters 4 through 9) provides an in-depth summary of the effects of perinatal injury across a range of behavioral domains. These chapters make up the heart of the book. They bring together data from a number of laboratories and summarize the mainly longitudinal findings on the behavioral effects of perinatal injury and its long-term consequences for this population of children. The behavioral data consistently point to the role of plasticity in the development of critical sensory, motor, cognitive, linguistic, and affective functions in this population of children, but the degree of plasticity and capacity for compensatory adaptation varies in important ways across domains. Thus, although the chapters are organized by behavioral domain, an important theme is the comparison and contrast of developmental effects across domains.

Part 3 (Chapters 10 and 11) of the book is a reflection on these issues. Chapter 10 considers the clinical implications of the data presented in this volume and asks the critical questions about whether and how specific interventions can support and promote behavioral development in children with perinatal injury. Chapter 11 provides a synthesis of all of the ideas and issues raised in the book. Critically, it offers a model of neurobehavioral development that captures the dynamic nature of change in both brain and behavioral systems, and provides a means of aligning theory and data from developmental neurobiology and developmental neuropsychology. At the heart of this model is the idea that neurobehavioral development, whether typical or following early pathology, involves an ongoing and robust series of interactions among biological and environmental factors. It views development as a continuous process of adaptation that is shaped by genetic, environmental, and temporal constraints. As such, the model returns to the fundamental question of the role of plasticity in brain development.

REFERENCES

Alberini CM. (2009). Transcription factors in long-term memory and synaptic plasticity. *Physiol Rev* 89(1):121–145.

Alajouanine, T., & Lhermitte, F. (1965). Acquired aphasia in children. *Brain*, 88, 553-562

Alvarado MC, Bachevalier J. (2000). Revisiting the maturation of medial temporal lobe memory functions in primates. *Learn Mem* 7(5):244–256.

Alvarado MC, Wright AA, Bachevalier J. (2002). Object and spatial relational memory in adult rhesus monkeys is impaired by neonatal lesions of the hippocampal formation but not the amygdaloid complex. *Hippocampus* 12(4):421–433.

Bachevalier J, Beauregard M, Alvarado MC. (1999). Long-term effects of neonatal damage to the hippocampal formation and amygdaloid complex on object discrimination and object recognition in rhesus monkeys (*Macaca mulatta*). *Behav Neurosci* 113(6):1127–1151.

Bachevalier J, Mishkin M. (1994). Effects of selective neonatal temporal lobe lesions on visual recognition memory in rhesus monkeys. *J Neurosci* 14(4):2128–2139.

Barker PA. (2009). Whither proBDNF? *Nat Neurosci* 12(2):105–106.

Bauman MD, Lavenex P, Mason WA, Capitanio JP, & Amaral DG. (2004). The development of social behavior following neonatal amygdala lesions in rhesus monkeys. *J Cogn Neurosci* 16(8):1388–1411.

Bavelier D, Dye MW, Hauser PC. (2006). Do deaf individuals see better? *Trends Cogn Sci* 10(11):512–518.

Bavelier D, Neville HJ. (2002). Cross-modal plasticity: where and how? *Nat Rev Neurosci* 3(6):443–452.

Bennett EL, Rosenzweig MR, Diamond MC. (1969). Rat brain: effects of environmental enrichment on wet and dry weights. *Science* 163(869):825–826.

Berlucchi G, Buchtel HA. (2009). Neuronal plasticity: historical roots and evolution of meaning. *Exp Brain Res* 192(3):307–319.

Black JE, Greenough WT. (1986). Induction of pattern in neural structure by experience: Implications for cognitive development. In Lamb ME, Brown AL, Rogoff B (Eds.), Advances in Developmental Psychology (Vol. 4, pp. 1–50). Hillsdale, NJ: Erlbaum.

Black JE, Sirevaag AM, Greenough WT. (1987). Complex experience promotes capillary formation in young rat visual cortex. *Neurosci Lett* 83(3):351–355.

Bowlby J. (1969). Attachment and Loss (Vol. 1). New York: Basic Books.

Briones TL, Klintsova AY, Greenough WT. (2004). Stability of synaptic plasticity in the adult rat visual cortex induced by complex environment exposure. *Brain Res* 1018(1):130–135.

Broca P. (1861). Remarques sur le siège de la faculté du language articulé; suivies d'une observation d'aphémie (perte de la parole). *Bulletins de la Société Anatomique* 6:330–357, 398–407.

Broca P. (1865). Du siège de la faculté du langage articulé dans l'hémisphère gauche du cerveau [On the site of articulated language in the left hemisphere]. Bulletin de la Société d'*Anthropologie* 6:377–393.

Brown, J. W., & Jaffe, J. (1975). Hypothesis on Cerebral Dominance. *Neuropsychologia, 13*(1), 107-110.

Brown TG. (1915). On the activities of the central nervous system of the unborn foetus of the cat; with a discussion of the question whether progression (walking, etc.) is a "learnt" complex. *J Physiol* 49:208–215.

Brown-Sequard, C.-E. (1877). Aphasia as an effect of brain-disease. *Dublin Journal of Medical Science, 63*, 209-225

Carlson, J., Netley, C., Hendrick, E., & Pritchard, J. (1968). A reexamination of intellectual abilities in hemidecorticated patients. *Transactions of the American Neurological Association,* 93, 198-201.

Chabot N, Charbonneau V, Laramee ME, Tremblay R, Boire D, Bronchti G. (2008). Subcortical auditory input to the primary visual cortex in anophthalmic mice. *Neurosci Lett* 433(2):129–134.

Chang FL, Greenough WT. (1982). Lateralized effects of monocular training on dendritic branching in adult split-brain rats. *Brain Res* 232(2):283–292.

Chebat DR, Chen JK, Schneider F, Ptito A, Kupers R, Ptito M. (2007). Alterations in right posterior hippocampus in early blind individuals. *Neuroreport* 18(4):329–333.

Clancy B, Darlington RB, Finlay BL. (2001). Translating developmental time across mammalian species. *Neuroscience* 105(1):7–17.

Collignon O, Voss P, Lassonde M, Lepore F. (2009). Cross-modal plasticity for the spatial processing of sounds in visually deprived subjects. *Exp Brain Res* 192(3):343–358.

Damasio A, Adolphs R, Damasio H. (2003). The contributions of the lesion method to the functional neuroanatomy of emotion. In Davidson RJ, Scherer KR, Goldsmith HH (Eds.), Handbook of Affective Sciences (pp. 66–92). Oxford: Oxford University Press.

Damasio H. (2000). The lesion method in cognitive neuroscience. In Boller F, Grafman J (Eds.), Handbook of Neuropsychology (2nd ed, pp. 77–102). New York: Elsevier.

Damasio H, Damasio AR. (2000). The lesion method in cognitive in cognitive neuroscience. In Farah MJ, Feinberg TE (Eds.), Patient-Based Approaches to Cognitive Neuroscience (pp. 21–34). Cambridge, MA: MIT Press.

Day, Patricia S., & Ulatowska, Hanna K. (1979). Perceptual, cognitive, and linguistic development after early hemispherectomy: Two case studies. *Brain & Language, 7*(1), 17-33.

Denenberg VH. (1981). Hemispheric laterality in animals and the effects of early experience. *Behav Brain Sci* 4(1):1–50.

Dennis, Maureen. (1980). Capacity and strategy for syntactic comprehension after left or right hemidecortication. *Brain & Language, 10*(2), 287-317.

Dennis, Maureen, & Kohn, Bruno. (1975). Comprehension of Syntax in Infantile Hemiplegics After Cerebral Hemidecortication: Left-Hemisphere Superiority. *Brain & Language, 2*(4), 472-482.

Emmorey K, Allen JS, Bruss J, Schenker N, Damasio H. (2003). A morphometric analysis of auditory brain regions in congenitally deaf adults. *Proc Natl Acad Sci U S A* 100(17):10049–10054.

Emmorey K, Grabowski T, McCullough S, Damasio H, Ponto LL, Hichwa RD, et al. (2003). Neural systems underlying lexical retrieval for sign language. *Neuropsychologia* 41(1):85–95.

Fellows LK, Heberlein AS, Morales DA, Shivde G, Waller S, Wu DH. (2005). Method matters: an empirical study of impact in cognitive neuroscience. *J Cogn Neurosci* 17(6):850–858.

Finger S. (1994). Origins of Neuroscience: A History of Explorations into Brain Function. New York: Oxford University Press.

Finger, S. Almli, R. (1988). Margaret Kennard and her "principle" in historical perspective. In Stanley Finger, T. E. LeVere, Robert Almli & D. G. Stein (Eds.), *Brain injury and recovery: Theoretical and controversial issues* (pp. 117-132). New York: Plenum.

Goldman PS. (1971). Functional development of the prefrontal cortex in early life and the problem of neuronal plasticity. *Exp Neurol* 32(3):366–387.

Goldman PS. (1974). Functional recovery after lesions of the nervous systems. 3. Developmental processes in neural plasticity. Recovery of function after CNS lesions in infant monkeys. *Neurosci Res Program Bull* 12(2):217–222.

Goldman PS, Rosvold HE, Mishkin M. (1970). Selective sparing of function following prefrontal lobectomy in infant monkeys. *Exp Neurol* 29(2):221–226.

Goldman-Rakic PS. (1981). Development and plasticity of primate frontal association cortex. In Schmitt FO, Worden FG, Adelman G, Dennis SG (Eds.), The Organization of the Cerebral Cortex: Proceedings of a Neurosciences Research Program Colloquium (pp. 69–97). Cambridge, MA: The MIT Press.

Goldman-Rakic PS. (1988). Topography of cognition: Parallel distributed networks in primate association cortex. *Ann Rev Neurosci* 11:137–156.

Goldman-Rakic PS, Leung H-C. (2002). Functional architecture of the dorsolateral prefrontal cortex in monkeys and humans. In Stuss DT, Knight RT (Eds.), Principles of Frontal Lobe Function (pp. 85–95). London: Oxford University Press.

Gott, Peggy S. (1973). Cognitive Abilities Following Right and Left Hemispherectomy. *Cortex, 9*(3), 266-274.

Gottlieb G. (1976). Conceptions of prenatal development: behavioral embryology. *Psychol Rev* 83(3):215–234.

Gottlieb G. (1998). Normally occurring environmental and behavioral influences on gene activity: from central dogma to probabilistic epigenesis. *Psychol Rev* 105(4):792–802.

Green CS, Bavelier D. (2008). Exercising your brain: a review of human brain plasticity and training-induced learning. *Psychol Aging* 23(4):692–701.

Greenough WT. (1993). Experience and brain development: An update. In Johnson MH (Ed.), Brain Development and Cognition: A Reader. Oxford: Blackwell.

Greenough WT, Black JE, Wallace CS. (1987). Experience and brain development. *Child Dev* 58(3):539–559.

Greenough WT, Chang FF. (1988). Plasticity of synapse structure and pattern in the cerebral cortex. In Peters A, Jones EG (Eds.), Cerebral Cortex (pp. 391–440). New York: Plenum.

Greenough WT, Hwang HM, Gorman C. (1985). Evidence for active synapse formation or altered postsynaptic metabolism in visual cortex of rats reared in complex environments. *Proc Natl Acad Sci U S A* 82(13):4549–4552.

Grossman AW, Churchill JD, Bates KE, Kleim JA, Greenough WT. (2002). A brain adaptation view of plasticity: is synaptic plasticity an overly limited concept? *Prog Brain Res* 138: 91–108.

Hammill, Donald, & Irwin, Orvis C. (1966). Iq Differences of Right and Left Spastic Hemiplegic Children. *Perceptual & Motor Skills, 22*(1), 193-194.

Hebb DO. (1949). The Organization of behavior; A Neuropsychological Theory. New York: Wiley.

Hubel, D. H., & Wiesel, T. N. (1964). Effects of Monocular Deprivation in Kittens. *Naunyn Schmiedebergs Arch Exp Pathol Pharmakol, 248*, 492-497.

Hubel, D. H., Wiesel, T. N., & LeVay, S. (1976). Functional architecture of area 17 in normal and monocularly deprived macaque monkeys. *Cold Spring Harb Symp Quant Biol, 40*, 581–589.

Hubel, D. H., Wiesel, T. N., & LeVay, S. (1977). Plasticity of ocular dominance columns in monkey striate cortex. *Philos Trans R Soc Lond B Biol Sci, 278*(961), 377–-409.

Izraeli R, Koay G, Lamish M, Heicklen-Klein AJ, Heffner HE, Heffner RS, et al. (2002). Cross-modal neuroplasticity in neonatally enucleated hamsters: structure, electrophysiology and behaviour. *Eur J Neurosci* 15(4):693–712.

Johnson MH. (2001). Functional brain development in humans. *Nat Rev Neurosci* 2(7):475–483.

Johnson MH. (2005). Sensitive periods in functional brain development: problems and prospects. *Dev Psychobiol* 46(3):287–292.

Jones TA, Greenough WT. (1996). Ultrastructural evidence for increased contact between astrocytes and synapses in rats reared in a complex environment. *Neurobiol Learn Mem* 65(1):48–56.

Kahn DM, Krubitzer L. (2002). Massive cross-modal cortical plasticity and the emergence of a new cortical area in developmentally blind mammals. *Proc Natl Acad Sci U S A* 99(17):11429–11434.

Kalia M. (2008). Brain development: anatomy, connectivity, adaptive plasticity, and toxicity. *Metabolism* 57 Suppl 2:S2–5.

Karlen SJ, Kahn DM, Krubitzer L. (2006). Early blindness results in abnormal corticocortical and thalamocortical connections. *Neuroscience* 142(3):843–858.

Kennard MA. (1936). Age and other factors in motor recovery from precentral lesions in monkeys. *Am J Physiol* 115:138–146.

Kennard MA. (1938a). Recovery of function in infant monkeys following cortical ablations. *Am J Physiol* 123:118.

Kennard MA. (1938b). Reorganization of motor function in the cerebral cortex of monkeys deprived of motor and premotor areas in infancy. *J Neurophysiol* 1:477–496.

Kennard MA, Fulton JF. (1942). Age and reorganization of central nervous system. *J Mount Sinai Hospital (New York)* 9:594–606.

Knudsen EI. (2004). Sensitive periods in the development of the brain and behavior. *J Cogn Neurosci* 16(8):1412–1425.

Kohn, Bruno. (1980). Right-hemisphere speech representation and comprehension of syntax after left cerebral injury. *Brain & Language*, 9(2), 350–361.

Kohn, Bruno, & Dennis, Maureen. (1974). Selective Impairments of Visuo-Spatial Abilities in Infantile Hemiplegics After Right Cerebral Hemidecortication. *Neuropsychologia, 12*(4), 505–512.

Kolb B. (1987). Recovery from early cortical damage in rats: I. Differential behavioral and anatomical effects of frontal lesions at different ages of neural maturation. *Behav Brain Res* 25(3):205–220.

Kolb B. (1995). Brain Plasticity and Behavior. Mahwah, NJ: Lawrence Erlbaum Associates, Inc.

Kolb B, Cioe J, Muirhead D. (1998). Cerebral morphology and function sparing after prenatal frontal cortex lesions in rats. *Behav Brain Res* 91(1–2):143–155.

Kolb B, Elliott W. (1987). Recovery from early cortical damage in rats: II. Effects of experience on anatomy and behavior following frontal lesions at 1 or 5 days of age. *Behav Brain Res* 26(1):47–56.

Kolb B, Holmes C, Whishaw IQ. (1987). Recovery from early cortical lesions in rats. III. Neonatal removal of posterior parietal cortex has greater behavioral and anatomical effects than similar removals in adulthood. *Behav Brain Res* 26(2–3):119–137.

Kolb B, Tomie JA. (1988). Recovery from early cortical damage in rats. IV. Effects of hemidecortication at 1, 5 or 10 days of age on cerebral anatomy and behavior. *Behav Brain Res* 28(3):259–274.

Kolb B, Whishaw IQ. (1989). Plasticity in the neocortex: mechanisms underlying recovery from early brain damage. *Prog Neurobiol* 32(4):235–276.

Kolb B, Whishaw IQ. (2000). Reorganization of function after cortical lesions in rodents. In Levin HS, Grafman J (Eds.), Cerebral Reorganization of Function after Brain Damage (pp. 109–129). New York: Oxford University Press.

Krashen, S. D. (1973). Lateralization, language learning, and the critical period: Some (Hammill & Irwin, 1966)new evidence. *Language Learning, 23*(1), 63–74.

Kuczewski N, Porcher C, Lessmann V, Medina I, Gaiarsa JL. (2009). Activity-dependent dendritic release of BDNF and biological consequences. *Mol Neurobiol* 39(1):37–49.

Laemle LK, Strominger NL, Carpenter DO. (2006). Cross-modal innervation of primary visual cortex by auditory fibers in congenitally anophthalmic mice. *Neurosci Lett* 396(2): 108–112.

Langworthy OR. (1924). Relation of onset of decerebrate rigidity to the time of myelination of tracts in the brain-stem and spinal cord of young animals. *Contrib Endocrinol* 17:127–140.

Lenneberg EH. (1967). Biological Foundations of Language. New York: Wiley.

LeVay, S., Wiesel, T. N., & Hubel, D. H. (1980). The development of ocular dominance columns in normal and visually deprived monkeys. *J Comp Neurol, 191*(1), 1–51

Levin AV. (2003). Congenital eye anomalies. *Pediatr Clin North Am* 50(1):55–76.

Lewis TL, Maurer D. (2005). Multiple sensitive periods in human visual development: evidence from visually deprived children. *Dev Psychobiol* 46(3):163–183.

Lorenz K. (1937/57). The conception of instinctive behavior. In Schiller CH (Ed.), Instinctive Behavior (pp. 129–175). New York: International Universities Press.

Malkova L, Mishkin M, Bachevalier J. (1995). Long-term effects of selective neonatal temporal lobe lesions on learning and memory in monkeys. *Behav Neurosci* 109(2):212–226.

Markham JA, Greenough WT. (2004). Experience-driven brain plasticity: beyond the synapse. *Neuron Glia Biol* 1(4):351–363.

Mattson MP. (2008). Glutamate and neurotrophic factors in neuronal plasticity and disease. *Ann N Y Acad Sci* 1144:97–112.

Maurer D, Lewis TL, Brent HP, Levin AV. (1999). Rapid improvement in the acuity of infants after visual input. *Science* 286(5437):108–110.

Maurer D, Lewis TL, Mondloch CJ. (2005). Missing sights: consequences for visual cognitive development. *Trends Cogn Sci* 9(3):144–151.

McFie, John. (1961). The Effects of Hemispherectomy on Intellectual Functioning in Cases of Infantile Hemiplegia. *Journal of Neurology, Neurosurgery & Psychiatry, 24*, 240–249.

Mehler MF. (2008). Epigenetics and the nervous system. *Ann Neurol* 64(6):602–617.

Michel GF, Tyler AN. (2005). Critical period: a history of the transition from questions of when, to what, to how. *Dev Psychobiol* 46(3):156–162.

Mishkin M. (1982). A memory system in the monkey. *Philos Trans R Soc Lond B Biol Sci* 298(1089):83–95.

Morita K. (2009). Computational implications of cooperative plasticity induction at nearby dendritic sites. *Sci Signal* 2(52):pe2.

Morris R. (1984). Developments of a water-maze procedure for studying spatial learning in the rat. *J Neurosci Methods* 11(1):47–60.

Moses P, Stiles J. (2002). The lesion methodology: contrasting views from adult and child studies. *Dev Psychobiol* 40(3):266–277.

Nithianantharajah J, Hannan AJ. (2006). Enriched environments, experience-dependent plasticity and disorders of the nervous system. *Nat Rev Neurosci* 7(9):697–709.

Noppeney U. (2007). The effects of visual deprivation on functional and structural organization of the human brain. *Neurosci Biobehav Rev* 31(8):1169–1180.

O'Leary DD, Stanfield BB. (1989). Selective elimination of axons extended by developing cortical neurons is dependent on regional locale: experiments utilizing fetal cortical transplants. *J Neurosci* 9(7):2230–2246.

Osler, William. (1987). *The cerebral palsies of children*. London: Mac Keith Press.

Oyama S. (2000). The Ontogeny of Information: Developmental Systems and Evolution (2nd ed.). Durham, NC: Duke University Press.

Pallas SL, Roe AW, Sur M. (1990). Visual projections induced into the auditory pathway of ferrets. I. Novel inputs to primary auditory cortex (AI) from the LP/pulvinar complex and the topography of the MGN-AI projection. *J Comp Neurol* 298(1):50–68.

Pascual-Leone A, Amedi A, Fregni F, Merabet LB. (2005). The plastic human brain cortex. *Annu Rev Neurosci* 28, 377–401.

Piche M, Chabot N, Bronchti G, Miceli D, Lepore F, Guillemot JP. (2007). Auditory responses in the visual cortex of neonatally enucleated rats. *Neuroscience* 145(3):1144–1156.

Piche M, Robert S, Miceli D, Bronchti G. (2004). Environmental enrichment enhances auditory takeover of the occipital cortex in anophthalmic mice. *Eur J Neurosci* 20(12):3463–3472.

Prather MD, Lavenex P, Mauldin-Jourdain ML, Mason WA, Capitanio JP, Mendoza SP, et al. (2001). Increased social fear and decreased fear of objects in monkeys with neonatal amygdala lesions. *Neuroscience* 106(4):653–658.

Ptito M, Schneider FC, Paulson OB, Kupers R. (2008). Alterations of the visual pathways in congenital blindness. *Exp Brain Res* 187(1):41–49.

Reed, J. C., & Reitan, R. M. (1969). Verbal and performance differences among brain-injured children with lateralized motor deficits. *Perceptual and Motor Skills, 29*(3), 747–752.

Rorden C, Karnath HO. (2004). Using human brain lesions to infer function: a relic from a past era in the fMRI age? *Nat Rev Neurosci* 5(10):813–819.

Rosenzweig MR, Bennett EL. (1972). Cerebral changes in rats exposed individually to an enriched environment. *J Comp Physiol Psychol* 80(2):304–313.

Rosenzweig MR, Krech D, Bennett EL, Diamond MC. (1962). Effects of environmental complexity and training on brain chemistry and anatomy: a replication and extension. *J Comp Physiol Psychol* 55(4):429–437.

Rosenzweig MR, Krech D, Bennett EL, Zolman JF. (1962). Variation in environmental complexity and brain measures. *J Comp Physiol Psychol* 55(6):1092–1095.

Rosenzweig MR, Love W, Bennett EL. (1968). Effects of a few hours a day of enriched experience on brain chemistry and brain weights. *Physiol Behav* 3(6):819–825.

Schiller, Francis. (1979). *Paul Broca, founder of French anthropology, explorer of the brain*. Berkeley: University of California Press.

Schlaggar BL, O'Leary DD. (1991). Potential of visual cortex to develop an array of functional units unique to somatosensory cortex. *Science* 252(5012):1556–1560.

Schneider GE. (1973). Early lesions of superior colliculus: factors affecting the formation of abnormal retinal projections. *Brain Behav Evol* 8(1):73–109.

Schuren JE. (1997). Interdisciplinary relationships: behavioral neurology. In Maruish ME (Ed.), Clinical Neuropsychology: Theoretical Foundations for Practitioners (pp. 21–34). Hillsdale, NJ: LEA.

Shimony JS, Burton H, Epstein AA, McLaren DG, Sun SW, Snyder AZ. (2006). Diffusion tensor imaging reveals white matter reorganization in early blind humans. *Cereb Cortex* 16(11):1653–1661.

Sirevaag AM, Greenough WT. (1987). Differential rearing effects on rat visual cortex synapses. III. Neuronal and glial nuclei, boutons, dendrites, and capillaries. *Brain Res* 424(2):320–332.

Stiles J. (2000). Neural plasticity and cognitive development. *Dev Neuropsychol* 18(2):237–272.

Stiles J. (2008). The Fundamentals of Brain Development: Integrating Nature and Nurture. Cambridge, MA: Harvard University Press.

Sur M, Angelucci A, Sharma J. (1999). Rewiring cortex: the role of patterned activity in development and plasticity of neocortical circuits. *J Neurobiol* 41(1):33–43.

Sur M, Garraghty PE, Roe AW. (1988). Experimentally induced visual projections into auditory thalamus and cortex. *Science* 242(4884):1437–1441.

Sur M, Leamey CA. (2001). Development and plasticity of cortical areas and networks. *Nat Rev Neurosci* 2(4):251–262.

Sur M, Pallas SL, Roe AW. (1990). Cross-modal plasticity in cortical development: differentiation and specification of sensory neocortex. *Trends Neurosci* 13(6):227–233.

Sur M, Rubenstein JL. (2005). Patterning and plasticity of the cerebral cortex. *Science* 310(5749): 805–810.

Szeligo F, Leblond CP. (1977). Response of the three main types of glial cells of cortex and corpus callosum in rats handled during suckling or exposed to enriched, control and impoverished environments following weaning. *J Comp Neurol* 172(2):247–263.

Teuber HL. (1974). Functional recovery after lesions of the nervous system. II. Recovery of function after lesions of the central nervous system: history and prospects. *Neurosci Res Program Bull*, 12(2):197–211.

Tropea D, Van Wart A, Sur M. (2009). Molecular mechanisms of experience-dependent plasticity in visual cortex. *Philos Trans R Soc Lond B Biol Sci* 364(1515):341–355.

Vargha-Khadem, F., & O'Gorman, A. M. (1983). *Aphasia in children with "prenatal" versus postnatal left hemisphere lesions: A clinical and CT scan study.* Paper presented at the 11th Meeting of the International Neuropsychological Soceity, Mexico City.

Vargha-Khadem, F., O'Gorman, A. M., & Watters, G. V. (1985). Aphasia and handedness in relation to hemispheric side, age at injury and severity of cerebral lesion during childhood. *Brain, 108*(Pt 3)(4), 677–696.

von Melchner L, Pallas SL, Sur M. (2000). Visual behaviour mediated by retinal projections directed to the auditory pathway. *Nature* 404(6780):871–876.

Webster MJ, Bachevalier J, Ungerleider LG. (1995). Transient subcortical connections of inferior temporal areas TE and TEO in infant macaque monkeys. *J Comp Neurol* 352(2):213–226.

Webster MJ, Ungerleider LG, Bachevalier J. (1991a). Connections of inferior temporal areas TE and TEO with medial temporal-lobe structures in infant and adult monkeys. *J Neurosci* 11(4):1095–1116.

Webster MJ, Ungerleider LG, Bachevalier J. (1991b). Lesions of inferior temporal area TE in infant monkeys alter cortico-amygdalar projections. *Neuroreport* 2(12):769–772.

Weed WK, Kennard MA. (1917). The reactions of kittens after decortication. *Am J Physiol* 43:131–157.

Wiesel TN, Hubel DH. (1963a). Effects of visual deprivation on morphology and physiology of cells in the cat's lateral geniculate body. *J Neurophysiol* 26:978–993.

Wiesel TN, Hubel DH. (1963b). Receptive fields of cells in striate cortex of very young, visually inexperienced kittens. *J Neurophysiol* 26:994–1002.

Wiesel TN, Hubel DH. (1963c). Single-cell responses in striate cortex of kittens deprived of vision in one eye. *J Neurophysiol* 26:1003–1017.

Wiesel TN, Hubel DH. (1965a). Comparison of the effects of unilateral and bilateral eye closure on cortical unit responses in kittens. *J Neurophysiol* 28(6):1029–1040.

Wiesel TN, Hubel DH. (1965b). Extent of recovery from the effects of visual deprivation in kittens. *J Neurophysiol* 28(6):1060–1072.

Witelson SF. (1985). On hemisphere specialization and cerebral plasticity from birth: Mark II. In Best CT (Ed.), Hemispheric Function and Collaboration in the Child (pp. 33–77). Orlando: Academic Press.

Woods, B. T., & Carey, S. (1979). Language deficits after apparent clinical recovery from childhood aphasia. *Annals of Neurology, 6*(5), 405–409.

Woods, Bryan T. (1980). The restricted effects of right-hemisphere lesions after age one: Wechsler test data. *Neuropsychologia, 18*(1), 65–70.

2

The Basics of Brain Development

THE HUMAN BRAIN is arguably the most complex of all biological systems. The mature brain is composed of more than 100 billion neurons that form more than 60 trillion connections (Pakkenberg & Gundersen, 1997). There are more than 20 billion neurons in the mature neocortex alone. The task of producing the basic neural elements in these numbers is daunting. At the height of corticogenesis (formation of the cortex) neurons are produced at the rate of 250,000 per minute. But brains are much more than simply the sum of their neural parts. Cells are produced, migrate to appropriate brain areas, and form molecular and cellular systems for communicating with each other. Networks of cells form information processing systems specialized for different functions. The information processing systems themselves are exquisitely tuned to the input from the environment. Given the complexity of this remarkable biological system, it should not be surprising that the processes that support the *development* of the human brain are comparably complex.

Human brain development is a protracted process that begins in the third week after conception with the differentiation of the neural progenitor (or neural stem) cells and extends at least through late adolescence. Indeed, studies documenting neural plasticity in the adult brain suggest that the capacity for developmental change is never entirely lost but may extend throughout the lifespan, though in a more limited form (Buonomano & Merzenich, 1998; Kaas, Merzenich, & Killackey, 1983; Kilgard & Merzenich, 1998). The processes that contribute to brain development over this extended period range from molecular events associated with gene expression to input from the outside world. Further, these very different sets of processes work in concert, interacting to support the ongoing series of events that define the milestones of brain development. Both gene expression and environmental input are essential for the generation of a normal brain, and disruption of either will alter the course of brain development. But neither is prescriptive nor determinative. Rather, brain development is well described as a complex series of dynamic and adaptive processes that operate at each point in development to promote the emergence and differentiation of new neural structures and functions. These processes operate within a highly constrained and genetically organized but constantly changing context (Morange, 2001; Stiles, 2008; Waddington,

1939) that, over time, supports the emergence of the complex and dynamic structure of the human brain.

This chapter will consider some of the major events that contribute to the development of the human brain from its early embryonic state through adolescence. It begins by reviewing the fundamental changes that occur during the embryonic period, which covers the first 8 weeks of gestation in humans. Development during the embryonic period results in an organism that, while only 25 to 30 mm long, is fully recognizable as human and possesses a rudimentary nervous system (Fig. 2.1). By gestational week 8 (GW8) the major compartments of the central and peripheral nervous system are well defined. The segmental organization of the spinal column and hindbrain has emerged, primitive midbrain and diencephalic structures are identifiable, and the neocortex has begun to form. The period of fetal development follows the embryonic period and extends through the end of gestation. It is a time of rapid growth and elaboration of both cortical and subcortical structures. Major fiber pathways form during this period. For example, thalamocortical and corticothalamic pathways are established by GW26, creating the major sensorimotor pathways of the brain (Kostovic & Jovanov-Milosevic, 2006; Kostovic & Judas, 2010). In addition, parcellation of the fetal neocortex becomes more refined as functional organization begins to emerge (Kostovic & Jovanov-Milosevic, 2006). Brain development continues for an extended period postnatally. The overall size of the brain increases fourfold through the preschool period, reaching approximately 90% of adult volume by age 6 (Courchesne et al., 2000; Iwasaki et al., 1997; Kennedy, Makris, Herbert, Takahashi, & Caviness, 2002; Kennedy & Dehay, 2001; Lenroot & Giedd, 2006; Paus et al., 2001; Reiss, Abrams, Singer, & Ross, 1996). But structural changes continue to be observed through childhood and adolescence, and these are accompanied by changes in functional organization that correspond systematically to changes in behavioral development.

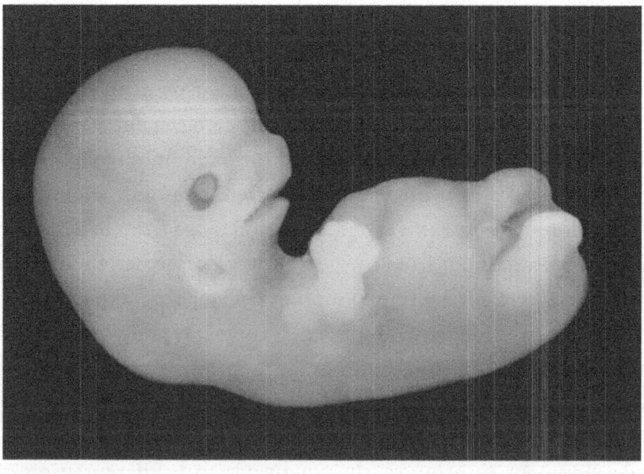

FIGURE 2.1 Human embryo at approximately 6 gestational weeks. It is approximately 25 mm long. (Image adapted with permission from Wikimedia Commons. en.wikipedia.org/wiki/File:Human_Embryo. This file is licensed under the Creative Commons Attribution 2.0 Generic license.)

The changes that are observed in the overall structure of the brain at different points in development are supported by dramatic changes occurring at the cellular level. Beginning on embryonic day 42 (E42; i.e., 42 days after conception) the first cortical neurons are produced by the neural progenitor cells (Bystron, Blakemore, & Rakic, 2008; Stiles, 2008). These cells migrate to different cortical areas. Neuron production is largely complete by mid-gestation and neuronal migration by the end of the prenatal period. Once in place, the neurons begin to differentiate, producing specific neurotransmitter substances and forming connections with other cells. The formation and stabilization of mature neural pathways is a protracted process that extends well into adolescence. Although synapse formation begins in the prenatal period, it rapidly accelerates immediately after birth. Indeed, the number of synapses in brains of infants and young children far exceeds that of adults (Huttenlocher & Dabholkar, 1997; Huttenlocher & de Courten, 1987). This exuberance of connectivity is an example of another important, if somewhat counterintuitive, hallmark of brain development, specifically the neural subtractive events. Two crucial subtractive processes are naturally occurring cell death, and synaptic exuberance and pruning. As impressive as the numbers of neurons in the mature brain are, the numbers initially produced are far higher, on the order of 30% to 80% across brain areas (Buss, Sun, & Oppenheim, 2006; Oppenheim, 1991; Rabinowicz, de Courten-Myers, Petetot, Xi, & de los Reyes, 1996). Similarly, connections among neurons in the developing brain are far more extensive than in the mature brain, again on the order of 50% higher in the young child than the adult (Innocenti & Price, 2005). The loss of neurons by non-pathological cell death processes and the retraction of exuberant connections by competitive processes provide important means of shaping and sculpting the emerging organization of the developing brain.

BRAIN DEVELOPMENT IN THE EMBRYONIC PERIOD

Brain development begins in GW3 on approximately E13 . Prior to this time the important events of fertilization, implantation, and cleavage have occurred. During fertilization the genetic contributions of the two parents are combined, triggering the initial development of the embryo. Implantation anchors the developing embryo to the wall of the uterus, an event necessary for its survival. Cleavage involves a series of symmetrical cell divisions that serve to increase the number of cells in the developing embryo (Larsen, 2001; Sadler, 2006; Sadler & Langman, 2010). By E4, the process of cleavage produces two cell groups, an inner cell mass that is surrounded by an outer cell mass (Fig. 2.2B). These two sets of cells together make up the blastocyst. The embryo will form from the inner cell mass, while extra-embryonic structures, such as the amnion and the yolk sac, will form from the outer cell mass. By E6, these two groups of cells separate, forming a large cavity in the center of the embryo called the blastocoel (Sadler & Langman, 2010). At this stage of development, the cells of the inner cell mass are pluripotent embryonic stem cells, which means they are capable of producing any cell line in the body (these are the cells that are the focus of much scientific research and political controversy). By E13, further differentiation of the inner cell mass is observed and two distinct cell layers emerge, the epiblast cell layer and the hypoblast cell layer (Fig. 2.3). The embryo will form from the epiblast layer, while the cells of the hypoblast will form additional extra-embryonic structures. Thus, by E13, the embryo has two layers and is shaped like a disk. The events involved in the first step of brain development—the induction of the neural progenitor cells—center on the cells of the epiblast layer of the two-layered embryo (Gilbert, 2006; Sadler, 2006; Sadler & Langman, 2010).

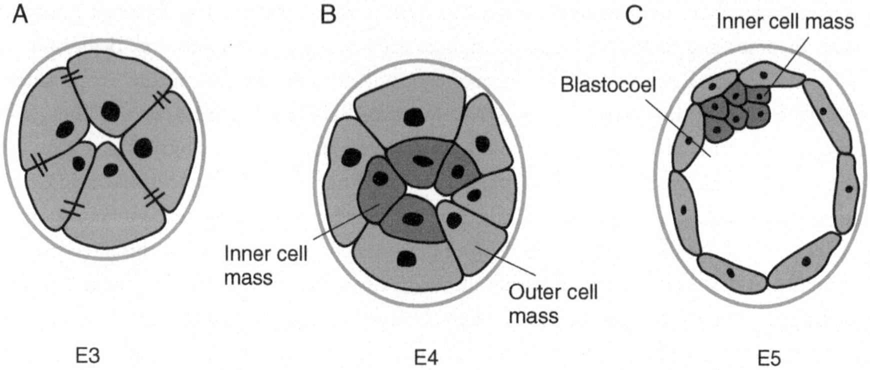

FIGURE 2.2 (A) During cleavage the embryonic cells divide and increase in number. (B) During the morula stage (E4), the embryonic cells differentiate into an inner cell mass that is surrounded by an outer cell mass. The inner cell mass will form the embryo; the outer cell mass will contribute to the placenta. (C) At the beginning of the blastocyst stage on E5, the blastocoel, or central cavity forms, separating the two cell lines. (Adapted with permission under the terms of the GNU Free Documentation License Version 1.2 or any later version published by the Free Software Foundation. A copy of the license is included in the section entitled *GNU Free Documentation License*. http://en.wikipedia.org/wiki/File:HumanEmbryogenesis.svg.)

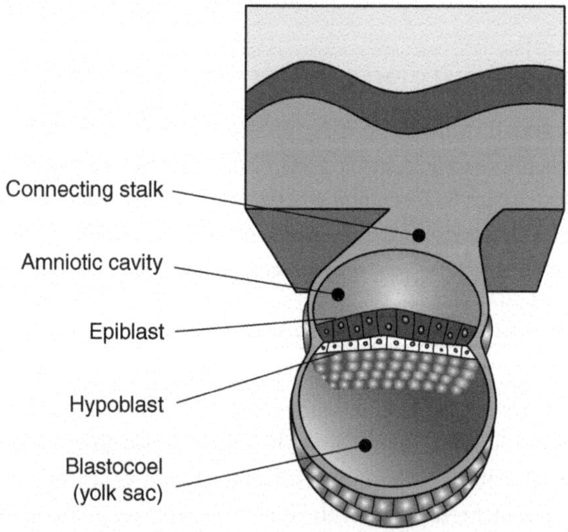

FIGURE 2.3 The human embryo at E13. Embryo within the context of extraembryonic structures. The connecting stalk anchors the embryo to the uterine wall. At this point in development the embryo is a two-layered structure that is positioned between the amniotic cavity and the blastocoel (primitive yolk sac). The epiblast layer of the embryo will give rise to all of the structures of the developing embryo, while the hypoblast layer will be displaced and will later give rise to extraembryonic structures. (Illustration by Matthew Stiles Davis; reproduced by permission of the publisher. From "The Fundamentals of Brain Development: Integrating Nature and Nurture" by Joan Stiles. Cambridge, MA: Harvard University Press Copyright © 2008 by the President and Fellows of Harvard College.)

Gastrulation and the Development of the Neural Stem Cells

As discussed earlier, at the end of the second week after conception, the embryo is a simple, oval structure that consists of two cell layers, the epiblast layer and the hypoblast layer. By the end of gastrulation the embryo will be transformed into a three-layered structure that is organized along three major spatial dimensions, rostral–caudal, dorsal–ventral, and right–left. Figure 2.4 A provides an overview of the major spatial dimensions of the embryo on E13. Figure 2.4B orients the embryo within the context of the embryonic placenta, and Figure 2.4C shows how the embryonic spatial axes relate to the major spatial dimensions of the infant (see figure caption for details).

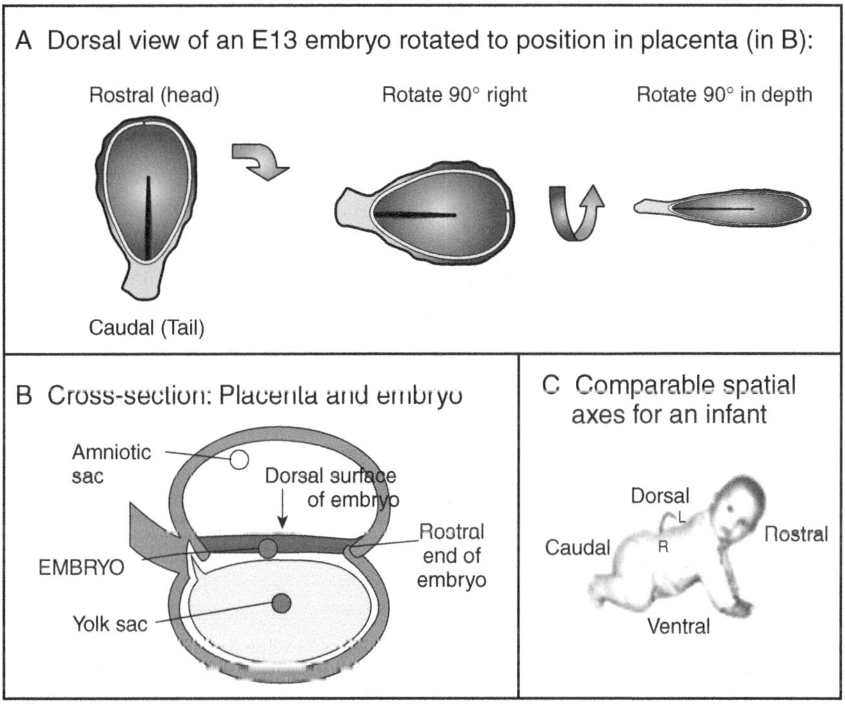

FIGURE 2.4 The major spatial dimensions of the E13 embryo. (A) The dorsal surface view of the embryo on E13 is shown in the first panel. The wall of the amniotic sac has been cut away to reveal the dorsal surface (epiblast layer) of the embryo. The rostral ("head") end of the embryo is on the top of this figure and the caudal ("tail") end is at the bottom. (B) A lateral cross-section of the embryo and placenta at E13. On E13, the two-layered embryo is located centrally between two major placental sacs. The amniotic sac (which later in development will surround the embryo) is located above the embryo and the yolk sac is located below. The rostral end of the embryo is to the right in this figure. To place the embryo shown in the first panel of A within the context of the lateral view of the embryo and placenta shown in B, it is necessary to first rotate the embryo so that the rostral end faces right (second panel of A), and then rotate the embryo in depth so that the dorsal surface faces up (last panel of A). (C) The comparable rostral–caudal and dorsal–ventral spatial axes of an infant. The spatial axes of a crawling infant are comparable to the position of the embryo in B. (Illustrations by Matthew Stiles Davis; adapted by permission of the publisher. From "The Fundamentals of Brain Development: Integrating Nature and Nurture" by Joan Stiles. Cambridge, MA: Harvard University Press Copyright © 2008 by the President and Fellows of Harvard College.)

During gastrulation, the two-layered embryo becomes three-layered, and at the end of gastrulation each layer contains one of the three primary stem cell lines (Gilbert, 2006; Sadler, 2006; Sadler & Langman, 2010). The bottom layer is called the endodermal layer, the middle layer the mesodermal layer, and the upper layer the ectodermal layer. Endodermal stem cells produce gut structures such as the gastrointestinal tract, respiratory tract, and parts of the liver and pancreas. Mesodermal cells produce structures such as muscle, bone, and the vascular system. There are two subgroups of ectodermal stem cells. One subgroup produces cells for things like epidermis, sweat glands, and tooth enamel, while the other gives rise to the cells of the brain and central nervous system. This neurectodermal cell line is made up of the neural progenitor cells. The neural progenitor cells will produce all of the neurons in the central nervous system, as well as many of the brain support cells, the astrocytes and oligodendrocytes. The key question, then, is what triggers this subset of epiblast cells to become neural stem cells.

The onset of gastrulation is signaled by the formation of the primitive streak on the surface of the epiblast layer of the embryo (Figure 2.5, left). A groove forms in the primitive streak that provides an opening in the epiblast layer. During gastrulation a subset of cells from the epiblast layer begins to migrate. First they move toward the opening in the primitive streak, then head down through the opening and under the epiblast layer (Fig. 2.5, center). The first cells to migrate move to the most anterior region of the embryo (top in Fig. 2.5, right), where they displace the cells of the anterior hypoblast layer to form the first part of the endodermal layer. Later-migrating cells form successively more posterior regions of the embryonic layers, with some completing the endodermal layer and others forming a new intermediate layer, the mesodermal layer. The migrating cells receive signals from cells in the hypoblast layer and other extra-embryonic tissue that induce them to become either endodermal or mesodermal cells. But how do the cells that remain in the epiblast layer receive signals to become ectodermal cells, and specifically what are the signals that induce the formation of neurectodermal cells?

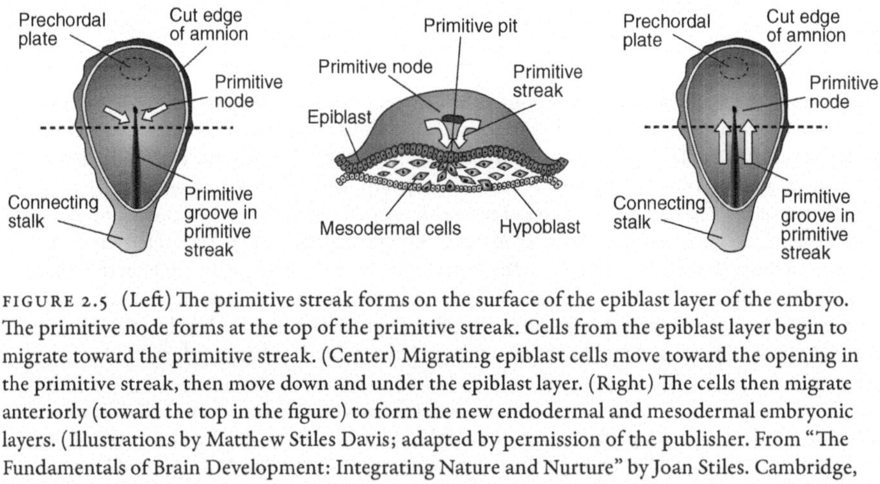

FIGURE 2.5 (Left) The primitive streak forms on the surface of the epiblast layer of the embryo. The primitive node forms at the top of the primitive streak. Cells from the epiblast layer begin to migrate toward the primitive streak. (Center) Migrating epiblast cells move toward the opening in the primitive streak, then move down and under the epiblast layer. (Right) The cells then migrate anteriorly (toward the top in the figure) to form the new endodermal and mesodermal embryonic layers. (Illustrations by Matthew Stiles Davis; adapted by permission of the publisher. From "The Fundamentals of Brain Development: Integrating Nature and Nurture" by Joan Stiles. Cambridge, MA: Harvard University Press Copyright © 2008 by the President and Fellows of Harvard College.)

The differentiation of the epiblast cells into neural progenitor cells is the result of complex molecular signaling that involves multiple gene products (i.e., proteins) that are produced by several different populations of embryonic cells. BMP4 is a secreted protein that is widely expressed in the deep layers of the embryo early in gastrulation. One function of BMP4 is to induce the cells that remain in the epiblast layer to become *epidural* ectodermal cells (Hemmati-Brivanlou & Melton, 1997a, 1997b; Niehrs, 2004). Recall that epiblast cells differentiate into one of two types of progenitor cell, neural progenitors and epidural progenitors. Any epiblast cell that receives a BMP4 signal will become an epidural progenitor. Thus, if the action of BMP4 is not blocked in critical regions of the epiblast layer of the embryo, the neural progenitor cells cannot form and brain development is arrested before it begins. The signals that protect the prospective neural progenitor cells from BMP4 signaling come from the migrating endodermal and mesodermal cells (collectively these cells are referred to as mesendodermal cells) that pass just beneath the subpopulation of epiblast cells that will become neurectodermal cells. These future neurectodermal cells are located along the axial midline of the epiblast layer of the embryo in a region that by the end of gastrulation will become the neural plate (Fig. 2.6). Cells that migrate just below this region of the epiblast send out protective signals that block BMP4 signaling, and allow the epiblast cells in the region of the emerging neural plate to differentiate in neurectodermal tissue. But what is the nature of these signals, and why are they produced by this population of migrating mesendodermal cells?

Just prior to the onset of migration of the mesendodermal cells, a structure called the primitive node forms at the top of the primitive streak in the epiblast layer of the

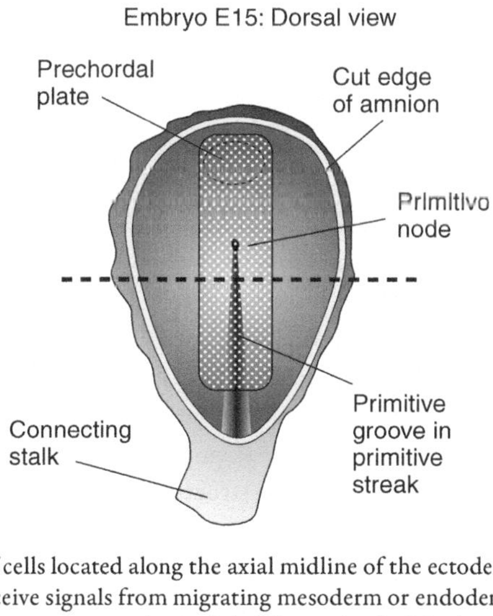

FIGURE 2.6 A subset of cells located along the axial midline of the ectodermal layer of the embryo (dotted area in figure) receive signals from migrating mesoderm or endoderm cells to become neurectodermal cells (i.e., neural progenitor cells). (Illustration by Matthew Stiles Davis, reprinted by permission of the publisher. From "The Fundamentals of Brain Development: Integrating Nature and Nurture" by Joan Stiles. Cambridge, MA: Harvard University Press Copyright © 2008 by the President and Fellows of Harvard College.)

embryo (see Fig. 2.5). The primitive node is a signaling center that provides molecular cues to the migrating mesendodermal cells that are critical for the differentiation of the neural progenitor cells. Specifically, signaling from the primitive node induces the migrating cells to express BMP4 antagonist proteins. BMP4 antagonists block the action of BMP4 by binding to critical receptors on the surface of the future neurectodermal cells. The blockade of BMP4 signaling prevents differentiation of these cells into epidural ectoderm, enabling other signaling pathways to induce a neurectodermal fate in this critical population of cells. Thus, one important function of nodal signaling is the preservation of the neural progenitor population. But nodal signaling is more complex and involves other signals that also serve to establish the initial anterior–posterior organization of the primitive nervous system.

Different subpopulations of neural progenitor cells produce neurons appropriate for forebrain, midbrain, or hindbrain and spinal cord structures. The initial signaling that establishes these subpopulations occurs during gastrulation. WNTs are another secreted protein widely expressed in deep layers of the embryo during gastrulation; they are associated with induction of "posterior fate" in neural progenitors. Similar to the effects of BMP4, preservation of cell lines capable of producing neurons for anterior brain regions requires blocking the signaling effects of WNTs. In very high concentrations WNTs induce progenitors that produce cells for the hindbrain and spinal column; in medium concentrations they induce midbrain progenitors; and when WNTs are blocked, forebrain progenitors emerge (Kiecker & Niehrs, 2001). Nodal signaling changes across the course of gastrulation such that the earliest-migrating cells, those that make up the most anterior region of the emerging neural plate, receive signals that induce the production of WNT antagonists in high concentrations. The concentration of antagonist production declines for later-migrating cells, and the last cells to migrate do not produce WNT antagonists, thus preserving posterior fate in appropriate regions of the neural plate. Thus, it is the temporal modulation of WNT antagonist signaling that arises from cells in the primitive node and is transmitted to migrating mesendodermal cells that provides the initial anterior–posterior patterning within the primitive nervous system.

In summary, by the end of gastrulation the first critical step in brain development is complete with the specification of the neural progenitor cells. These cells are located in the embryonic neural plate, which runs along the extent of the anterior–posterior midline of the most dorsal layer of the three-layered embryonic disk. In addition, very primitive patterning within the population of neural progenitors has been introduced such that the anterior–posterior axis of the primitive neural plate has been established. The kinds of interactive signaling processes observed during gastrulation provide the first illustration of the dynamic and interactive nature of brain development. It is the interaction among cells from different populations that induces the differentiation and development of the emerging embryonic structures. The events of gastrulation set the stage for the next step in brain development, which is the formation of the first true neural structure, the neural tube.

Neurulation and Segmentation of the Neural Tube

The neural tube is the earliest and most primitive manifestation of the nervous system. The process of neural tube formation is called neurulation. Neurulation begins with the induction of the neural progenitor cells during gastrulation, but the major changes that define neural tube formation occur immediately after gastrulation, between E18 and E28. Neurulation begins with the formation of two ridges that bracket the two sides of the neural plate (Fig. 2.7A). The outside of each ridge is composed of *epidural* ectodermal tissue, and the inside of *neuoectodermal* tissue. Over the course of several days, the ridges rise, fold inward, and fuse to form a hollow tube (Copp, Greene, & Murdoch, 2003; Greene & Copp, 2009). The outer layer of the closed tube is composed of epidural ectodermal cells, while neuroectodermal cells line the center of the tube. Soon after tube closure, an intermediate layer of mesodermal cells fills in between the two original layers, creating a tube with three concentric cell layers that surround a hollow cylindrical core called the lumen (Finnell, Junker, Wadman, & Cabrera, 2002). Fusion begins in the center of the emerging neural tube and then proceeds in both the anterior and posterior directions (Fig. 2.7B). The ends of the tube, the anterior and posterior neuropores, are the last segments to close. The anterior neuropore closes on approximately E25 and the posterior neuropore on E27.

Once neurulation is complete, the neural progenitor cells form a single layer that lines the center of the neural tube. Thus, the progenitor cell population is positioned immediately adjacent to the lumen of the neural tube. As the embryo develops, this central opening will become more complex in shape and will eventually become the ventricular system of the mature brain. Because the neural progenitor cell layer that gives rise to most of the neurons in the brain and central nervous system is positioned immediately next to the ventricles, this important neural proliferative region is often referred to as the "ventricular zone."

Although the basic three-dimensional organization of the embryo is evident by the end of neurulation, over the next month the embryo undergoes rapid growth. At the end of neurulation the embryo is 3 to 5 mm long, and by the end of GW8 it will have grown to 27 to 31 mm, a tenfold increase. During this period the shape of the primitive nervous system changes

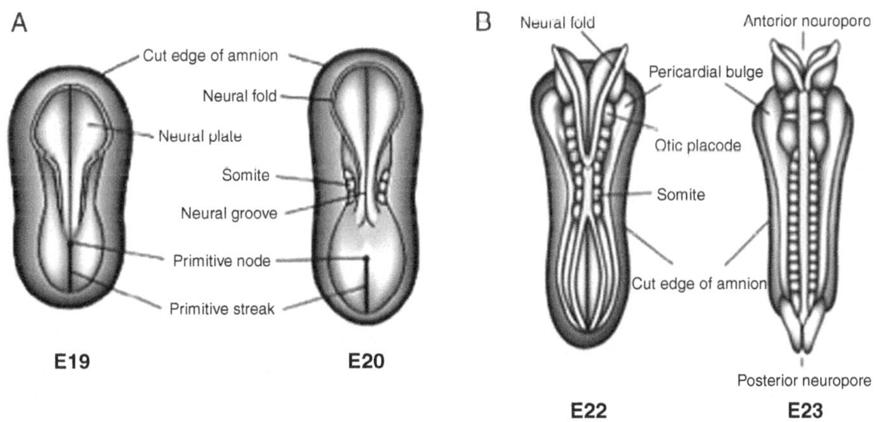

FIGURE 2.7 (A) Closure of the neural tube begins with the formation of two neural ridges that run along the anterior–posterior axis of the neural plate. (B) Closure of the neural tube begins in the center and extend to the neuropores at the two ends of the neural tube. (Illustrations by Matthew Stiles Davis, reprinted by permission of the publisher. From "The Fundamentals of Brain Development: Integrating Nature and Nurture" by Joan Stiles. Cambridge, MA: Harvard University Press Copyright © 2008 by the President and Fellows of Harvard College.)

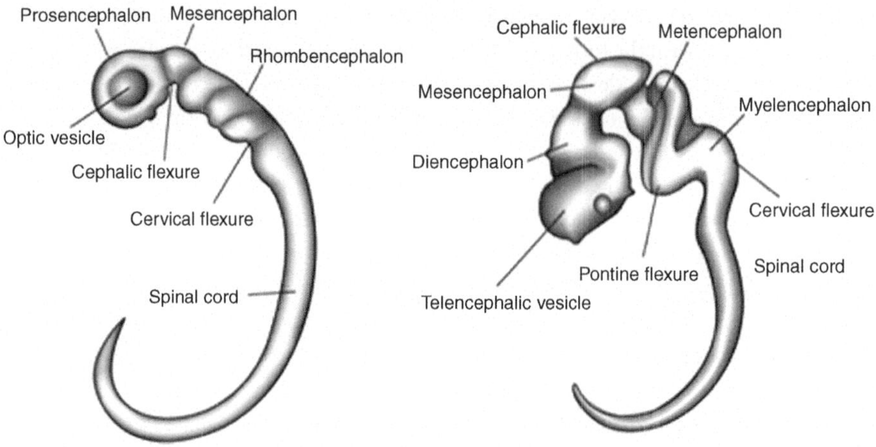

FIGURE 2.8 (Left) The primary vesicles of the developing embryo. (Right) The secondary vesicles at the end of the embryonic period. (Illustrations by Matthew Stiles Davis, reprinted by permission of the publisher. From "The Fundamentals of Brain Development: Integrating Nature and Nurture" by Joan Stiles. Cambridge, MA: Harvard University Press Copyright © 2008 by the President and Fellows of Harvard College.)

dramatically. Just before closure of the anterior neuropore (E25), the anterior end of the tube begins to expand, forming the three primary "brain vesicles," or pouches (Fig. 2.8A). The most anterior of these embryonic brain vesicles is called the prosencephalon, which is the embryonic precursor of the forebrain. The middle vesicle is the mesencephalon, which is the precursor of midbrain structures, and the most posterior is the rhombencephalon, which will become the hindbrain. These three segments further subdivide, and by the end of embryonic period the five secondary brain vesicles are present (Fig. 2.8B). The prosencephalon divides into the telencephalon and the diencephalon, and the rhombencephalon divides into the metencephalon and myelencephalon. The mesencephalon does not further divide. These five subdivisions are aligned along the anterior–posterior axis of the embryo and establish the primary organization of the central nervous system (Stiles, 2008; Vieira et al., 2010). Table 2.1 provides a summary of the major brain structures that are derived from each of the major brain vesicles.

Neural Patterning in the Embryonic Period

The changes observed in the gross morphology of the developing embryonic nervous system reflect more specific changes in neural patterning within brain regions. Hallmarks of brain development include both the progressive differentiation of new structures, and the elaboration and progressive functional commitment of existing ones. Thus, the process of neural patterning is gradual and follows an ongoing course of continuous specification and refinement (Sur & Rubenstein, 2005). The patterning observed during gastrulation provides only a primitive map of emerging nervous system organization. By the end of the embryonic period, neural patterning within the developing nervous system is much more elaborate, and involves patterning in all three spatial dimensions. Patterning beyond the embryonic period

TABLE 2.1 PRIMARY AND SECONDARY SUBDIVISION OF THE NEURAL TUBE

Primary Vesicle	Secondary Vesicle	Mature Derivatives	Central Cavity
Prosencephalon	Telencephalon	Cerebral cortex Basal ganglia Basal forebrain	Lateral ventricles
	Diencephalon	Thalamus Hypothalamus	Third ventricle
Mesencephalon	Mesencephalon	Midbrain—tectum	Cerebral aqueduct
Rhombencephalon	Metencephalon	Hindbrain—pons Cerebellum	Fourth ventricle
	Myelencephalon	Medulla	
Spinal cord	Spinal cord	Spinal cord	Central canal

only serves to contribute to the complexity of the developing brain. Space does not permit an extended discussion of embryonic neural patterning. One example, focused on very early patterning within the developing neocortex, will serve both to define the construct of neural patterning and to illustrate the idea of continuous specification and refinement of brain areas.

The mature neocortex is partitioned into well-defined structurally and functionally distinct areas that are differentiated by their cellular organization and patterns of neuronal connectivity. Brodmann (1909) provided one of the first systematic account of cortical areas in the human brain. His system of specifying cortical areas is still widely used (Fig. 2.9). Initial patterning of neocortex into cortical areas results from different molecular signals present in different regions of the neocortical proliferative zone. Early studies identified two signaling molecules, Emx2 and Pax6, that play an essential role in the early patterning of the presumptive neocortex. These two signaling molecules are expressed in opposite concentration gradients along the anterior–posterior extent of the neocortical proliferative zone (Fig. 2.10, top panel). The concentration of Emx2 is highest in posterior and medial regions and lowest in anterior lateral regions; Pax6 has the opposite expression pattern. The interaction of these two gradients contributes to early patterning of the neocortex (Bishop, Rubenstein, & O'Leary, 2002; Hamasaki, Leingartner, Ringstedt, & O'Leary, 2004). A high concentration of Pax6 combined with a low concentration of Emx2 induces progenitors to produce neurons appropriate for motor cortex, while the reverse concentrations induce production of neurons for visual cortex. At intermediate levels of both factors, somatosensory cortices emerge. Studies of mutant mice, for which expression of either *Emx2* or *Pax6* is blocked (thus altering the balance of signals across the cortical proliferative zone), show systematic shifts in the organization of cortical areas, documenting that it is the interaction of these two signaling molecules that induces change in the surrounding cell populations (Fig. 2.10). When *Emx2* is blocked, visual areas shrink and somatosensory and motor areas enlarge; when *Pax6* is blocked, visual areas enlarge while somatosensory and motor

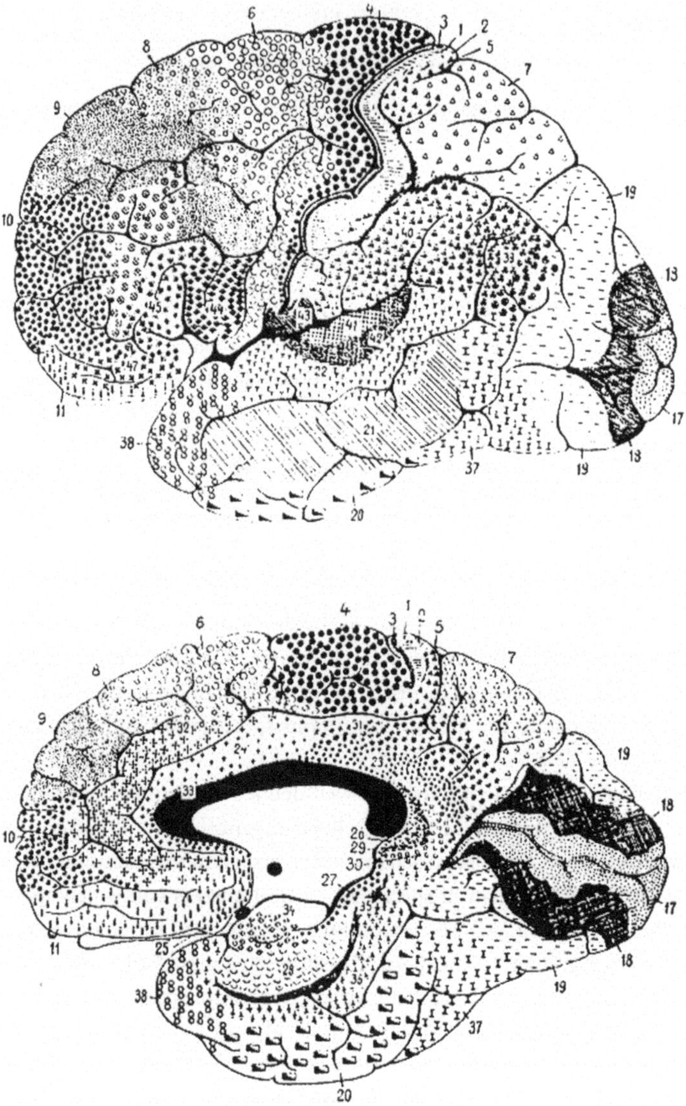

FIGURE 2.9 Brodmann areas on the lateral surface of the human brain are shown in the top figure and on the medial surface in the bottom figure. Based on cytoarchitectonic studies, Brodmann identified 47 unique structural areas in the human brain. Most have subsequently been associated with different functions.

areas shrink. Thus, it is the effect of the particular level of one molecular signal in combination with the particular level of another signal that produces the classical pattern of sensorimotor organization in the developing cortex.

Since these original reports of the role of Pax6 and Emx2 signaling in neocortical patterning, it has become clear that the interactions are more complex. At least two additional molecules have been identified, Coup-TF1 and SP8. Both are produced in gradients.

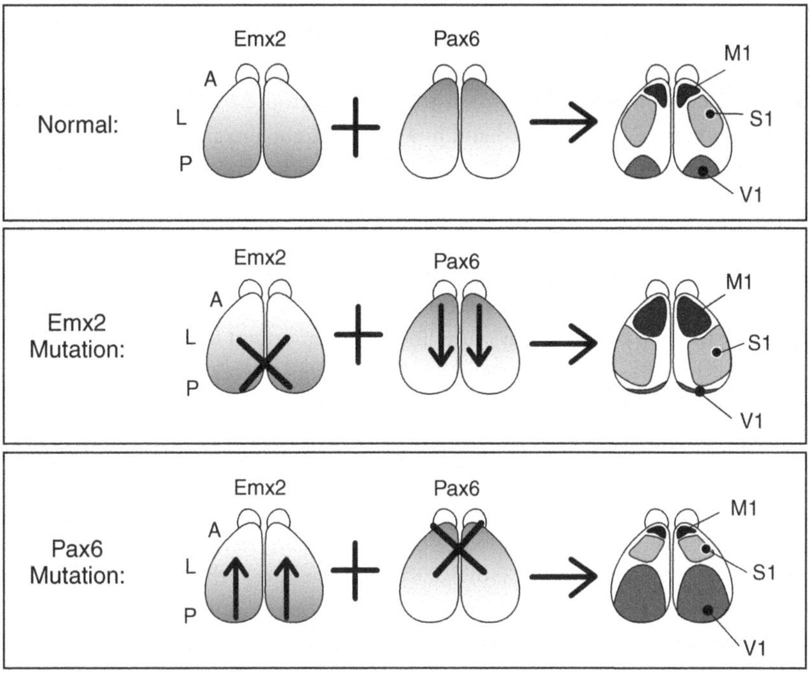

FIGURE 2.10 The effects of different concentrations of Emx2 and Pax6 on the development of sensorimotor cortical areas. It is the combination of the specific concentration of each molecule that determines the identity of the cortical region. Mutations that affect the quantities of either molecule alter cortical patterning. (Adapted with permission from Bishop KM, Rubenstein JL, et al. (2002). Distinct actions of Emx1, Emx2, and Pax6 in regulating the specification of areas in the developing neocortex. *J Neurosci* 22(17) 7627–7638, Figure 1.)

Coup-TF1 is expressed in greatest concentration in caudal–lateral regions, while SP8 is expressed in rostral–medial regions. As was the case with Pax6 and Emx2, blocking the expression of these genes results in dramatic alteration in the sensorimotor organization of the neocortex (O'Leary, Chou, Hamasaki, et al., 2007; O'Leary, Chou, & Sahara, 2007; O'Leary & Sahara, 2008; Sansom & Livesey, 2009; Zembrzycki, Griesel, Stoykova, & Mansouri, 2007).

Areal patterning arising from these molecular signaling pathways occurs during GW6, at the very beginning of corticogenesis. This patterning of sensorimotor areas occurs in regions of the neocortical proliferative zone that during gastrulation had been specified as "anterior." Thus, this later patterning constitutes an elaboration or refinement of an earlier phase of neural patterning. As will be discussed later, patterning within these regions is far from complete in GW6. Fundamental organizational features of the sensory and motor cortices will not arise until the late fetal period, and across the period of fetal and early postnatal development, the structural and functional identity of these basic brain areas remains malleable and subject to the effects of input and experience.

NEURONS: PRODUCTION, MIGRATION, DIFFERENTIATION

To appreciate the nature and significance of the changes in the gross anatomy of the embryonic and fetal brain, it is necessary to understand something about how the basic neural elements, the neurons, are produced and how they become integrated into the functional information processing systems of the brain. Different populations of neurons form gray matter structures in many regions of the brain, including hindbrain and spinal column, cerebellum, midbrain structures, deep subcortical nuclei, and the neocortex (Fig. 2.11A). Regions of the brain that contain the cell bodies of neurons are gray (hence the name). White matter regions contain the major fiber pathways that connect neurons in different parts of the brain. The fiber pathways contain axons that extend from the cell body of neurons and act as transmission lines for sending electrochemical signals to other populations of neurons. The fiber pathways form the primary information processing networks in the brain. The efficiency of information transmission in the pathways is greatly enhanced by myelin, which ensheaths the axons, something like insulation on telephone wires. Myelin is a fatty substance that is white (hence the name).

Although all of the gray matter regions form essential parts of the information processing networks of the brain, one structure is of particular importance—the neocortex. The remainder of this section will focus on the production of neurons destined for the neocortex. The neocortex is the thin mantle of cells that covers the surface of the mammalian brain, something like the rind on an orange (Fig. 2.11B). In species with very small brains such as mice, the surface of the neocortex is smooth and lacks the characteristic pattern of gyral and sulcal enfolding that characterizes primate brains (see Fig. 2.11A). This difference reflects the dramatic evolutionary expansion in the size of the neocortical mantle. A flattened and unfolded human neocortex is roughly 2,500 cm^2 (~2.7 ft^2, approximately the size of an open newspaper), whereas the neocortex of a rat is 6 cm^2 (<1 in^2, the size of a postage stamp). Despite the

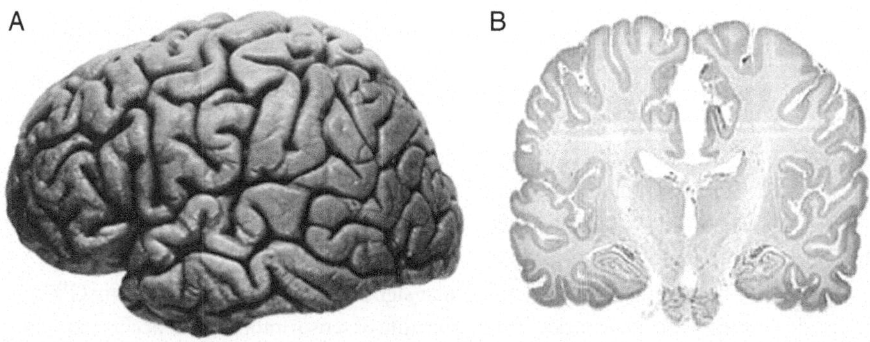

FIGURE 2.11 Two views of the human brain. (A) Lateral view (rostral end is left, caudal is right) shows a surface marked by gyri and sulcal folds (right hemisphere of J. Piłsudski's brain, lateral view, image in the public domain). (B) Coronal cross-section stained for cell bodies that mark neurons. The neocortex is the thin mantel layer (dark gray) on the surface of the brain. The white areas are connecting fiber pathways. (Image reproduced with permission from http://www.brains.rad.msu.edu, which is supported by the U.S. National Science Foundation. Images obtained with permission from Wiki Commons http://commons.wikimedia.org/wiki.)

large differences in the horizontal expanse of the cortex across species, the thickness is remarkably well preserved. The thickness of the cortex ranges between 2 and 5 mm across regions in humans, and between 1 and 2 mm in rat. Further, the organization of the cortex in the vertical dimension is also well preserved. Across brain areas and species the neocortex is a uniformly six-layered structure. The layers are differentiated by the types of neurons they contain and the kinds of connections they make. Across species, the deepest layers of cortex (layers 5 and 6) project principally to subcortical areas, layer 4 in sensory cortices is the primary input layer receiving information from the outside world via the thalamus (vision, audition, sensation), and layers 2 and 3 form association networks among cortical areas. Thus, the laminar organization of the neocortex is essential for establishing the major information processing networks in the brain, and that is well preserved across species.

Across the period of cortical neurogenesis, most neurons are produced in the ventricular zone (VZ) deep in the brain, and they migrate radially toward the surface of the brain to form the neocortical mantle. It is an orderly and elegant process that requires mechanisms for both producing the right neural elements at the right time and for guiding migration of neurons to the appropriate regions of cortex. Once in place in the cortex, the neurons receive signals that influence their specific pattern of differentiation and support the emergence of information processing networks. The rest of this section considers the basic processes of neuron production, migration, and differentiation.

Neuron Production

As discussed earlier, the human cerebrum contain billions of neurons, most of which are produced by mid-gestation (Bayer, Altman, Russo, & Zhang, 1993; Rakic, 1995a). The pool of neural progenitor cells that is specified at the end of gastrulation is far too small to accommodate neuron production at this scale. Thus, the first step in neuron production involves increasing the size of the neural progenitor cell population. Neural progenitors are a "mitotic" population of cells—that is, they can divide to form new cells. Neurons are post mitotic cells; once formed they are no longer capable of dividing and producing new cells.

From the end of gastrulation through approximately E42 in humans, the population of neural progenitor cells divides by what is described as a "symmetrical" mode of cell division (Bystron et al., 2008). Symmetrical cell division produces two identical cells, which in the case of the neural progenitors is two neural progenitor cells. Over multiple of rounds of cell division between E25 and E42, symmetrical cell division provides the means for augmenting the size of the neural progenitor pool. Indeed, it has been suggested that one elegant explanation for the tenfold increase in the size of the neocortex between rhesus macaque and man is a simple extension of the time period for symmetrical cell division (Rakic, 1995b). In monkey this period ends on E40 rather than E42. Since each round of cell division doubles the size of the progenitor pool, even a few extra rounds of cell division at the end of the process of symmetrical cell division would have a dramatic impact on the number of available progenitor cells, the number of neurons produced, and thus the size of the cortex.

Beginning on approximately E42, the mode of cell division begins to shift from symmetrical to asymmetrical. During asymmetrical cell division, two different types of cells are produced. In neural progenitors, asymmetrical cell division produces one neural progenitor and one neuron (Wodarz & Huttner, 2003). The new progenitor cell remains in the proliferative zone and continues to divide and produce new neurons. The post-mitotic neuron leaves the proliferative zone to take its place in the developing neocortex. The shift to asymmetrical cell division among the progenitor population is gradual and initially includes only a small proportion of progenitors, but those numbers increase dramatically by the end of cortical neurogenesis. Cortical neurogenesis in humans is complete by approximately E108 (Clancy, Darlington, & Finlay, 2001).

Neuron Migration

Most neurons are produced in the VZ and a somewhat later-emerging proliferative zone immediately adjacent to the VZ, the subventricular zone (SVZ). From there they migrate radially out to the developing neocortex. Very early in neocortical development the distances the neuron must traverse are small. Thus, the earliest-produced neurons can use a mode of migration referred to as "somal translocation." In somal translocation the neuron extends a long basal process, which is an extension of the cell's body, just beyond the edge of the VZ into the outer region of the brain compartment (Fig. 2.12A). The basal process attaches to the pial surface, which is the outer surface of the developing brain (Miyata, Kawaguchi, Okano, & Ogawa, 2001). The nucleus of the cell then moves through the cytoplasm of the basal process. As the nucleus moves up the process becomes shorter and thicker but remains attached to the pial surface. At the end of somal translocation the nucleus of the cell has moved out of the VZ and into the embryonic cortex.

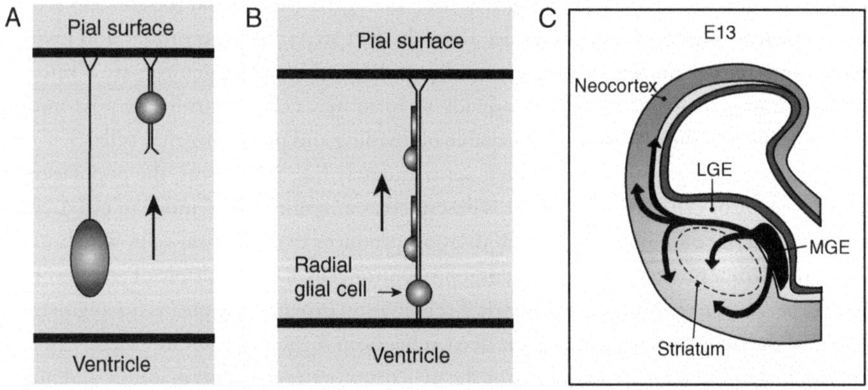

FIGURE 2.12 (A) Neuron migration by somal translocation. The new neuron extends a cytoplasmic process and attaches to the outside of the brain compartment (pial surface), and then the nucleus moves up into the brain area. (B) Neuron migration by radial glial guide. Radial glia provide a scaffold for neurons to migrate along. (C) Neuron migration from second proliferative zone in ganglionic eminences by tangential migration (arrows indicate direction of migration for different neuron populations). (A and B adapted with permission from Nadarajah, Alifragis, Wong, and Parnavelas (2003). Neuronal migration in the developing cerebral cortex: observations based on real-time imaging. Cerebral Cortex 13:607–611, Figure 5. C adapted from illustrations by Matthew Stiles Davis, reprinted by permission of the publisher. From "The Fundamentals of Brain Development: Integrating Nature and Nurture" by Joan Stiles. Cambridge, MA: Harvard University Press Copyright © 2008 by the President and Fellows of Harvard College.)

As development proceeds, the brain becomes larger and the primary mode of neuronal migration from the VZ/SVZ changes. Because of the greater distances, neurons require what was originally identified as a special population of cells within the VZ called radial glial guides to support their migration (Rakic, 1972). Much like neurons migrating via somal translocation, radial glial guides extend a basal process that attaches to the pial surface of the brain. However, the nucleus of the radial glial cells remains in the VZ, and the basal process forms a kind of scaffolding along which neurons can migrate (Fig. 2.12B). The migrating neurons attach themselves to the radial glial guide and move along the cellular scaffold out into the developing cortical plate. Each glial scaffold can support the migration of many neurons. Although the radial glial guides were originally thought to be a special, transient population of cells, it has recently been discovered that the cells that provide the scaffolding are actually the neural progenitor cells (Noctor, Flint, Weissman, Dammerman, & Kriegstein, 2001; Noctor et al., 2002; Parnavelas, Alifragis, & Nadarajah, 2002; Weissman, Noctor, Clinton, Honig, & Kriegstein, 2003).

Recent studies have identified a second proliferative zone located in the region of the ventral telencephalon that will later develop into the basal ganglia (Fig. 2.12C, coronal view of one cerebral hemisphere). During embryonic and fetal development three compartments in this region, the medial, lateral, and caudal ganglionic eminences, are the source of an important class of inhibitory cortical interneurons (Anderson, Marin, Horn, Jennings, & Rubenstein, 2001; Corbin, Nery, & Fishell, 2001; Nery, Fishell, & Corbin, 2002). Unlike neurons migrating from the VZ/SVZ, these neurons traverse long distances using a mode of migration that has been termed "tangential migration" because the route of migration traverses the contour of developing cortical mantle tangentially. Tangential migration involves a variety of signaling pathways not seen in radial migration. Neurons use a number of guidance molecules produced in local regions along their migratory route to direct their movement into the cortex (Marin & Rubenstein, 2001).

The migration of neurons into the developing neocortex results in the formation of an orderly six-layered structure. With one exception, earlier-migrating neurons form deepest layers of cortex and later-migrating neurons form successively more superficial layers (Fig. 2.13) such that the order of migration has been described as inside-out. The exception to the inside-out rule is the earliest set of migrating neurons. These first neurons to leave the proliferative zone initially form a primitive structure called the preplate (Fig. 2.14, left). Once the preplate is complete, the next wave of migrating neurons splits the preplate into two separate regions, the marginal zone (MZ) and the subplate (SP). These neurons begin to form a new region between the MZ and SP, which is the emerging cortical plate (CP; Fig. 2.14, middle). The first neurons to arrive in the CP are the cells that will form cortical layer 6, the deepest layer of cortex; subsequently migrating cells will form progressively more superficial layers of cortex.

Both the MZ and the SP are transient brain layers that play a critical role in the development of the cortex, but both disappear by the end of the fetal period (Fig. 2.14, right). The MZ contains an important class of cells, the Cajal-Retzius (CR) cells. CR cells play a critical role in the positioning of neurons into the correct layers of cortex. The CR cells produce a molecular signal, called Reelin, that is part of the pathway that signals neurons when to stop migrating and take up their position in cortex (Bielle et al., 2005; Huang, 2009). Each new wave of migrating neurons bypasses the previous wave of neurons such that each new wave

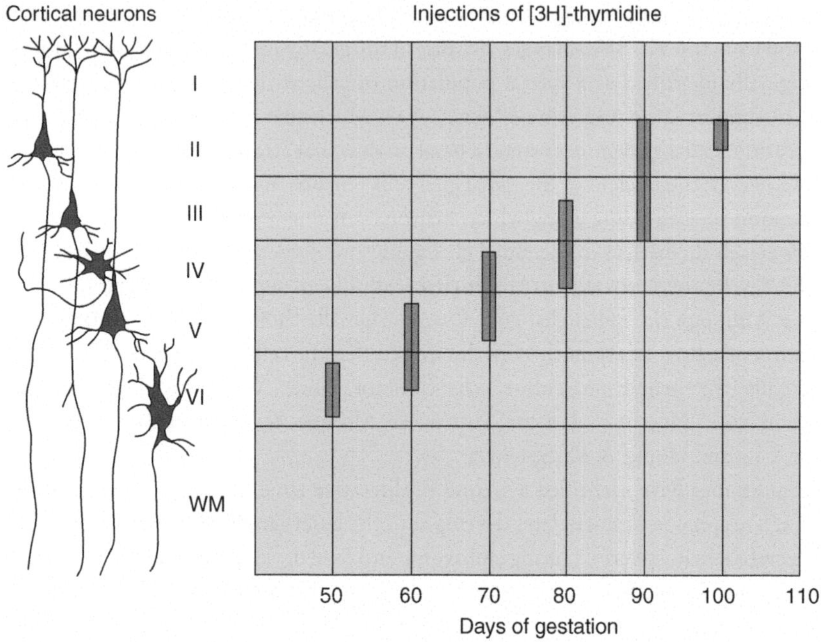

FIGURE 2.13 The earliest-produced neurons migrate to the deepest cortical layers, while later-produced neurons migrate to successively more superficial layers, creating an inside-out order of migration. (Adapted with permission from Sanes DH, Reh TA, Harris WA. (2006). "Development of the Nervous System" (2nd ed.). Burlington, MA: Elsevier Academic Press. Figure 3.18, p. 74.)

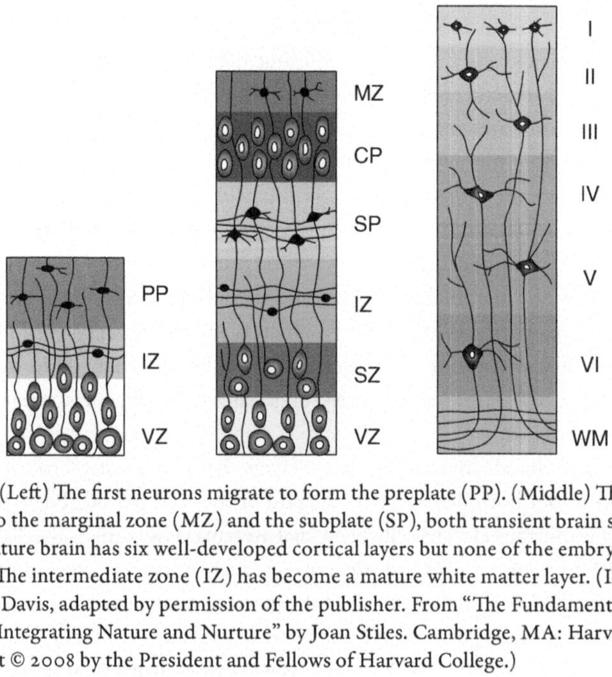

FIGURE 2.14 (Left) The first neurons migrate to form the preplate (PP). (Middle) The next neurons split the PP into the marginal zone (MZ) and the subplate (SP), both transient brain structures. (Right) The mature brain has six well-developed cortical layers but none of the embryonic structures (MZ, SP, VZ). The intermediate zone (IZ) has become a mature white matter layer. (Illustrations by Matthew Stiles Davis, adapted by permission of the publisher. From "The Fundamentals of Brain Development: Integrating Nature and Nurture" by Joan Stiles. Cambridge, MA: Harvard University Press Copyright © 2008 by the President and Fellows of Harvard College.)

of migrating cells takes its place in the most superficial position within the developing cortex. As each new wave of neurons reaches the top of the cortical plate, it moves into the zone of Reelin signaling and receives the cue to stop. The cortex of animals with defects in Reelin signaling lacks laminar structure; the preplate fails to split, and the neurons simply conglomerate under the abnormal preplate (Rice & Curran, 2001). Neurons in the subplate layer do not participate in the formation of cortical layers, but, as will be discussed later, they are essential for establishing the primary sensory inputs to the developing neocortex.

Neuron Differentiation

The different layers of cortex contain different types of neurons. One question is how these different classes of neurons are derived. This question was addressed by McConnell et al. (Desai & McConnell, 2000; Frantz & McConnell, 1996; McConnell & Kaznowski, 1991) in a series of studies that asked whether different subsets of progenitor cells produce specific kinds of neurons, or whether the same progenitor is capable of producing multiple neuron types. They found that early in corticogenesis, neural progenitor cells are capable of producing any neuron type, but that with development they became more and more restricted in the types of neurons they can produce. McConnell et al. used progenitor cell transplant studies to examine this question. They took dividing progenitor cells from a host fetus of a particular age and transplanted the cells into a donor animal of a different age. The key question was: What kinds of neurons do the transplanted progenitors produce in the *host* environment? In the first experiment, progenitor cells were taken from young donor animals (if left in the donor these progenitors would produce neurons for layer 6 of cortex) and were transplanted into an older host (whose progenitors were producing layer 2 and 3 neurons). The transplanted progenitors produced layer 2 and 3, neurons suggesting a shift to production of neurons that are appropriate for the host neocortex. However, when the timing was reversed and progenitors from an older host were transplanted to a younger animal, the progenitors continued to produce cells appropriate for the donor animal. It appears that early in corticogenesis, progenitor cells can receive signals to produce any neural cell line, but as development proceeds and these early cell types are no longer needed, the progenitor loses the capacity to generate those cells, exhibiting what is termed fate restriction. Further studies suggest that the signals to the progenitor cells that determine the type of neuron produced during a particular point in corticogenesis may, in part, emanate from the developing neocortex itself. As each cortical layer is completed, signaling from the cortical neurons inhibits the production of neurons for that cortical layer.

Once they have reached their target region of cortex, the young neurons need to become part of information processing networks. To become integrated into neural networks, the neurons need to develop neuronal processes (axons and dendrites) that allow them to communicate with other neurons. Axons are the principal means of sending signals from the neuron, while dendrites are major sites for receiving input from other neurons. Each cell has many dendrites that form dense "arbors" in the immediate vicinity of the cell, and a single axon that can extend for some distance away from the cell. At the tip of each axon is a structure called a growth cone. The growth cone is the site of axon elongation and extension (Brown, Keynes, & Lumsden, 2001). As the axon is extended, the growth cone samples the local environment for guidance molecules that direct the axon toward its target.

Some guidance cues are attractive and signal movement toward a source; others are repulsive and guide movement away. Once the axon has reached its target, a connection is formed with the target cell. At the point of connection, a synapse is formed that provides a means of transmitting the electrochemical information that is the essential means of communication in the brain.

Two of the most important pathways in the brain are the ones that transmit sensorimotor information, the thalamocortical (TC) and corticothalamic (CT) pathways. The TC relays sensory and motor information from the receptors in the retina, cochlea, muscle, or skin to the sensorimotor regions of the neocortex via the major subcortical sensorimotor relay, the thalamus. The CT pathway completes the feedback loop by transmitting information from cortex back to the thalamus. These essential pathways begin to form in the later part of the second trimester in humans and are complete by GW26 (Judas, Sedmak, Pletikos, & Jovanov-Milosevic, 2010; Kostovic & Jovanov-Milosevic, 2006). The cells of the transient subplate layer of the developing brain (see Fig. 2.14, middle) play an essential role in establishing these pathways. When TC axons arrive at the developing cortex during GW22 they do not immediately make connections with neurons in the primary input layer of cortex (layer 4). Rather, they stop and make connections with the neurons of the subplate layer. The TC–subplate connections last for approximately 4 weeks, during which time the subplate neurons make connections with neurons in cortical layer 4. The subplate neurons appear to provide instructive input to the TC neurons during this period. In the absence of subplate neuron signaling, normal patterns of connectivity between TC axons and layer 4 cortical neurons do not emerge. A similar pattern of instructive connectivity is seen in the development of the CT pathway. Prior to the establishment of connections between neurons from the deep layers of cortex (layers 5 and 6) and the thalamus, subplate neurons extend and establish connections with thalamic neurons. It is thought that the subplate connections may serve to guide the CT axons to their position in the thalamus. Once the TC and CT pathways are complete, the subplate neurons retract their connections and the cells themselves gradually die off.

BRAIN DEVELOPMENT IN THE FETAL PERIOD

The events of the embryonic period set the stage for rapid changes in the structure and organization of the fetal brain. The proliferation, migration, and differentiation of neuron populations provide the foundation for changes in the fetal period. The production of these neural elements is reflected in increases in overall brain volume, but also in systematic changes observed in the separate white and gray matter compartments of the brain. Given the dramatic growth that is observed, it is somewhat surprising that regressive events also play an important role in brain development during this period. In the prenatal brain, naturally occurring cell death is observed on a large scale involving 50% or more of cells across regions, and it is seen in all cell populations, including neurons, neural progenitors, and glial populations.

Changes in the Morphology of the Fetal Brain

The gross morphology of the developing neocortex undergoes striking change during the prenatal period. The human neocortex begins as a smooth, lissencephalic structure (much like rat cortex) and gradually develops the characteristic mature pattern of gyral and sulcal folding. The formation of gyri and sulci follows an orderly sequence. Primary sulci are first seen as grooves positioned in specifically targeted brain regions; secondary branches then begin to form off the primary sulci, followed later by the tertiary branches. The first fissure to form is the longitudinal fissure that separates two cerebral hemispheres. Its development begins in rostral regions as early as GW8 (Chi, Dooling, & Gilles, 1977) and proceeds caudally until it is complete at GW22. Other primary sulci form between GW14 and 26. These include sylvian, cingulate, and parieto-occipital calcarine (GW14–16); central and superior temporal (GW20–24); and superior frontal, precentral, inferior frontal, postcentral, and intraparietal (GW25 and 26). Secondary sulci emerge between GW30 and 35; formation of tertiary sulci begins during GW36 and extends well into the postnatal period.

Brain volumes also undergo rapid change in the pre- and postnatal periods. Average whole brain volume (including cerebral hemispheres, brain stem, and cerebellum) is approximately 150 mL (9 in^3) at GW29 (beginning of the third prenatal trimester). By term it reaches 400 mL (24 in^3), which is about 25% of average adult volume (Huppi et al., 1998). By age 6, brain volume reaches 90% of adult levels (Courchesne et al., 2000; Iwasaki et al., 1997; Kennedy et al., 2002; Kennedy & Dehay, 2001; Lenroot & Giedd, 2006; Paus et al., 2001; Reiss et al., 1996) and then increases very gradually through early adolescence (Courchesne et al., 2000).

The more protracted changes in brain morphology are seen in the very gradual development of the gray and white matter compartments of the brain. At GW30, cortical gray matter volume is approximately 40 mL (2.4 in^3) and increases to 160 mL (9.8 in^3) at term, a 400% increase in the last trimester. Gray matter volumes continue to increase in the preschool period and early school-age period. Between birth and 6 years gray matter volume doubles, but after that the pace declines such that between 6 and 9 years only an additional 13% increase is observed (Courchesne et al., 2000; Giedd et al., 1999). After approximately age 10, gray matter volumes begin to decline in a linear fashion at the rate of about 5% per decade across the lifespan. White matter volumes undergo much slower rates of change in the prenatal period. Unmyelinated white matter volume is approximately 100 mL (6 in^3) at GW30, rising to 150 mL (9.1 in^3) at term. There is very little myelinated white matter in the preterm brain. At GW30 myelinated white matter volume is 5 mL (0.3 in^3), increasing to 20 mL (1.2 in^3) by term. During the preschool and school-age period white matter volume changes in a linear fashion, increasing by 74%, with more modest increases continuing through adolescence (Courchesne et al., 2000; Giedd et al., 1999).

Regressive Events in the Fetal Brain: Naturally Occurring Cell Death in Neuronal Cell Populations

Development is usually associated with the addition of new structures and augmentation of functions. It is somewhat counterintuitive, then, that two very important processes in brain development involve the large-scale loss of neural elements. These two processes include naturally occurring cell death, which involves the normal loss of 50% or more of the neurons and glial cells within a brain region, and synaptic exuberance and pruning, in which there is massive excess production of connections followed by the systematic elimination of up to 50% of those connections. Both of these processes reflect nonpathological events that play an essential role in establishing the complex networks of the developing brain. The timescales of these two sets of events are different. Most naturally occurring cell death in neuronal populations occurs prenatally, while both production and pruning of connections within the developing brain and cell death in glial populations are largely postnatal events. This section will examine the role of prenatal cell death in neuronal populations during the fetal period. The postnatal regressive events will be discussed in the next section of this chapter.

There are two broad categories of cell death. Necrotic cell death is a pathological process that follows insult or injury to a population of cells and is a mechanism for eliminating damaged tissue from the biological system. Apoptosis is a distinct form of cell death that reflects a highly regulated sequence of physiological events. Apoptosis is a well-understood cell-intrinsic process. It involves a cascade of gene expression that ultimately results in the breakdown of nuclear chromatin (DNA and support proteins) and the fragmenting of the cell. All neurons and neural progenitor cells (as well as many other types of cells) have this intrinsic "suicide" program. The set of genes involved in the apoptotic cascade is large but very specific, with each molecular signal triggering the next step in the cascade. A wide variety of cell-intrinsic and environmental factors can influence the apoptotic process. Some trigger cell death, while others protect the cell by preventing the cascade. Across brain regions, the rate of apoptosis within all cortical layers is high, reaching 70% in some regions (Rabinowicz et al., 1996).

One factor that protects against the apoptosis cascade is a class of neurotrophic (or "nourishing") substances. The first neurotrophic factor was discovered by Levi-Montalchini (Levi-Montalcini, 1964) in her studies of cell death in neuronal populations. She called the substance "nerve growth factor" (NGF). Levi-Montalchini was able to modulate the survival of neurons by experimentally increasing or decreasing the amount of NGF available in the vicinity of the neurons. Subsequent work has identified a number of other neurotrophic factors, each of which is effective in different subpopulations of neurons. Neurotrophic factors are produced by neurons, but the available quantity is affected by the level of activity of the cell: the more active the cell, the more neurotrophin it produces. Neurotrophins are produced by neurons in target cell populations, and they are taken up at the synapse by the neurons that make connections with the target (Huang & Reichardt, 2001). The survival of a neuron depends on its ability to establish connections with other neurons and obtain neurotrophic factors. Apoptosis is often the consequence of a neuron's failure to establish functional connections and become integrated into a neural system.

During development it is thought that neurons from different brain regions compete for neurotrophic resources in target brain areas. Some connections are more functional or better suited to a particular pathway than others (e.g., they fire more reliably or efficiently, or integrate more effectively with other parts of the neural network). Neurons that establish effective connections are able to obtain more neurotrophic factor and thus are more likely to survive. Thus, one important function of cell death in brain development is its role in regulating the establishment of effective and functional neural circuits. Cells that make more effective connections are protected from cell death and the pathways they are a part of stabilize, while cells that fail to make connections or that make less optimal connections are lost.

A number of other functions for cell death have also been proposed. It may serve as a mechanism for correcting errors in neuronal production or migration. It may also play an essential role in eliminating cell populations that serve only a transient function in brain development. These would include the cells of the MZ or SP. Importantly, there is substantial evidence of high levels of cell death in the neural progenitor population (de la Rosa & de Pablo, 2000; Yeo & Gautier, 2004). Rates of apoptosis in the VZ increase across the period of corticogenesis, suggesting gradual elimination of this important largely but transient cell population. Note that the mechanism for triggering cell death in the MZ, SP, or progenitor cell populations must differ from those discussed for neurons. None of these populations contain cells that enter neural networks; thus, the specific effects of neurotrophin availability are not likely associated with the apoptotic pathways in these cells groups.

BRAIN DEVELOPMENT IN THE POSTNATAL PERIOD

Brain development is a protracted event that extends for many years after the birth of the child. Changes are observed at all levels, from cells to complex neural systems. This section will examine a number of important aspects of development in the postnatal period. First, though most neurons are produced prenatally, glial development extends well into postnatal development. One important aspect of glial development is the formation of myelin-producing cells that serve to insulate axons and make neural circuits more efficient. Recent work suggests that glia may also play a more extended role in the establishment of neural circuitry, serving as source of signaling. Second, advances in vivo imaging technologies are beginning to inform the study of postnatal brain development in humans. Much, though not all, of what is know about prenatal mammalian brain development derives from animal studies, leaving the specifics of the human developmental course less certain. However, in the postnatal period brain imaging of children is providing important clues about the time course of age-related biological and functional alterations in the brain. These data derive from both anatomical studies of brain structure as well as functional neuroimaging. Data from both of these imaging modalities provide an opportunity to link these changes to evolving behavior. Finally, experience plays an increasingly prominent role in brain development in the postnatal period. Experience is not an incidental player in the complex processes that underlie brain development; rather, the emergence of many systems relies on the right input being available at the right developmental moment.

Postnatal Proliferation and Migration of Neurons and Support Cells

As discussed earlier, cortical neurogenesis is largely a prenatal event. In the postnatal period, neurogenesis continues to only a very limited degree in the cerebrum. In the SVZ, new neurons continue to emerge and migrate to the olfactory bulb. Neurons are also produced in the dentate gyrus of the hippocampus, where they migrate from the subgranular layer of the dentate only as far as the nearby granular layer (Cayre, Canoll, & Goldman, 2009). Recent work indicates that this late neuron production in the dentate gyrus may be associated with memory functions in adults (Aimone, Deng, & Gage, 2010; Deng, Aimone, & Gage, 2010). These exceptional forms of neurogenesis appear to continue throughout adult life but produce only a small percentage of the neuronal population (Gage, 2002).

Although the production and migration of neurons are largely prenatal events, proliferation and migration of glial progenitors, while beginning prenatally, continue for a protracted period as oligodendrocytes and astrocytes differentiate. In fact, glial progenitors (particularly oligodendrocyte progenitor cells [OPCs]) appear to persist indefinitely in the adult brain in a wide anatomical distribution, and can differentiate in response to injury. Glial progenitors proliferate in the forebrain SVZ and migrate radially and laterally into the overlying white matter and cortex, striatum, and hippocampus, where they differentiate into oligodendrocytes and astrocytes. Unlike neural progenitors, glial progenitors continue to proliferate as they migrate (Cayre et al., 2009).

Upon reaching its destination, an OPC begins to differentiate by extending processes and upregulating myelin protein expression. The processes then begin to form membrane wraps around nearby axons. Eventually the oligodendrocyte forms tightly wrapped multilayered sheaths from which most of the cytoplasm has been extruded. The dramatic increase in axonal conduction velocity associated with myelination is well known. However, recent research suggests that functional interactions between oligodendrocytes and neurons extend far beyond the effects of the electrically insulating sheath. Oligodendrocytes synthesize a number of trophic factors that appear to contribute to the maintenance of axonal integrity and neuronal survival, and neuron–oligodendrocyte interactions have been shown to influence neuronal size and axon diameter (McTigue & Tripathi, 2008). They also induce the clustering of sodium channels along the axon, which plays an important role in signal conduction. Finally, recent studies suggest that a subset of the OPCs dispersed throughout the brain form excitatory and inhibitory connections with neurons, and thus may contribute actively and directly to neural signaling (Lin & Bergles, 2004). Although the full scope of neuron–glia interactions is still poorly defined, it is clear that these interactions play an important role in the functional organization of neural circuits during postnatal life (Bradl & Lassmann, 2010).

Regressive Events in the Postnatal Period

Regressive events continue to play an important role in postnatal brain development. Two major classes of regressive events are prominent postnatally. First, widespread cell death is prominent in glial cell populations. In addition, the exuberant production followed by extensive retraction of synapses is observed throughout the brain during a protracted period of postnatal development that extends at least through adolescence.

Cell Death in Glial Populations

As described above, brain development involves overproduction of neurons and glial cells, neural processes, and synapses. Although neural apoptosis has its peak during prenatal life, apoptosis in glial cell populations has a time course corresponding to the protracted postnatal time course of differentiation from glial precursors. During the period of initial myelination, many excess oligodendrocytes undergo apoptosis a few days after differentiating, and there is evidence that this process depends on signals from nearby axons, such that the number of surviving oligodendrocytes matches the local axonal surface area (see McTigue & Tripathi, 2008, for review).

Synaptic Exuberance and Pruning

The development of neural networks requires that precise sets of connections be made between developing neurons and their targets. However, initial patterns of connectivity in the developing brain lack this precision. Early connectivity is exuberant in terms of both the number of connections and their topography. Rakic et al. (Bourgeois, Goldman-Rakic, & Rakic, 1994; Bourgeois & Rakic, 1993; Zecevic, Bourgeois, & Rakic, 1989) first documented very rapid and exuberant synapse production in a wide range of cortical areas during the first postnatal months in rhesus macaque. The number of synapses in visual, motor, and prefrontal brain areas reaches a maximum at 2 months after birth and plateaus at levels nearly twice as high as observed in the adult brain. The number of connections slowly declines between 2 months and 3 years (the age of maturity in macaque), when adult levels of synaptic connectivity are obtained. Thus, synaptic exuberance and pruning appears to be the norm in the primate brain.

Similar studies have been reported for humans using autopsy material from individual brains obtained from the prenatal period through adulthood (Huttenlocher & Dabholkar, 1997; Huttenlocher & de Courten, 1987). As was the case with the monkey studies, synapse production throughout the human brain increases rapidly beginning at birth, and peaks at levels far higher than observed in the mature brain. The period of synaptic exuberance is followed by a slow decline in synapse numbers that continues for years and eventually stabilizes at typical adult levels (Fig. 2.15). Unlike the data reported for monkeys, the timing of peak production differs across brain regions. Exuberant synapse production peaks in sensory areas in the second half of the first year of life, while in frontal cortices the peak occurs in the mid-preschool period.

Exuberant connectivity in the developing brain reflects more than simply increased synapse numbers. Within the developing neural system, transient connections form among many brain regions that are not found in the mature brain. This exuberant connectivity

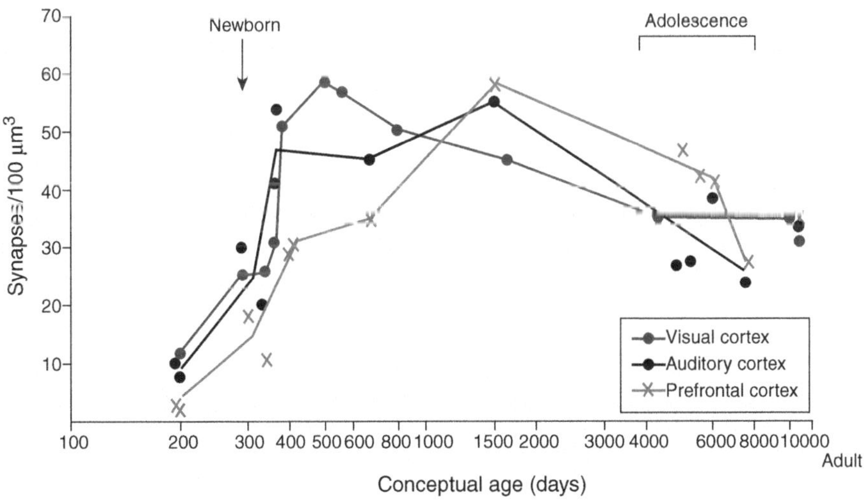

FIGURE 2.15. Number of synapses in a constant volume of tissue across the human lifespan. Synapse numbers increase dramatically at birth and peak in early childhood at levels far higher than in adults. Gradual pruning back of exuberant connections occurs over many years. The period of peak production differs for different brain areas. (Adapted with permission from Huttenlocher PR, Dabholkar AS (1997). Regional differences in synaptogenesis in human cerebral cortex. *J Comp Neurol* 387:167–178, Figure 2.)

creates a very different topography of brain connectivity early in development (Innocenti & Price, 2005; Stanfield & O'Leary, 1985; Stanfield, O'Leary, & Fricks, 1982). Connections across the corpus callosum are initially widespread and acquire the typical mapping across homologous brain regions only with extended development. Exuberant connectivity is observed in early development throughout the brain, including pathways as diverse as the thalamocortical pathways, corticospinal tract, and pathways linking the temporal lobe and the limbic system. The stabilization or elimination of pathways is affected by a wide range of factors. Competition for resources such as neurotrophic factors plays a significant role in selection of pathways. Afferent input plays a critical role in system activity and acts as a powerful modulator of stabilization or elimination of pathways. As discussed below, the dynamic processes associated with the exuberant production of synapses and their elimination are important factors in the normal pattern of activity-driven modulation of brain organization and neural plasticity.

Anatomical Imaging Studies of Postnatal Brain Development

For many years, structural MRI has been an important tool for investigating human brain development in the postnatal period. These studies have provided important data on changes in the major gray and white tissue compartments of the brain. More recently studies have begun to focus on another measure of cortical morphology that appears to undergo systematic change with development: specifically, regional cortical thickness. Another important aspect of neural change that has recently begun to be explored using MRI technologies is the maturation of brain fiber tracts. Diffusion-weighted imaging has begun to provide a detailed account of regional change in the maturation of the major fiber tracts in the developing brain.

MRI Studies of Changes in Brain Morphology

Over the past two decades, MRI studies have revealed dramatic changes in the tissues of the developing brain during the postnatal brain growth spurt. These MRI signal changes reflect alterations in tissue chemistry that are presumed to mark the proliferation of oligodendrocytes and deposition of myelin, and they reveal much about the timing and anatomical distribution of these processes (Barkovich, 2000, 2005). The visual appearance of the brain on MR images changes appreciably over the first 2 to 3 years of life, mirroring an orderly pattern of myelination in white matter regions. However, the changes in gross brain structure that continue past this age are subtler and were fully appreciated only after quantitative morphometry techniques were applied. Early MR morphometry studies comparing brain morphology in children and adults showed that gray matter volumes, both in the cerebral cortex and in subcortical nuclei, were considerably larger in school-age children than in young adults (Jernigan, Hesselink, Sowell, & Tallal, 1991; Jernigan & Tallal, 1990; Jernigan, Trauner, Hesselink, & Tallal, 1991; Pfefferbaum et al., 1994). This suggested that tissue alterations related to brain maturation might be much more protracted during childhood than was generally supposed, and that some of these alterations might be regressive; that is, they might involve tissue loss. These findings were confirmed and extended by later studies (see Toga, Thompson, & Sowell, 2006, for a review), but the underlying tissue alterations remain a matter of speculation. The size of the cranial vault increases dramatically after birth but very little after the first decade. However, the MRI results suggest that throughout childhood and adolescence effects of waning progressive changes, associated with continuing maturation of glial populations and neurotrophic effects, are opposed by concurrent regressive changes, perhaps associated with pruning of neuronal processes. These observations are consistent with ample histological evidence for ongoing myelination across this period (Yakovlev & Lecours, 1967) and more limited, but persuasive, evidence for reduction of synaptic density in cortex during childhood (Huttenlocher & Dabholkar, 1997), but it remains unclear to what extent these factors, and perhaps others, contribute to the changing morphology observed with MRI. Data shown in Figure 2.16, plotting estimated volumes of brain structures across the lifespan, illustrate that during childhood and adolescence changes in brain structure are at least as dramatic as those at the end of life. The plots illustrate results from an extended age range for volumes of particular brain structures (from Jernigan & Gamst, 2005). Shown are continuous age-related decreases in volume of frontal cortex and thalamus across the lifespan, and increases in cerebral white matter volume during childhood and early adulthood that give way to decreases later in life. All volumes are normalized for cranial volume—which does not change appreciably over this age range.

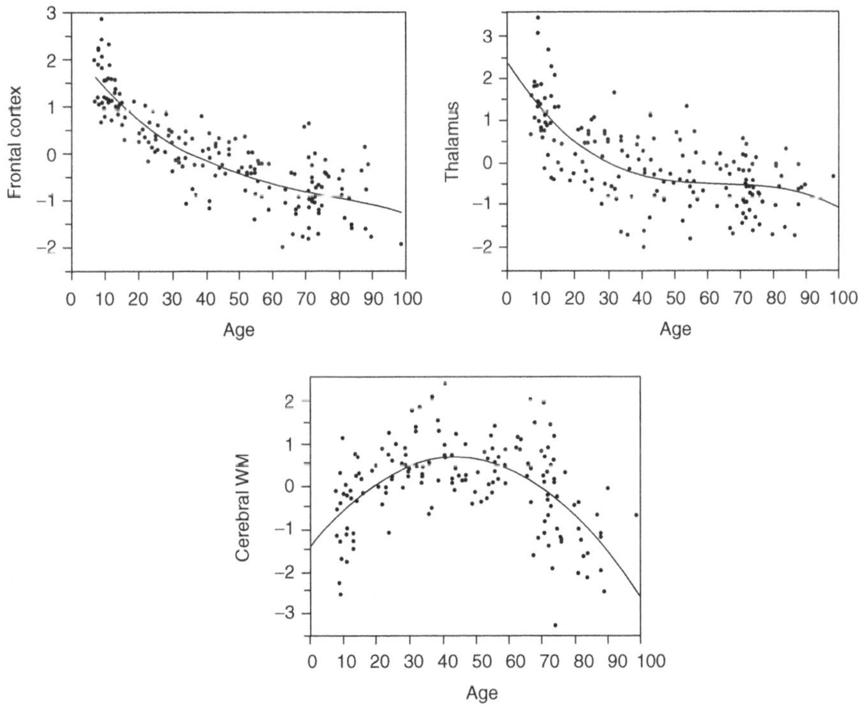

FIGURE 2.16 Estimated volumes of brain structures in normal volunteers are plotted against age for frontal cortex, thalamus, and cerebral white matter. Note the rapid age-related change (and striking individual differences) in the childhood and adolescent age range. (Adapted with permission from Jernigan TL, Gamst AC (2004). Changes in volume with age—consistency and interpretation of observed effects. *Neurobiol Aging* 26(9):1275–1278.)

More recent MR morphometry studies have provided more anatomical detail by employing mapping methods for visualizing the pattern of age-related change (Giedd et al., 1996; Sowell et al., 1999; Sowell, Trauner, Gamst, & Jernigan, 2002). Studies of developing children describe the protracted course of postnatal white matter growth and establish that the volume of tissue with the MR signal characteristics of gray matter declines concurrently in locations throughout the brain (e.g., in cerebral cortex and deep nuclei). The most detailed studies, employing both high-resolution mapping techniques and longitudinal assessments (Gogtay et al., 2004; Sowell et al., 2004), have revealed a modal pattern of childhood and adolescent change in the cerebral cortex that includes not only widespread, regionally specific, apparent cortical thinning, but more limited areas of cortical thickening as well (Fig. 2.17). On average, cortical thinning appears to occur first in primary sensory-motor cortex and then to progress into secondary, then multimodal, and then supramodal cortical areas throughout childhood and adolescence. A recent study (Østby et al., 2009) confirmed these observations in a large cross-sectional sample and provided concurrent estimates of cortical surface area and cortical thickness. This is an important contribution since studies of cortical volume conflate these factors, and no previous studies had addressed whether the changes in cortical thickness are accompanied by alterations of surface area as well. Østby et al. (2009) reported that between the ages of 8 and 30 years more modest decreases in cortical surface area accompany the dramatic decreases in cortical thickness.

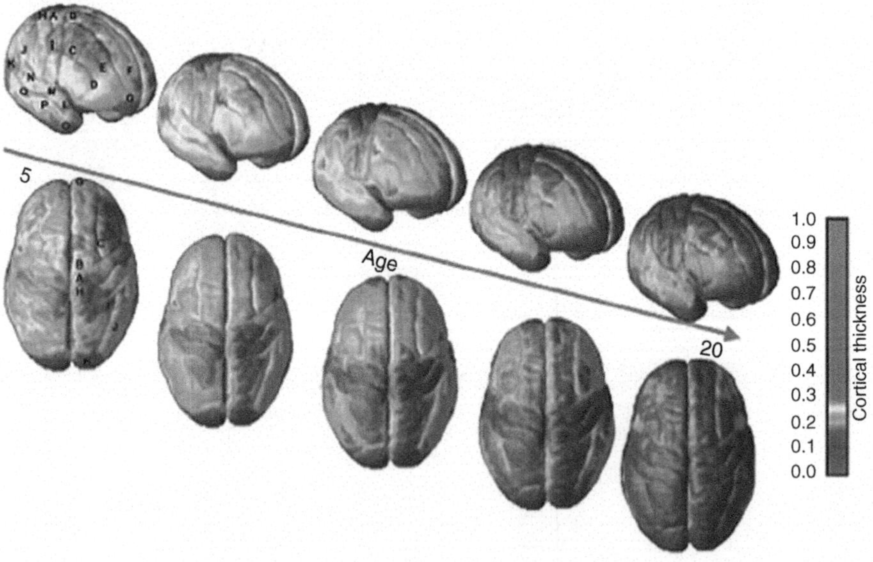

FIGURE 2.17 Systematic regional change in cortical thickness emerges with development. Dark areas indicate thinner regions of cortex. The changes are very systematic, beginning in sensorimotor areas and then extending to progressively higher-order cognitive systems. (Reprinted with permission from Gogtay N, Giedd JN, Lusk L, Hayashi KM, Greenstein D, Vaituzis AC, Nugent TF 3rd, Herman DH, Clasen LS, Toga AW, Rapoport JL, Thompson PM (2004). Dynamic mapping of human cortical development during childhood through early adulthood. *Proc Natl Acad Sci U S A* 101(21):8174–8179, Figure 3.) (See color insert.)

An important issue germane to the interpretation of these effects is their relationship to myelination. At the most basic level, cortical "thinning" could simply reflect increased myelination in the white matter tracts coursing within and near the deepest layer of cortex. In other words, the "gray" signal of the unmyelinated fibers could simply be becoming more "white" as myelin is deposited. This is clearly a part of what is measured as cortical thinning with morphometry, especially in younger children. However, there is evidence that true regressive changes also occur in some structures—probably due to loss or simplification of neuronal processes (dendrites and/or axons). This can be inferred from the fact that the progressive changes that would be expected to result from continuing myelination do not seem to increase cranial volume in late childhood (as though they were opposed by some regressive factor) and from the fact that there are modest but significant cerebrospinal fluid volume increases adjacent to the cortical surface and in the ventricular system over this age range, as might be expected in the wake of the loss of neural elements in the adjacent tissues (Jernigan, Trauner, et al., 1991; Sowell et al., 2002). In summary, MR morphometry studies reveal a complex pattern of development in brain structure during childhood and hint that ongoing maturation of fiber tracts likely plays a key role. Only recently, however, has it been possible to examine the maturation of fiber tracts directly, using diffusion tensor imaging (DTI) (Basser, Mattiello, & LeBihan, 1994; Mori & van Zijl, 1995).

Diffusion Imaging of Fiber Tract Development

Diffusion imaging measures the diffusion of water molecules through the tissue. A common use of diffusion imaging involves estimating the movement, or diffusion, of water molecules along three primary spatial axes. The diffusion of water molecules in fluids such as cerebrospinal fluid has been described as isotropic, which means that the molecules move, or diffuse, freely and equally in all spatial directions. Diffusion in gray matter is lower but also relatively isotropic. However, in tissue containing fiber bundles, diffusion has been described as an anisotrophic, reflecting the preponderance of movement along the long axis of the fibers. The measure of anisotrophy usually employed in DTI studies assesses the disproportionate movement of water molecules in one spatial direction, and is termed fractional anisotropy (FA).

Diffusion in the cerebral white matter of human newborns is high, and exhibits low anisotropy (Hermoye et al., 2006). As the brain matures and myelination increases, there is a generalized decline in diffusivity along all spatial directions in all tissue compartments. However, the degree of decline along the long axis of fiber tracts is less pronounced, and thus the measure of FA increases within fiber tracts. These increases in FA provide a measure of fiber tract maturation in the developing brain (Suzuki, Matsuzawa, Kwee, & Nakada, 2003). There is accumulating evidence that alterations reflected in DTI measures continue throughout childhood and adolescence (Barnea-Goraly et al., 2005; Schleussner et al., 2004; Snook, Paulson, Roy, Phillips, & Beaulieu, 2005). The data suggest that developmental change in FA reaches asymptote earliest in long projection, then commissural, and finally association fibers (see Cascio, Gerig, & Piven, 2007; Huppi & Dubois, 2006; Mukherjee & McKinstry, 2006, for reviews).

Lebel et al. (Lebel & Beaulieu, 2011; Lebel, Walker, Leemans, Phillips, & Beaulieu, 2008) reported diffusion imaging results from a large group of typically developing children and young adults. Robust increases in FA across the 5- to 12-year age range were observed within a wide range of fiber tracts. In Figure 2.18 the cross-sectional results are shown for four major tracts: the corpus callosum (splenium), the inferior and superior longitudinal fasciculi, and the inferior fronto-occipital fasciculi. These plots reveal the rapid change in FA in young school-age children for all tracts. But the rates of change also vary considerably. The splenium and the inferior longitudinal fasciculi reach asymptotic levels of FA comparable to adults long before the superior longitudinal and the inferior fronto-occipital fasciculi. More recently this group also reported individual trajectories of fiber tract FA using a longitudinal imaging protocol. These data clearly demonstrate that over this age range substantial increases in FA occur within individual children, and they suggest wide individual differences in the pace of these changes.

Functional Imaging Studies of Developmental Change in Brain Organization

Advances in functional imaging technologies make it possible to characterize developmental change in the functional organization of brain regions and networks. Although there are a

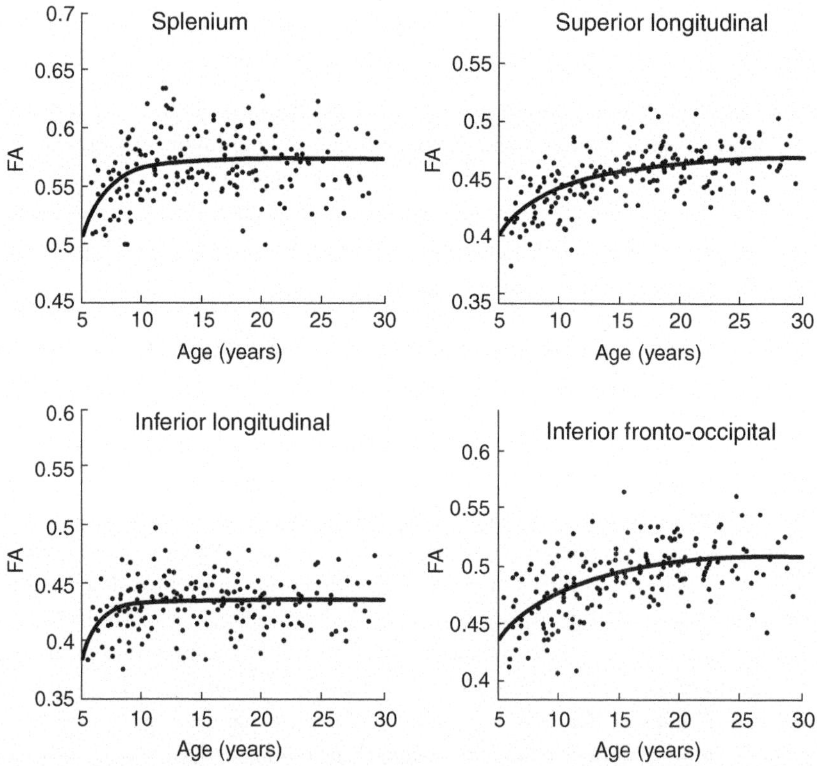

FIGURE 2.18 Cross-sectional data showing robust FA increases in four major fiber tracts; note rapid change in FA in young school-age children and variability in the pace at which FA in the different tracts approaches asymptote. (Adapted with permission from Lebel C, Walker L, et al. (2008). Microstructural maturation of the human brain from childhood to adulthood. *NeuroImage* 40(3):1044–1055.)

number of functional imaging modalities, including multiple modalities using MRI methods, MRI of the blood oxygenation level-dependent (BOLD) signal, often simply referred to a functional magnetic resonance imaging (fMRI), has become one of the most widely used techniques for mapping brain function to brain anatomy. BOLD imaging measures subtle changes in the magnetic field arising from changes in the ratio of oxygenated and deoxygenated blood caused by neuronal activity in brain tissue. Activity within brain tissue initially consumes oxygen in hemoglobin, producing deoxygenated hemoglobin, a paramagnetic substance that degenerates local BOLD signal. In addition, local activity initiates a cascade of signals that increases arterial blood flow into the region, thereby increasing the ratio of oxygenated blood to deoxygenated blood, and that increases BOLD signal in proportion to the hemodynamic response. This hemodynamic response function and associated changes in the BOLD signal rise over several seconds to a peak response approximately 4 to 8 seconds following the neuronal activation. It is the BOLD signal increase that is generally observed in fMRI studies. Task-specific BOLD functional activity is measured by acquiring a time series images of the brain that document specific activation states of the brain over time. At each point in the time series a set of 30 to 40 sequential planar images that encompass the whole brain are acquired. Each whole-brain acquisition takes approximately 2 seconds, so a typical 5-minute functional imaging task generates a time series of approximately 150 whole-brain images. This series captures regional fluctuations in the local BOLD signal over time. Most analyses use signal averaging to minimize random noise factors and produce a mean estimated BOLD response to specific task-related factors (i.e., stimuli, response). A common means of manipulating local brain activity is to ask participants to engage in a specific task for a brief period of time, and to compare patterns of task-specific brain activity to activity during either rest or during a control task.

The great majority of studies to date have focused on single cognitive domains such as language or attention. Moreover, most studies tend to focus on a single or small set of cortical regions, so called regions of interest (ROIs), that are believed to be most important for the execution of the function. This parallels the vast majority of work in adults. More recently, the focus of both adult and developmental studies has begun to shift from ROI-based analytic designs to studies of whole-brain functional networks. This work provides the opportunity to examine brain–behavior relationships in a more comprehensive fashion by considering not simply componential functioning of subsystems, but also interactions among multiple components and even across networks. This section begins with brief overviews of the two major approaches to fMRI, ROI-based studies and whole-brain analyses of neural systems. It then considers the major developmental findings from three of the most widely studied cognitive domains—visuospatial processing of faces, cognitive control, and language. The great majority of these studies have used ROI-based approaches to describe developmental change in the components of the neural processing systems for each domain. Important and globally consistent patterns of data have emerged from these studies; however, inconsistencies persist in the findings from each domain. These inconsistencies arise, at least in part, from the limited definition of the neural substrate that arises from ROI approaches. Thus, each section will consider available findings about developmental change in functional connectivity for each of the three cognitive domains.

ROI-based studies of neuroimaging focus on functional activity from one to a limited number of regions within a targeted neurocognitive domain. Developmental studies often define the brain regions to be studies based on adult neuroimaging findings. The developmental studies typically ask whether children activate the adult brain region, whether the extent or distribution of activation is comparable to adults (e.g., volume of activation), or whether there is evidence of change in the intensity of activation relative to adults (e.g., percent signal change). In general, across each of the three domains discussed below, this adult-guided ROI approach has produced mixed findings on the patterns of developmental change. An alternative to the ROI-based approach is whole-brain analysis of task-related activation. In these analyses, reports include functional activation throughout the brain, sometimes in conjunction with activity within predefined ROIs. Within development, the ratio of ROI to whole-brain studies weighs heavily in favor of ROI studies.

A newer approach to brain activation analysis is to examine patterns of coherent signal that define coordinated activation between brain regions, so-called functional connectivity. Within fMRI studies, functional connectivity is typically determined by calculating the correlation of fMRI BOLD signal between numerous brain areas, either during task performance or, more commonly, from periods when no task is performed. In its simplest form, connectivity analysis produces maps of regions that are correlated to a specific ROI or "seed region" (Biswal, Yetkin, Haughton, & Hyde, 1995; Fair, Schlaggar, et al., 2007) In more complex analyses, connectivity is defined by various network structures determined, for example, by the degree of interconnectivity between local modules and hubs connecting distributed modules (Bullmore & Sporns, 2009; Rubinov & Sporns, 2010).

Functional connectivity of the developing brain has been characterized in a number of recent studies as reflecting strengthening of long-range network connectivity with age, accompanied by pruning of local network connectivity (Uddin, 2010). These changes are observed for both task-related networks as well as the so-called default network, which is defined as a neural network that increases in activity during periods without goal-directed tasks. While some elements of mature default and task-related networks can be detected in the neonate (Fransson, Aden, Blennow, & Lagercrantz, 2011; Gao et al., 2009; Lin et al., 2008; Liu, Flax, Guise, Sukul, & Benasich, 2008; Smyser, Snyder, & Neil, 2011), ongoing change in both the elements of the networks and their patterns of functional connectivity is observed throughout the childhood period. Further, the timescale for development of neural networks also differs by domain, with sensory networks maturing ahead of networks for higher cognitive functions (Supekar, Uddin et al., 2010; Lopez-Larson, Anderson et al., 2011; Zielinski, Gennatas, Zhou, & Seeley, 2010). A number of studies have used resting-state functional connectivity (rs-fcMRI) (i.e., data from fMRI scans during which the participant is not engaging is specific goal-directed behavior) to study the development of the default network in young children. Fair et al. (Fair et al., 2008, 2009) report that the default networks of 7-year-old children exhibit strong interhemispheric connectivity but only sparse connectivity across regions. Adult-like default network structure is not observed until late adolescence.

FMRI Studies of Face Processing

Virtually all adults are experts in face processing. However, developmental studies of behavior show that adult expertise is acquired slowly over a protracted period that begins in early infancy and extends well into adolescence (Bushnell, Sai, & Mullin, 1989; Cassia, Turati, &

Simion, 2004; Johnson & Morton, 1991; Turati, Simion, Milani, & Umilta, 2002). The protracted behavioral development is mirrored in the development of the neural systems for face processing insofar that adult levels of maturity are not achieved until late adolescence (Cohen Kadosh & Johnson, 2007, de Haan, Johnson, & Halit, 2003; de Haan, Pascalis, & Johnson, 2002; Grill-Spector, Golarai, & Gabrieli, 2008; Taylor, 2004).

Most adult face processing studies have focused on a core brain network within ventral temporal-occipital (VOT) cortices that is responsible for processing perceptual aspects of faces. The brain regions of the core network include the middle aspects of the lateral fusiform gyrus, often referred to as the fusiform face area (FFA); the inferior occipital gyrus in Brodmann's area 18, often referred to as the occipital face area (OFA); and the posterior superior temporal sulcus (pSTS). The core network tends to show a strong right hemisphere bias. The FFA and OFA are associated with processing invariant features of face stimuli, while the pSTS is associated with dynamic feature processing such as eye gaze direction. The core face processing networks are activated both by tasks making specific demands, such remembering a specific face (Epstein, Higgins, Parker, Aguirre, & Cooperman, 2006; Gauthier, Curby, Skudlarski, & Epstein, 2005; Mazard, Schiltz, & Rossion, 2006; Xu, 2005; Yovel & Kanwisher, 2004, 2005), and by tasks without specific demands, such as passive viewing tasks (Grill-Spector, Knouf, & Kanwisher, 2004; Kanwisher, McDermott, & Chun, 1997; Kanwisher, Stanley, & Harris, 1999; Rhodes, Byatt, Michie, & Puce, 2004; Wojciulik, Kanwisher, & Driver, 1998).

A small but growing number of studies have used fMRI to explore the development of the neural basis of face processing. The majority of studies explored developmental changes in the FFA specifically. The findings are mixed on the question of when children produce a reliable FFA; some studies suggest that young school-age children fail to produce reliable FFA activation to faces (Gathers, Bhatt, Corbly, Farley, & Joseph, 2004). By contrast, one study reported adult-like levels of FFA activation by age 7 (Pelphrey, Lopez, & Morris, 2009). Nevertheless, the preponderance of evidence indicates that school-age children produce reliable FFA activation, but the patterns of activation within the fusiform gyrus region vary considerably from those observed among adults. Systematic increases in fMRI BOLD signal activation both in terms of the extent or size of activation (Brambati, Benoit, Monetta, Belleville, & Joubert, 2010; Golarai et al., 2007; Peelen, Glaser, Vuilleumier, & Eliez, 2009) and intensity or percent signal change (Brambati et al., 2010; Cohen Kadosh, Cohen Kadosh, Dick, & Johnson, 2010; Golarai et al., 2007; Joseph, Gathers, & Bhatt, 2011) have been reported from the early school-age period through adulthood. These developmental activation changes correlate with improvement in recognition memory for faces (Golarai et al., 2007; Golarai, Liberman, Yoon, & Grill-Spector, 2010) and with task demand (Scherf, Luna, Avidan, & Behrmann, 2011).

An even smaller number of studies explored developmental changes in core network components other than the FFA. In the very limited number of studies exploring development within the OFA, the results appear more consistent than those obtained for the FFA. Three studies reported no activation in the OFA for 7- and 8-year-olds (Aylward et al., 2005; Joseph et al., 2011; Scherf, Behrmann, Humphreys, & Luna, 2007), and one reported increases in activation in the right OFA by early adolescence (Aylward et al., 2005). Reports for the STS are mixed: one study reported no activation in children (Scherf et al., 2007), while a second found adult levels of activation as early as age 7 (Golarai et al., 2007).

In summary, the ROI approach applied to questions of developmental trajectories for the core face network has provided varied patterns across the school-age period into adolescence. A fair reading of the pattern of findings is that the core network shows protracted development, although the precise relationship for the development of components within the network is unclear.

While some studies have examined whole-brain patterns of activation, only a few have used measures of functional connectivity to examine the development of brain networks for face processing. One study explicitly examined developmental change in the core network (Cohen Kadosh et al., 2010). They studied children between 7 and 12 years, and adults, and found very similar patterns of dynamic connectivity across ages; specifically, they found that activation of the region of the inferior occipital gyrus (IOG), a region that includes the OFA, influenced activation in regions of both the fusiform gyrus (FG), the region encompassing the FFA, and the STS. However, the magnitude of effects differed with age. In contrast to adults, both the child groups exhibited weaker connectivity between IOG and FG, and no significant connectivity between IOG and STS. Furthermore, unlike adults, for whom specific task demands altered network activity, Cohen Kadosh et al. found no task-selective effects for the child groups.

There is a growing body of evidence that the brain network for face processing extends considerably beyond the core network (Fairhall & Ishai, 2007; Gobbini & Haxby, 2007; Haxby et al., 2001; Haxby, Hoffman, & Gobbini, 2000; Ishai, Schmidt, & Boesiger, 2005). In addition to the components of the core system, the extended face processing system includes the amygdala for processing of emotional expressions, inferior frontal gyrus for semantic processing, orbitofrontal and nucleus accumbens as part of the reward system (Haxby et al., 2000, 2001; Ishai et al., 2005), the anterior paracingulate cortex for processing of attitudes and mental states, the pSTS (posterior superior temporal sulcus)–temporal parietal junction for intentions, anterior temporal regions for personal identity and biographical information, and precuneus/posterior cingulate for episodic memory (Brambati et al., 2010; Gobbini & Haxby, 2007). In studies of adults, different components of the extended network activate in a task-dependent fashion. Thus, during passive viewing only the core network activates, and additional components of the extended network emerge depending on task demand.

One recent study (Joseph et al., 2011) explicitly examined age-related change in the organization of the extended face processing network. They reported both progressive changes, in which a brain region shows increasing face-preferential activation, and regressive changes, where responsiveness to faces declines. Progressive changes were observed in critical regions of the core face network, suggesting the gradual specialization of brain regions for face processing. Complementary regressive changes in more widespread brain areas suggested that children initially recruit a broader range of brain regions than adults, including more left hemisphere components as well as areas in the frontal, temporal, and parietal lobes, when engaged in face processing. These data suggest that with development the face processing network is gradually pruned and refined as expertise expands. Haist et al. (Haist, Adamo, Han, Lee, & Stiles, submitted) used ICA analyses to examine change in the brain networks engaged during a passive face processing task. Like Josephs (Joseph et al., 2011), they reported much more extensive activation in young children. Interestingly, many of the exuberantly activated areas found for children corresponded to the components of the extended face network in adults. For adults activation was limited to the core face processing network, consistent with the fact that the task was simple passive viewing. However, children nonselectively recruit the entire extended network, reflecting their immaturity and lack of expertise with face processing.

FMRI Studies of Cognitive Control

Cognitive control refers to a range of behaviors that work in concert to voluntarily guide behavior. They include planning, filtering of information, and impulse control, and they engage processes of response inhibition, working memory, and focused attention (Bunge & Wright, 2007; Luna, Padmanabhan, & O'Hearn, 2010). They are often referred to as executive processes. The development of cognitive control processes is protracted and extends at least into adolescence (Luna, Garver, Urban, Lazar, & Sweeney, 2004). Very young children show some facility across the range of executive functions; with development, increasing flexibility and consistency in the execution of task control responses are observed (Luna, 2009).

Although the neural systems for cognitive control are complex and distributed, prefrontal systems play a particularly important role. Thus, prefrontal cortex (PFC) has been the focus of many of the developmental fMRI studies. However, the findings from this work have been somewhat mixed. A number of studies have reported increasing activation in prefrontal regions with age (Bunge, Dudukovic, Thomason, Vaidya, & Gabrieli, 2002; Luna et al., 2001; Rubia et al., 2000; Rubia, Smith, Taylor, & Brammer, 2007), while others have reported activation declines (Booth et al., 2003; Casey et al., 1997; Durston et al., 2002).

Luna (Luna, 2009; Luna et al., 2010) has suggested that neural changes observed across development reflect both widespread change in the neural components of cognitive control, and critically their efficient integration and coordination into a smoothly operating and consistent system. Thus, she argues that a more complete account of developmental change in the neural networks for cognitive control is essential for understanding the development of these abilities. Indeed, very recent work examining developmental change in the brain networks for cognitive control supports this idea and provides a possible means for integrating the diverse data focused on individual brain regions (Fair, Dosenbach, et al., 2007). Those studies are discussed in greater detail below.

A small number of studies have examined changes in functional connectivity within task control networks. They suggest a developmental shift in functional connectivity yielding cognitive control networks that are both more segregated and internally better integrated (Fair et al., 2009; Fair, Dosenbach, et al., 2007). These studies examined two brain networks believed to be associated with cognitive control—specifically, a frontoparietal network that is engaged for adaptive online control of processing on a trial-by-trial basis, and a cingulo-opercular network that provides sustained task control over a longer timescale. The emergence of these two systems as independent networks occurs slowly and is the product of a developmental shift in organization that involves the segregation of the components of the cingulo-opercular system from the frontoparietal system, coupled with integration of the components within the cingulo-opercular system. The findings from these studies suggest that mature brain networks emerge over a protracted period of time and presumably reflect the experience of the developing organism.

Finally, changes in the control networks for working memory were examined by Finn et al. (Finn, Sheridan, Kam, Hinshaw, & D'Esposito, 2010). In adults, simple delayed match to sample tasks activate a frontal network centered in the lateral PFC. When tasks require processing of novel stimuli or construction of relations among stimuli, the hippocampus is also recruited. In a longitudinal study of younger (15 years of age) and older adolescents (18 years of age), Finn et al. (Finn et al., 2010) found that lateral PFC is recruited during delayed match to sample tasks at both ages, but the hippocampus activates only at younger ages. Further, the activity of the right hippocampus is correlated with lateral PFC activity in younger but not older adolescents. To further assess the effects of task demand, both high- and low-load conditions were examined separately at both time points. Consistent with the overall analyses, strong correlations between hippocampal and PFC activations were observed in the younger adolescents for both low- and high-load trials. For the older adolescents, a correlation between hippocampal and PFC activity was also observed, but only for the high-load trials. These findings suggest that even in middle adolescence the working memory network is expanded to include brain regions that are employed only during complex memory demand task in adults. With development these networks gradually become more specialized.

FMRI Studies Language

Imaging studies of brain organization for language have shown that for most adults the major components of language are primarily mediated by a left lateralized frontotemporal network (Rasmussen & Milner, 1977). The majority of brain imaging studies of children have tried to determine whether these same core brain regions support language in children and whether there is any change with age in the patterns of activation within these regions. A central question has concerned the degree of left laterality in children as compared to adults.

While most studies support a general pattern of increasing lateralization with development, there are both task- and age-related differences in the findings. Patterns of activation for lexical processing tasks tend to show earlier left lateralization (Balsamo, Xu, & Gaillard, 2006; Everts et al., 2009; Gaillard et al., 2003; Lidzba, Schwilling, Grodd, Krageloh-Mann, & Wilke, 2011) than those involving more complex aspects of language, such as verb generation (Holland et al., 2001; Ressel, 2008; Szaflarski, Holland, Schmithorst, & Byars, 2006). However, even on lexical tasks, there are significant changes in the amount of activation within traditional language areas, particularly in frontal regions (Brown et al., 2005; Gaillard et al., 2003). There is also evidence for a developmental decline in language task-related activation for non-language areas such as the ventral visual pathway (Balsamo et al., 2006; Schmithorst, Holland, & Plante, 2007) and right frontal regions (Brown et al., 2005).

On more complex tasks the findings of robust increases in left lateralization are consistent. Verb generation tasks yield both increasing activation with age in traditional left hemisphere language areas (Holland et al., 2001; Ressel, 2008; Szaflarski et al., 2006) as well as decreasing activation in right hemisphere regions associated with attention and task performance (Szaflarski et al., 2006). Finally, a recent study using story comprehension tasks reported increasingly focal activation with age in the superior temporal gyrus bilaterally, but there was no evidence of age-related increases in laterality (Lidzba et al., 2011).

A small number of studies have begun to examine developmental change in the brain networks for language. Karunanayaka et al. (Karunanayaka et al., 2010, 2011) used ICA and structural equation modeling on a large sample of child data. They reported age-related increases in connectivity between the left medial temporal and frontal regions. They also found increasing lateralization with age in some components of the network, particularly in anterior brain regions, but little change within posterior regions, particularly the superior temporal gyrus. These data thus support the idea of systematic changes with age in both long-range ipsilateral and at least some aspects of interhemispheric connectivity.

Other support for these kinds of change comes from a recent study examining the development of frontotemporal pathways that are important for syntactic processing. Friederici et al. employed a correlational analysis of low-frequency fluctuations in the fMRI data (Friederici, Brauer, & Lohmann, 2011) to explore differences in the left hemisphere networks for complex syntactic processing in adults and children. The principal language pathway has both a dorsal component extending from left dorsal inferior frontal gyrus to left posterior superior temporal gyrus/sulcus (STS/STG) that is associated with working memory resources for syntactic processing, and a ventral component extending from left ventral inferior frontal gyrus to the anterior-to-mid portion of the STG that is associated with complex syntactic processing. The patterns of network correlations suggest strikingly different patterns of organization for adults and children. While adults showed strong frontotemporal correlations for both the dorsal and ventral components of the pathway, correlations for children were weak for all components, and weakest for the dorsal component. Further, the children showed strong interhemispheric correlations that were not observed in adults both in superior temporal regions and between the left inferior frontal sulcus and the right pSTG. Finally, while children exhibited weak or nonexistent long-range frontotemporal connectivity, they had a strong level of local connectivity. These data are consistent with data from both resting state and other task domains and suggest that the functional connectivity of the developing brain is well characterized as reflecting strengthening of long-range network connectivity with age, accompanied by pruning of local network connectivity.

The Role of Experience in Postnatal Brain Development

As discussed throughout this chapter, the events of the prenatal period serve to establish the core compartments of the developing nervous system from the spinal cord and hindbrain to the cortical structures of the telencephalon. These early events also provide initial patterning within each of the major subdivisions of the brain. Both the segmental organization of the hindbrain–spinal column and the initial patterning of neocortical somatosensory areas emerge by the end of the embryonic period. But this early patterning, particularly in the neocortex, is both underspecified and malleable. The mature organization of the neocortex emerges over a protracted time during the postnatal period, and it requires diverse forms of input. Some of this input arises from within the organism in the form of molecular signaling and cross-regional activity. But the specific experience of the individual organism also plays an essential role in establishing the mature organization of the neocortex. The development of normal brain organization requires input via all of the major sensorimotor systems. When specific aspects of input are lacking, alternative patterns of brain organization can and do emerge. These alternative patterns of organization reflect the effects of altered profiles of neural competition and capture a fundamental property of mammalian brain development, the capacity for plastic adaptation. Chapter 1 discussed the issue of neural plasticity in considerable detail, and the particulars of that discussion will not be repeated here. Rather, a summary of data documenting the effects of altered early experience on the development of neural systems will be presented.

Greenough has used the term "experience expectant" development to capture the idea that the early experience of the organism plays an essential role in normal brain development, particularly in the early postnatal period (Greenough, Black, & Wallace, 1987). The development of typical visual or auditory neocortical areas requires—"expects"—particular types of input. When that input is lacking, brain areas develop differently, and the specific pattern of development reflects the kinds of input that organism actually received. Later in development, the developing—and even the mature—nervous system continues to require input to acquire new knowledge and to develop functional neural systems. Greenough has termed this later phase of development "experience dependent" learning. These two important constructs suggest that throughout development, experience plays an essential role in establishing and refining neural organization in ways that allow the organism to adapt to the contingences of the world in which it lives. Studies that systematically manipulate the specific experience of the young organism provide insight into the dynamic and adaptive nature of brain development.

The experience of the young organism can be altered in a number of ways. In the simplest form, the input to the developing neural system can be changed either by manipulating the complexity of the surrounding environment or by restricting input from specific systems via sensory deprivation. Both of these manipulations have a dramatic effect on the structural and functional organization of the developing brain. Greenough has shown that simply rearing animals in either impoverished (standard laboratory cage) or enriched environments (large enclosures with interesting and changing landmarks and multiple littermates) has dramatic effects on a wide range of brain structures and functions (Black, Sirevaag, & Greenough, 1987; Greenough & Chang, 1988; Jones & Greenough, 1996; Markham & Greenough, 2004). Animals reared in complex environments show enhancement in density of cortical synapses, increases in the number of brain support cells, and even augmentation of the complexity of the brain vascular system. Further, many of the effects of rearing in the complex environment persist even when the animal is returned to more impoverished conditions.

Sensory deprivation has more selective effects that target particular cortical sensory systems. The seminal studies by Hubel and Weisel (Hubel & Freeman, 1977; Hubel & Wiesel, 1977) showed that monocular visual deprivation in the early postnatal period can substantially alter basic patterns of organization within primary visual cortex (PVC). One important feature of PVC organization is the ocular dominance columns. Within the typical primary visual pathway, inputs from the two eyes remain segregated from the retina to the thalamus to PVC. In PVC the inputs from the two eyes form a distinctive banded pattern, giving the input layer of PVC a striped appearance (Fig. 2.19A). When patterned input to one eye is blocked by suturing the eyelid closed, the effect on ocular dominance column organization is striking. The bands representing the active eye widen and expand into the territory of the deprived eye, while the bands representing the deprived eye shrink to thin stripes (Fig. 2.19B). These changes in PVC represent an adaptive response to the altered

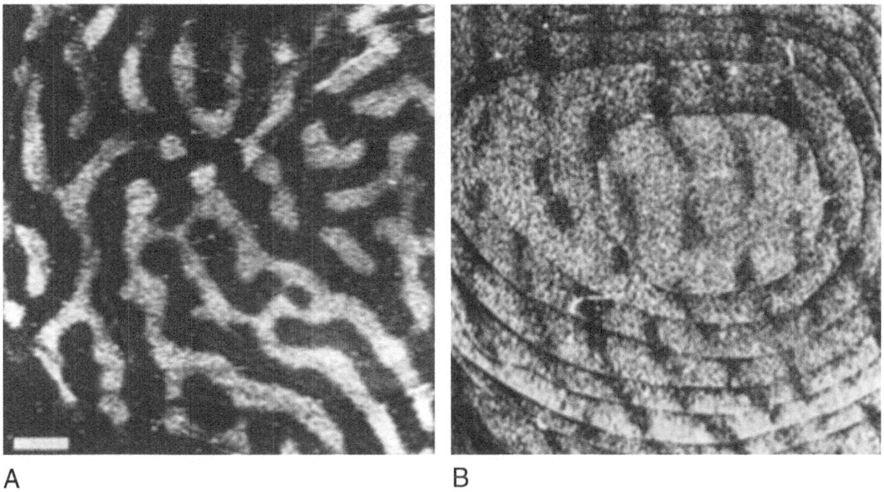

FIGURE 2.19 Autoradiographs of the ocular dominance columns (ODCs) in two young monkeys. A radioactive dye was injected into one eye and taken up by neurons in the input layer of primary visual cortex (PVC). (A) The normal patterning of the ODC in a 6-week-old monkey. ODCs from each eye are equal and adult-like. (B) ODC patterning from an animal that was monocularly deprived at 2 weeks of age. The nondeprived eye was injected with the tracer at 18 months of age. ODCs for the nondeprived eye (light bands) expand while those of the deprived eye (dark bands) shrink, showing clear dominance of the nondeprived eye in PVC. (Adapted with permission from LeVay S, Wiesel TN, Hubel DH. (1980). The development of ocular dominance columns in normal and visually deprived monkeys. *J Comp Neurol* 191:1–51, Figures 5 and 6.)

experience of the organism—in the wild the animal would not likely have the advantage of having the monocular suturing process reversed.

The enriched experience and visual deprivation studies provide powerful evidence of the role of experience on brain development. The enrichment studies suggest widespread effects of experience on the complexity and function of the developing system, while the deprivation studies document the capacity for neural reorganization *within* particular sensory systems. But the experimental studies can be more invasive, introducing procedures that directly affect, and often eliminate, targeted brain areas. These studies provide evidence that plasticity in the developing neural system can extend to the capacity to develop fundamentally different patterns of organization and function in the face of injury. For example, Sur et al. (Pallas, Roe, & Sur, 1990; Sur, Garraghty, & Roe, 1988) surgically eliminated the major input pathway to primary auditory cortex (PAC) in 1-day-old ferrets. The central question was what would happen to this important basic sensory area: would it simply atrophy in the absence of normal auditory input, or would it adopt a new function? In the normal course of early development, the visual pathway from the retina extends what are typically transient connections to PAC, in addition to the normal connections to PVC. The retina–PAC connections are typically pruned as part of normal competitive processes (i.e., the inputs from the cochlea form a more efficient and robust pathway than the inputs from the retina). However, in the absence of competition, the inputs from the retina stabilize and form a functional visual pathway to PAC. PAC takes on patterns of internal organization that, while cruder, are characteristic of PVC (Sur & Leamey, 2001), and the "rewired" PAC functions as a visual area in behavioral testing (von Melchner, Pallas, & Sur, 2000). Thus, the altered early experience of the organism results in fundamental functional and structural reorganization of a primary sensory area, providing robust evidence for the role of neural plasticity in early brain development. Functional imaging studies of humans with congenital sensory loss confirm that similar patterns of functional reassignment of cortical area are possible in humans.

BRAIN DEVELOPMENT AS A DYNAMIC AND ADAPTIVE PROCESS

As suggested by the data presented in this chapter, the processes that underlie and guide brain development involve the ongoing interplay of genetic and environmental factors. At each point in development, an organism's intrinsic and environmental factors interact to support the increasingly complex and elaborate structures and functions of the brain. During the embryologic period, the interactive processes are most prominent at the level of cell–cell interactions, where one population of cells generates molecular signals that alter the developmental course of another population of cells. However, even during this earliest period, interactions involving factors in the external environment also play essential roles in the development of the embryonic brain. During the fetal and postnatal periods, organism intrinsic factors continue to play a critical role in development, but across this extended period a wide array of factors in the external world influence the course of brain development in increasingly prominent ways.

The integrity of the developmental process depends absolutely upon the availability of the right neural elements appearing at the appropriate moment in developmental time. Often the emergence of a new element depends upon developmental events that immediately precede its appearance. Although nothing in neural development appears to be "predetermined," the process of development is nonetheless orderly and follows regular patterns over time. The constructs of "progressive differentiation" and "progressive commitment" capture important aspects of the temporal nature of brain development and can account for the regularities that are observed (Stiles, 2008). At all levels of the neural system, progressive differentiation of specific elements and structures and progressive commitment of those elements to functional systems appear to be the governing principles of brain development. The timescales for differentiation and commitment vary both at different levels of the system and across subsystems within a neural level. The coordination and integration of these multiple levels of change happening on multiple timescales is an essential element of brain development.

Organisms (and nervous systems) are initially simple and relatively undifferentiated, and over time become more complex and elaborate. Patterning within neural regions undergoes continuous refinement and specification. During gastrulation this is evident in the emergence of new cell lines. Initially pluripotent stem cells are induced to more specific fates and functions. This increasing specification is accompanied by spatial parcellation of cell populations: the three primary germ lines are segregated into the three embryonic layers; neuroectodermal cells are confined to the axial midline of the ectodermal layer; neuroectodermal cells in different regions of the neural plate differentiate to produce cells appropriate for more anterior or posterior brain regions. But the patterning observed during gastrulation reflects only the earliest and most primitive forms of brain organization. A hallmark of brain development is the continuing elaboration, modification, and refinement of brain areas and pathways. In the fetal period pathways and neural networks begin to emerge, setting up distant signaling within the developing brain that influences both the differentiation of cortical areas, and commitment to new functions. In the postnatal period the role of experience becomes an essential player both in the adaptation to new circumstances and in the commitment of functional systems to their mature patterns of organization.

The model of brain development presented here differs significantly from older maturational models in which systems were thought to appear in a predetermined linear fashion (Stiles, 2008). But this more dynamic model fits the growing body of data on brain development from the early embryologic period through postnatal development. Critically, it is a model that allows for adaptation and can account for profiles of neurocognitive development that diverge from the "typical" pathway. The study of children with perinatal brain injury provides an important means for exploring the capacity for neural plasticity and adaptive change during early development that are the hallmarks of a dynamic model of brain development. They also present opportunities for examining questions about the limits on plasticity, and for defining how alterations of the neural system can fit within the constraints of the developmental process.

REFERENCES

Aimone JB, Deng W, Gage FH. (2010). Adult neurogenesis: integrating theories and separating functions. *Trends Cognitive Sci* 14(7):325–337.

Anderson SA, Marin O, Horn C, Jennings K, Rubenstein JL. (2001). Distinct cortical migrations from the medial and lateral ganglionic eminences. *Development* 128(3):353–363.

Aylward EH, Park JE, Field KM, Parsons AC, Richards TL, Cramer SC, et al. (2005). Brain activation during face perception: evidence of a developmental change. *J Cogn Neurosci* 17(2): 308–319.

Balsamo LM, Xu B, Gaillard WD. (2006). Language lateralization and the role of the fusiform gyrus in semantic processing in young children. *NeuroImage* 31(3):1306–1314.

Barkovich AJ. (2000). Concepts of myelin and myelination in neuroradiology. *AJNR Am J Neuroradiol* 21(6):1099–1109.

Barkovich AJ. (2005). Magnetic resonance techniques in the assessment of myelin and myelination. *J Inherited Metabolic Dis* 28(3):311–343.

Barnea-Goraly N, Menon V, Eckert M, Tamm L, Bammer R, Karchemskiy A, et al. (2005). White matter development during childhood and adolescence: a cross-sectional diffusion tensor imaging study. *Cereb Cortex* 15(12):1848–1854.

Basser PJ, Mattiello J, LeBihan D. (1994). MR diffusion tensor spectroscopy and imaging. *Biophysical J* 66(1):259–267.

Bayer SA, Altman J, Russo RJ, Zhang X. (1993). Timetables of neurogenesis in the human brain based on experimentally determined patterns in the rat. *Neurotoxicology* 14(1):83–144.

Bielle F, Griveau A, Narboux-Neme N, Vigneau S, Sigrist M, Arber S, et al. (2005). Multiple origins of Cajal-Retzius cells at the borders of the developing pallium. *Nat Neurosci* 8(8):1002–1012.

Bishop KM, Rubenstein JL, O'Leary DD. (2002). Distinct actions of Emx1, Emx2, and Pax6 in regulating the specification of areas in the developing neocortex. *J Neurosci* 22(17):7627–7638.

Biswal B, Yetkin FZ, Haughton VM, Hyde JS. (1995). Functional connectivity in the motor cortex of resting human brain using echo-planar MRI. *MR in Medicine* 34(4):537–541.

Black JE, Sirevaag AM, Greenough WT. (1987). Complex experience promotes capillary formation in young rat visual cortex. *Neurosci Lett* 83(3):351–355.

Booth JR, Burman DD, Meyer JR, Lei Z, Trommer BL, Davenport ND, et al. (2003). Neural development of selective attention and response inhibition. *NeuroImage* 20(2):737–751.

Bourgeois JP, Goldman-Rakic PS, Rakic P. (1994). Synaptogenesis in the prefrontal cortex of rhesus monkeys. *Cerebral Cortex* 4(1):78–96.

Bourgeois JP, Rakic P. (1993). Changes of synaptic density in the primary visual cortex of the macaque monkey from fetal to adult stage. *J Neurosci* 13(7):2801–2820.

Bradl M, Lassmann H. (2010). Oligodendrocytes: biology and pathology. *Acta Neuropathol* 119(1):37–53.

Brambati SM, Benoit S, Monetta L, Belleville S, Joubert S. (2010). The role of the left anterior temporal lobe in the semantic processing of famous faces. *NeuroImage* 53(2):674–681.

Brown M, Keynes R, Lumsden A. (2001). The Developing Brain. Oxford: Oxford University Press.

Brown TT, Lugar HM, Coalson RS, Miezin FM, Petersen SE, Schlaggar BL. (2005). Developmental changes in human cerebral functional organization for word generation. *Cerebral Cortex* 15(3):275–290.

Bullmore E, Sporns O. (2009). Complex brain networks: graph theoretical analysis of structural and functional systems. *Nature Rev Neurosci* 10(3):186–198.

Bunge SA, Dudukovic NM, Thomason ME, Vaidya CJ, Gabrieli JD. (2002). Immature frontal lobe contributions to cognitive control in children: evidence from fMRI. *Neuron* 33(2): 301–311.

Bunge SA, Wright SB. (2007). Neurodevelopmental changes in working memory and cognitive control. *Current Opin Neurobiol* 17(2):243–250.

Buonomano DV, Merzenich MM. (1998). Cortical plasticity: from synapses to maps. *Annu Rev Neurosci* 21, 149–186.

Bushnell IW, Sai F, Mullin JT. (1989). Neonatal recognition of the mother's face. *Br J Dev Psychol* 7(1):3–15.

Buss RR, Sun W, Oppenheim RW. (2006). Adaptive roles of programmed cell death during nervous system development. *Annu Rev Neurosci* 29, 1–35.

Bystron I, Blakemore C, Rakic P. (2008). Development of the human cerebral cortex: Boulder Committee revisited. *Nat Rev Neurosci* 9(2):110–122.

Cascio CJ, Gerig G, Piven J. (2007). Diffusion tensor imaging. *J Am Acad Child Adolesc Psychiatry* 46(2):213–223.

Casey BJ, Trainor RJ, Orendi JL, Schubert AB, Nystrom LEJ, Giedd JN, et al. (1997). A developmental functional MRI study of prefrontal activation during performance of a go-no-go task. *J Cogn Neurosci* 9(6):835–847.

Cassia VM, Turati C, Simion F. (2004). Can a nonspecific bias toward top-heavy patterns explain newborns' face preference? *Psychol Sci* 15(6):379–383.

Cayre M, Canoll P, Goldman JE. (2009). Cell migration in the normal and pathological postnatal mammalian brain. *Progress Neurobiol* 88(1):41–63.

Chi JG, Dooling EC, Gilles FH. (1977). Gyral development of the human brain. *Ann Neurol* 1(1):86–93.

Clancy B, Darlington RB, Finlay BL. (2001). Translating developmental time across mammalian species. *Neuroscience* 105(1):7–17.

Cohen Kadosh K, Cohen Kadosh R, Dick F, Johnson MH. (2010). Developmental changes in effective connectivity in the emerging core face network. *Cerebral Cortex Nov. 2 [e-pub].*

Cohen Kadosh K, Johnson MH. (2007). Developing a cortex specialized for face perception. *Trends Cogn Sci* 11(9):367–369.

Copp AJ, Greene ND, Murdoch JN. (2003). The genetic basis of mammalian neurulation. *Nat Rev Genet* 4(10):784–793.

Corbin JG, Nery S, Fishell G. (2001). Telencephalic cells take a tangent: non-radial migration in the mammalian forebrain. *Nat Neurosci* 4 Suppl 1177–1182.

Courchesne E, Chisum HJ, Townsend J, Cowles A, Covington J, Egaas B, et al. (2000). Normal brain development and aging: quantitative analysis at in vivo MR imaging in healthy volunteers. *Radiology* 216(3):672–682.

de Haan M, Johnson MH, Halit H. (2003). Development of face-sensitive event-related potentials during infancy: A review. *Intl J Psychophysiol [Special Issue: Where and when in the developing brain: Neurophysiology of cognition in infants and children]* 51(1):45–58.

de Haan M, Pascalis O, Johnson MH. (2002). Specialization of neural mechanisms underlying face recognition in human infants. *J Cogn Neurosci* 14(2):199–209.

de la Rosa EJ, de Pablo F. (2000). Cell death in early neural development: beyond the neurotrophic theory. *Trends Neurosci* 23(10):454–458.

Deng W, Aimone JB, Gage FH. (2010). New neurons and new memories: how does adult hippocampal neurogenesis affect learning and memory? Nature Rev *Neurosci* 11(5):339–350.

Desai AR, McConnell SK. (2000). Progressive restriction in fate potential by neural progenitors during cerebral cortical development. *Development* 127(13):2863–2872.

Durston S, Thomas KM, Yang Y, Ulug AM, Zimmerman RD, Casey BJ. (2002). A neural basis for the development of inhibitory control. *Dev Sci* 5(4):F9–F16.

Epstein RA, Higgins JS, Parker W, Aguirre GK, Cooperman S. (2006). Cortical correlates of face and scene inversion: a comparison. *Neuropsychologia* 44(7):1145–1158.

Everts R, Lidzba K, Wilke M, Kiefer C, Mordasini M, Schroth G, et al. (2009). Strengthening of laterality of verbal and visuospatial functions during childhood and adolescence. *Human Brain Mapping* 30(2):473–483.

Fair DA, Cohen AL, Dosenbach NU, Church JA, Miezin FM, Barch DM, et al. (2008). The maturing architecture of the brain's default network. *Proc Natl Acad Sci U S A* 105(10): 4028–4032.

Fair DA, Cohen AL, Power JD, Dosenbach NU, Church JA, Miezin FM, et al. (2009). Functional brain networks develop from a "local to distributed" organization. *PLoS Computational Biol* 5(5):e1000381.

Fair DA, Dosenbach NU, Church JA, Cohen AL, Brahmbhatt S, Miezin FM, et al. (2007). Development of distinct control networks through segregation and integration. *Proc Natl Acad Sci U S A* 104(33):13507–13512.

Fair DA, Schlaggar BL, Cohen AL, Miezin FM, Dosenbach NU, Wenger KK, et al. (2007). A method for using blocked and event-related fMRI data to study "resting state" functional connectivity. *Neuroimage* 35(1):396–405.

Fairhall SL, Ishai A. (2007). Effective connectivity within the distributed cortical network for face perception. *Cerebral Cortex* 17(10):2400–2406.

Finn AS, Sheridan MA, Kam CL, Hinshaw S, D'Esposito M. (2010). Longitudinal evidence for functional specialization of the neural circuit supporting working memory in the human brain. *J Neurosci* 30(33):11062–11067.

Finnell RH, Junker WM, Wadman LK, Cabrera RM. (2002). Gene expression profiling within the developing neural tube. *Neurochem Res* 27(10):1165–1180.

Fransson P, Aden U, Blennow M, Lagercrantz H. (2011). The functional architecture of the infant brain as revealed by resting-state FMRI. *Cerebral Cortex* 21(1):145–154.

Frantz GD, McConnell SK. (1996). Restriction of late cerebral cortical progenitors to an upper-layer fate. *Neuron* 17(1):55–61.

Friederici A, Brauer J, Lohmann G. (2011). Maturation of the language network: from inter- to intrahemispheric connectivities. *PLoS ONE* 6(6):e20726.

Gage FH. (2002). Neurogenesis in the adult brain. *J Neurosci* 22(3):612–613.

Gaillard WD, Sachs BC, Whitnah JR, Ahmad Z, Balsamo LM, Petrella JR, et al. (2003). Developmental aspects of language processing: fMRI of verbal fluency in children and adults. *Human Brain Mapping* 18(3):176–185.

Gao W, Zhu H, Giovanello KS, Smith JK, Shen D, Gilmore JH, et al. (2009). Evidence on the emergence of the brain's default network from 2-week-old to 2-year-old healthy pediatric subjects. *Proc Natl Acad Sci U S A* 106(16):6790–6795.

Gathers AD, Bhatt R, Corbly CR, Farley AB, Joseph JE. (2004). Developmental shifts in cortical loci for face and object recognition. *Neuroreport* 15(10):1549–1553.

Gauthier I, Curby KM, Skudlarski P, Epstein RA. (2005). Individual differences in FFA activity suggest independent processing at different spatial scales. *Cogn Affect Behav Neurosci* 5(2):222–234.

Giedd JN, Blumenthal J, Jeffries NO, Castellanos FX, Liu H, Zijdenbos A, et al. (1999). Brain development during childhood and adolescence: a longitudinal MRI study. *Nat Neurosci* 2(10):861–863.

Giedd JN, Rumsey JM, Castellanos FX, Rajapakse JC, Kaysen D, Vaituzis AC, et al. (1996). A quantitative MRI analysis of the corpus callosum in children and adolescents. *Dev Brain Res* 91:274–280.

Gilbert SF. (2006). Developmental Biology (8th ed.). Sunderland, MA: Sinauer Associates Inc.

Gobbini MI, Haxby JV. (2007). Neural systems for recognition of familiar faces. *Neuropsychologia* 45(1):32–41.

Gogtay N, Giedd JN, Lusk L, Hayashi KM, Greenstein D, Vaituzis AC, et al. (2004). Dynamic mapping of human cortical development during childhood through early adulthood. *Proc Natl Acad Sci U S A* 101(21):8174–8179.

Golarai G, Ghahremani DG, Whitfield-Gabrieli S, Reiss A, Eberhardt JL, Gabrieli JDE, et al. (2007). Differential development of high-level visual cortex correlates with category-specific recognition memory. *Nature Neurosci 10(4):512–522.*

Golarai G, Liberman A, Yoon JM, Grill-Spector K. (2010). Differential development of the ventral visual cortex extends through adolescence. *Frontiers Human Neurosci* 3:80.

Greene ND, Copp AJ. (2009). Development of the vertebrate central nervous system: formation of the neural tube. *Prenatal Diagnosis* 29(4):303–311.

Greenough WT, Black JE, Wallace CS. (1987). Experience and brain development. *Child Dev* 58(3):539–559.

Greenough WT, Chang FF. (1988). Plasticity of synapse structure and pattern in the cerebral cortex. In Peters A, Jones EG (Eds.), Cerebral Cortex (pp. 391–440). New York: Plenum.

Grill-Spector K, Golarai G, Gabrieli J. (2008). Developmental neuroimaging of the human ventral visual cortex. *Trends Cogn Sci* 12(4):152–162.

Grill-Spector K, Knouf N, Kanwisher N. (2004). The fusiform face area subserves face perception not generic within-category identification. *Nat Neurosci* 7(5):555–562.

Haist F, Adamo M, Han J, Lee K, Stiles J. (submitted). On the development of visual processing for faces.

Hamasaki T, Leingartner A, Ringstedt T, O'Leary DD. (2004). EMX2 regulates sizes and positioning of the primary sensory and motor areas in neocortex by direct specification of cortical progenitors. *Neuron* 43(3):359–372.

Haxby JV, Gobbini MI, Furey ML, Ishai A, Schouten JL, Pietrini P. (2001). Distributed and overlapping representations of faces and objects in ventral temporal cortex. *Science* 293(5539):2425–2430.

Haxby JV, Hoffman EA, Gobbini MI. (2000). The distributed human neural system for face perception. *Trends Cogn Sci* 4(6):223–233.

Hemmati-Brivanlou A, Melton D. (1997a). Vertebrate embryonic cells will become nerve cells unless told otherwise. *Cell* 88(1):13–17.

Hemmati-Brivanlou A, Melton D. (1997b). Vertebrate neural induction. *Annu Rev Neurosci* 20, 43–60.

Hermoye L, Saint-Martin C, Cosnard G, Lee SK, Kim J, Nassogne MC, et al. (2006). Pediatric diffusion tensor imaging: normal database and observation of the white matter maturation in early childhood. *NeuroImage* 29(2):493–504.

Holland SK, Plante E, Weber Byars A, Strawsburg RH, Schmithorst VJ, Ball WS, Jr. (2001). Normal fMRI brain activation patterns in children performing a verb generation task. *NeuroImage* 14(4):837–843.

Huang EJ, Reichardt LF. (2001). Neurotrophins: roles in neuronal development and function. *Annu Rev Neurosci* 24:677–736.

Huang Z. (2009). Molecular regulation of neuronal migration during neocortical development. *Mol Cell Neurosci* 42(1):11–22.

Hubel DH, Freeman DC. (1977). Projection into the visual field of ocular dominance columns in macaque monkey. *Brain Res* 122(2):336–343.

Hubel DH, Wiesel TN. (1977). Ferrier Lecture. *Functional architecture of macaque monkey visual cortex. Proc R Soc Lond B Biol Sci* 198(1130):1–59.

Huppi PS, Dubois J. (2006). Diffusion tensor imaging of brain development. *Semin Fetal Neonatal Med* 11(6):489–497.

Huppi PS, Maier SE, Peled S, Zientara GP, Barnes PD, Jolesz FA, et al. (1998). Microstructural development of human newborn cerebral white matter assessed in vivo by diffusion tensor magnetic resonance imaging. *Pediatr Res* 44(4):584–590.

Huttenlocher PR, Dabholkar AS. (1997). Regional differences in synaptogenesis in human cerebral cortex. *J Comp Neurol* 387(2):167–178.

Huttenlocher PR, de Courten C. (1987). The development of synapses in striate cortex of man. *Human Neurobiol* 6(1):1–9.

Innocenti GM, Price DJ. (2005). Exuberance in the development of cortical networks. *Nat Rev Neurosci* 6(12):955–965.

Ishai A, Schmidt CF, Boesiger P. (2005). Face perception is mediated by a distributed cortical network. *Brain Res Bull* 67(1–2):87–93.

Iwasaki N, Hamano K, Okada Y, Horigome Y, Nakayama J, Takeya T, et al. (1997). Volumetric quantification of brain development using MRI. *Neuroradiology* 39: 841–846.

Jernigan TL, Gamst AC. (2005). Changes in volume with age—consistency and interpretation of observed effects. *Neurobiol Aging* 26(9):1271–1278.

Jernigan TL, Hesselink JR, Sowell E, Tallal PA. (1991). Cerebral structure on magnetic resonance imaging in language- and learning-impaired children. *Arch Neurol* 48:539–545.

Jernigan TL, Tallal P. (1990). Late childhood changes in brain morphology observable with MRI. *Dev Med Child Neurol* 32(5):379–385.

Jernigan TL, Trauner DA, Hesselink JR, Tallal PA. (1991). Maturation of human cerebrum observed in vivo during adolescence. *Brain* 114 (Pt 5):2037–2049.

Johnson MH, Morton J. (1991). Biology and Cognitive Development: The Case of Face Recognition. Cambridge, MA: Blackwell Press.

Jones TA, Greenough WT. (1996). Ultrastructural evidence for increased contact between astrocytes and synapses in rats reared in a complex environment. *Neurobiol Learn Mem* 65(1): 48–56.

Joseph JE, Gathers AD, Bhatt RS. (2011). Progressive and regressive developmental changes in neural substrates for face processing: testing specific predictions of the Interactive Specialization account. *Dev Sci 14(2):227–241.*

Judas M, Sedmak G, Pletikos M, Jovanov-Milosevic N. (2010). Populations of subplate and interstitial neurons in fetal and adult human telencephalon. *J Anat* 217(4):381–399.

Kaas JH, Merzenich MM, Killackey HP. (1983). The reorganization of somatosensory cortex following peripheral nerve damage in adult and developing mammals. *Annu Rev Neurosci* 6: 325–356.

Kanwisher N, McDermott J, Chun MM. (1997). The fusiform face area: a module in human extrastriate cortex specialized for face perception. *J Neurosci* 17(11):4302–4311.

Kanwisher N, Stanley D, Harris A. (1999). The fusiform face area is selective for faces not animals. *Neuroreport* 10(1):183–187.

Karunanayaka P, Schmithorst VJ, Vannest J, Szaflarski JP, Plante E, Holland SK. (2010). A group independent component analysis of covert verb generation in children: a functional magnetic resonance imaging study. *NeuroImage* 51(1):472–487.

Karunanayaka P, Schmithorst VJ, Vannest J, Szaflarski JP, Plante E, Holland SK. (2011). A linear structural equation model for covert verb generation based on independent component analysis of FMRI data from children and adolescents. *Frontiers Systems Neurosci* 5:29.

Kennedy DN, Makris N, Herbert MR, Takahashi T, Caviness VS Jr. (2002). Basic principles of MRI and morphometry studies of human brain development. *Dev Sci* 5(3):268–278.

Kennedy H, Dehay C. (2001). Gradients and boundaries: limits of modularity and its influence on the isocortex. *Dev Sci* 4(2):147–148.

Kiecker C, Niehrs C. (2001). A morphogen gradient of Wnt/beta-catenin signalling regulates anteroposterior neural patterning in Xenopus. *Development* 128(21):4189–4201.

Kilgard MP, Merzenich MM. (1998). Plasticity of temporal information processing in the primary auditory cortex. *Nature Neurosci* 1(8):727–731.

Kostovic I, Jovanov-Milosevic N. (2006). The development of cerebral connections during the first 20–45 weeks' gestation. *Semin Fetal Neonatal Med* 11(6):415–422.

Kostovic I, Judas M. (2010). The development of the subplate and thalamocortical connections in the human foetal brain. *Acta Paediatr* 99(8):1119–1127.

Larsen WJ. (2001). Human Embryology (3rd ed.). New York: Churchill Livingstone.

Lebel C, Beaulieu C. (2011). Longitudinal development of human brain wiring continues from childhood into adulthood. *J Neurosci* 31(30):10937–10947.

Lebel C, Walker L, Leemans A, Phillips L, Beaulieu C. (2008). Microstructural maturation of the human brain from childhood to adulthood. *NeuroImage* 40(3):1044–1055.

Lenroot RK, Giedd JN. (2006). Brain development in children and adolescents: Insights from anatomical magnetic resonance imaging. *Neurosci Biobehav Rev* 30(6):718–729.

Levi-Montalcini R. (1964). The nerve growth factor. *Ann N Y Acad Sci* 118:149–170.

Lidzba K, Schwilling E, Grodd W, Krageloh-Mann I, Wilke M. (2011). Language comprehension vs. language production: Age effects on fMRI activation. *Brain Language* March 29 [e-pub].

Lin SC, Bergles DE. (2004). Synaptic signaling between GABAergic interneurons and oligodendrocyte precursor cells in the hippocampus. *Nature Neurosci* 7(1):24–32.

Lin W, Zhu Q, Gao W, Chen Y, Toh CH, Styner M, et al. (2008). Functional connectivity MR imaging reveals cortical functional connectivity in the developing brain. *AJNR Am J Neuroradiol* 29(10):1883–1889.

Liu WC, Flax JF, Guise KG, Sukul V, Benasich AA. (2008). Functional connectivity of the sensorimotor area in naturally sleeping infants. *Brain Res* 1223:42–49.

Lohmann G, Hoehl S, Brauer J, Danielmeier C, Bornkessel-Schlesewsky I, Bahlmann J, et al. (2010). Setting the frame: the human brain activates a basic low-frequency network for language processing. *Cerebral Cortex* 20(6):1286–1292.

Lopez-Larson, M. P., Anderson, J. S., Ferguson, M. A., & Yurgelun-Todd, D. (2011). Local Brain Connectivity and Associations with Gender and Age. *Developmental cognitive neuroscience : a journal for cognitive, affective and social developmental neuroscience, 1*(2), 187–197.

Luna B. (2009). Developmental changes in cognitive control through adolescence. *Adv Child Dev Behav* 37:233–278.

Luna B, Garver KE, Urban TA, Lazar NA, Sweeney JA. (2004). Maturation of cognitive processes from late childhood to adulthood. *Child Dev* 75(5):1357–1372.

Luna B, Padmanabhan A, O'Hearn K. (2010). What has fMRI told us about the development of cognitive control through adolescence? *Brain Cognition* 72(1):101–113.

Luna B, Thulborn KR, Munoz DP, Merriam EP, Garver KE, Minshew NJ, et al. (2001). Maturation of widely distributed brain function subserves cognitive development. *NeuroImage* 13(5): 786–793.

Marin O, Rubenstein JL. (2001). A long remarkable journey: tangential migration in the telencephalon. *Nat Rev Neurosci* 2(11):780–790.

Markham JA, Greenough WT. (2004). Experience-driven brain plasticity: beyond the synapse. *Neuron Glia Biol* 1(4):351–363.

Mazard A, Schiltz C, Rossion B. (2006). Recovery from adaptation to facial identity is larger for upright than inverted faces in the human occipito-temporal cortex. *Neuropsychologia* 44(6):912–922.

McConnell SK, Kaznowski CE. (1991). Cell cycle dependence of laminar determination in developing neocortex. *Science* 254(5029):282–285.

McTigue DM, Tripathi RB. (2008). The life death and replacement of oligodendrocytes in the adult CNS. *J Neurochemistry* 107(1):1–19.

Miyata T, Kawaguchi A, Okano H, Ogawa M. (2001). Asymmetric inheritance of radial glial fibers by cortical neurons. *Neuron* 31(5):727–741.

Morange M. (2001). The Misunderstood Gene (M. Cobb, Trans.). Cambridge MA: Harvard University Press.

Mori S, van Zijl PC. (1995). Diffusion weighting by the trace of the diffusion tensor within a single scan. *MR Medicine* 33(1):41–52.

Mukherjee P, McKinstry RC. (2006). Diffusion tensor imaging and tractography of human brain development. *Neuroimaging Clin North Am* 16(1):19–47.

Nery S, Fishell G, Corbin JG. (2002). The caudal ganglionic eminence is a source of distinct cortical and subcortical cell populations. *Nat Neurosci* 5(12):1279–1287.

Niehrs C. (2004). Regionally specific induction by the Spemann-Mangold organizer. *Nature Rev Genetics* 5(6):425–434.

Noctor SC, Flint AC, Weissman TA, Dammerman RS, Kriegstein AR. (2001). Neurons derived from radial glial cells establish radial units in neocortex. *Nature* 409(6821):714–720.

Noctor SC, Flint AC, Weissman TA, Wong WS, Clinton BK, Kriegstein AR. (2002). Dividing precursor cells of the embryonic cortical ventricular zone have morphological and molecular characteristics of radial glia. *J Neurosci* 22(8):3161–3173.

O'Leary DD, Chou SJ, Sahara S. (2007). Area patterning of the mammalian cortex. *Neuron* 56(2):252–269.

O'Leary DD, Chou SJ, Hamasaki T, Sahara S, Takeuchi A, Thuret S, et al. (2007). Regulation of laminar and area patterning of mammalian neocortex and behavioural implications. *Novartis Found Symp* 288:141–159; discussion 159–164, 276–181.

O'Leary DD, Sahara S. (2008). Genetic regulation of arealization of the neocortex. *Current Opinion Neurobiol* 18(1):90–100.

Oppenheim RW. (1991). Cell death during development of the nervous system. *Annu Rev Neurosci* 14:453–501.

Østby Y, Tamnes CK, Fjell AM, Westlye LT, Due-Tonnessen P, Walhovd KB. (2009). Heterogeneity in subcortical brain development: A structural magnetic resonance imaging study of brain maturation from 8 to 30 years. *J Neurosci* 29(38):11772–11782.

Pakkenberg B, Gundersen HJ. (1997). Neocortical neuron number in humans: effect of sex and age. *J Comp Neurol* 384(2):312–320.

Pallas SL, Roe AW, Sur M. (1990). Visual projections induced into the auditory pathway of ferrets. I. Novel inputs to primary auditory cortex (AI) from the LP/pulvinar complex and the topography of the MGN-AI projection. *J Comp Neurol* 298(1):50–68.

Parnavelas JG, Alifragis P, Nadarajah B. (2002). The origin and migration of cortical neurons. *Prog Brain Res* 136:73–80.

Paus T, Collins DL, Evans AC, Leonard G, Pike B, Zijdenbos A. (2001). Maturation of white matter in the human brain: a review of magnetic resonance studies. *Brain Res Bull* 54(3): 255–266.

Peelen MV, Glaser B, Vuilleumier P, Eliez S. (2009). Differential development of selectivity for faces and bodies in the fusiform gyrus. *Dev Sci* 12(6):F16–25.

Pelphrey KA, Lopez J, Morris JP. (2009). Developmental continuity and change in responses to social and nonsocial categories in human extrastriate visual cortex. *Frontiers Human Neurosci* 3:25.

Pfefferbaum A, Mathalon DH, Sullivan EV, Rawles JM, Zipursky RB, Lim KO. (1994). A quantitative magnetic resonance imaging study of changes in brain morphology from infancy to late adulthood. *Arch Neurol* 51:874–887.

Rabinowicz, T, de Courten-Myers GM, Petetot JM, Xi G, de los Reyes E. (1996). Human cortex development: estimates of neuronal numbers indicate major loss late during gestation. *J Neuropathol Exp Neurol* 55(3):320–328.

Rakic P. (1972). Mode of cell migration to the superficial layers of fetal monkey neocortex. *J Comp Neurol* 145(1):61–83.

Rakic P. (1995a). Corticogenesis in human and nonhuman primates. In Gazzaniga MS (Ed.), The Cognitive Neurosciences (pp. 127–145). Cambridge, MA: The MIT Press.

Rakic P. (1995b). A small step for the cell a giant leap for mankind: a hypothesis of neocortical expansion during evolution. *Trends Neurosci* 18(9):383–388.

Rasmussen T, Milner B. (1977). The role of early left-brain injury in determining lateralization of cerebral speech functions. *Ann N Y Acad Sci* 299:355–369.

Reiss AL, Abrams MT, Singer HS, Ross JL. (1996). Brain development gender and IQ in children: A volumetric imaging study. *Brain* 119(5):1763–1774.

Ressel V. (2008). Increases in language lateralization in normal children as observed using magnetoencephalography. *Brain Language* 106(3):167–176.

Rhodes G, Byatt G, Michie PT, Puce A. (2004). Is the fusiform face area specialized for faces individuation or expert individuation? *J Cogn Neurosci* 16(2):189–203.

Rice DS, Curran T. (2001). Role of the reelin signaling pathway in central nervous system development. *Annu Rev Neurosci* 24:1005–1039.

Rubia K, Overmeyer S, Taylor E, Brammer M, Williams SC, Simmons A, et al. (2000). Functional frontalisation with age: mapping neurodevelopmental trajectories with fMRI. *Neurosci Biobehav Rev* 24(1):13–19.

Rubia K, Smith AB, Taylor E, Brammer M. (2007). Linear age-correlated functional development of right inferior fronto-striato-cerebellar networks during response inhibition and anterior cingulate during error-related processes. *Human Brain Mapping* 28(11):1163–1177.

Rubinov M, Sporns O. (2010). Complex network measures of brain connectivity: uses and interpretations. *NeuroImage* 52(3):1059–1069.

Sadler TW. (2006). Langman's Medical Embryology (10th ed.). Philadelphia: Lippincott Williams Wilkins.

Sadler TW, Langman J. (2010). Langman's Medical Embryology (11th ed.). Philadelphia: Lippincott William Wilkins.

Sansom SN, Livesey FJ. (2009). Gradients in the brain: the control of the development of form and function in the cerebral cortex. *Cold Spring Harb Perspect Biol* 1(2):a002519.

Scherf KS, Behrmann M, Humphreys K, Luna B. (2007). Visual category-selectivity for faces places and objects emerges along different developmental trajectories. *Dev Sci* 10(4):F15–30.

Scherf KS, Luna B, Avidan G, Behrmann M. (2011). "What" precedes "which": developmental neural tuning in face- and place-related cortex. *Cerebral Cortex Jan. 21 [e-pub].*

Schleussner E, Schneider U, Arnscheidt C, Kahler C, Haueisen J, Seewald HJ. (2004). Prenatal evidence of left-right asymmetries in auditory evoked responses using fetal magnetoencephalography. *Early Human Dev* 78(2):133–136.

Schmithorst VJ, Holland SK, Plante E. (2007). Object identification and lexical/semantic access in children: a functional magnetic resonance imaging study of word-picture matching. *Human Brain Mapping* 28(10):1060–1074.

Smyser CD, Snyder AZ, Neil JJ. (2011). Functional connectivity MRI in infants: exploration of the functional organization of the developing brain. *NeuroImage* 56(3):1437–1452.

Snook L, Paulson LA, Roy D, Phillips L, Beaulieu C. (2005). Diffusion tensor imaging of neurodevelopment in children and young adults. *NeuroImage* 26(4):1164–1173.

Sowell ER, Thompson PM, Holmes CJ, Batth R, Jernigan TL, Toga AW. (1999). Localizing age-related changes in brain structure between childhood and adolescence using statistical parameter mapping. *NeuroImage* 9:587–597.

Sowell ER, Thompson PM, Leonard CM, Welcome SE, Kan E, Toga AW. (2004). Longitudinal mapping of cortical thickness and brain growth in normal children. *J Neurosci* 24(38): 8223–8231.

Sowell ER, Thompson PM, Rex D, Kornsand D, Tessner KD, Jernigan TL, et al. (2002). Mapping sulcal pattern asymmetry and local cortical surface gray matter distribution in vivo: maturation in perisylvian cortices. *Cerebral Cortex* 12(1):17–26.

Sowell ER, Trauner DA, Gamst A, Jernigan TL. (2002). Development of cortical and subcortical brain structures in childhood and adolescence: a structural MRI study. *Dev Med Child Neurol* 44(1):4–16.

Stanfield BB, O'Leary DD, Fricks C. (1982). Selective collateral elimination in early postnatal development restricts cortical distribution of rat pyramidal tract neurones. *Nature* 298(5872):371–373.

Stanfield BB, O'Leary DD. (1985). The transient corticospinal projection from the occipital cortex during the postnatal development of the rat. *J Comp Neurol* 238(2):236–248.

Stiles J. (2008). The Fundamentals of Brain Development: Integrating Nature and Nurture. Cambridge, MA: Harvard University Press.

Supekar, K., Uddin, L. Q., Prater, K., Amin, H., Greicius, M. D., & Menon, V. (2010). Development of functional and structural connectivity within the default mode network in young children. *NeuroImage, 52*(1), 290-301.

Sur M, Garraghty PE, Roe AW. (1988). Experimentally induced visual projections into auditory thalamus and cortex. *Science* 242(4884):1437–1441.

Sur M, Leamey CA. (2001). Development and plasticity of cortical areas and networks. *Nat Rev Neurosci* 2(4):251–262.

Sur M, Rubenstein JL. (2005). Patterning and plasticity of the cerebral cortex. *Science* 310(5749):805–810.

Suzuki Y, Matsuzawa H, Kwee IL, Nakada T. (2003). Absolute eigenvalue diffusion tensor analysis for human brain maturation. *NMR Biomedicine* 16(5):257–260.

Szaflarski JP, Holland SK, Schmithorst VJ, Byars AW. (2006). fMRI study of language lateralization in children and adults. *Human Brain Mapping* 27(3):202–212.

Taylor, M. J., Batty, M., & Itier, R. J. (2004). The faces of development: a review of early face processing over childhood. *J Cogn Neurosci, 16*(8), 1426–1442.

Toga AW, Thompson PM, Sowell ER. (2006). Mapping brain maturation. *Trends Neurosci* 29(3):148–159.

Turati C, Simion F, Milani I, Umilta C. (2002). Newborns' preference for faces: What is crucial? *Dev Psychol* 38(6):875–882.

Uddin LQ. (2010). Typical and atypical development of functional human brain networks: insights from resting-state fMRI. *Frontiers Systems Neurosci* 4:21.

Vieira C, Pombero A, Garcia-Lopez, R, Gimeno L, Echevarria D, Martinez S. (2010). Molecular mechanisms controlling brain development: an overview of neuroepithelial secondary organizers. *Intl J Dev Biol* 54(1):7–20.

von Melchner L, Pallas SL, Sur M. (2000). Visual behaviour mediated by retinal projections directed to the auditory pathway. *Nature* 404(6780):871–876.

Waddington CH. (1939). An Introduction to Modern Genetics. New York: Macmillan.

Weissman T, Noctor SC, Clinton BK, Honig LS, Kriegstein AR. (2003). Neurogenic radial glial cells in reptile rodent and human: from mitosis to migration. *Cerebral Cortex* 13(6): 550–559.

Wodarz A, Huttner WB. (2003). Asymmetric cell division during neurogenesis in Drosophila and vertebrates. *Mech Dev* 120(11):1297–1309.

Wojciulik E, Kanwisher N, Driver J. (1998). Covert visual attention modulates face-specific activity in the human fusiform gyrus: fMRI study. *J Neurophysiol* 79(3):1574–1578.

Xu Y. (2005). Revisiting the role of the fusiform face area in visual expertise. *Cerebral Cortex* 15(8):1234–1242.

Yakovlev PI, Lecours AR. (1967). The myelogenetic cycles of regional maturation of the brain. In Mankowski A (Ed.), Regional Development of the Brain in Early Life (pp. 3–69). Philadelphia: Davis.

Yeo W, Gautier J. (2004). Early neural cell death: dying to become neurons. *Dev Biol* 274(2): 233–244.

Yovel G, Kanwisher N. (2004). Face perception: domain specific not process specific. *Neuron* 44(5):889–898.

Yovel G, Kanwisher N. (2005). The neural basis of the behavioral face-inversion effect. *Curr Biol* 15(24):2256–2262.

Zecevic N, Bourgeois JP, Rakic P. (1989). Changes in synaptic density in motor cortex of rhesus monkey during fetal and postnatal life. *Brain Res Dev Brain Res* 50(1):11–32.

Zembrzycki A, Griesel G, Stoykova A, Mansouri A. (2007). Genetic interplay between the transcription factors Sp8 and Emx2 in the patterning of the forebrain. *Neural Dev* 2:8.

Zielinski BA, Gennatas ED, Zhou J, Seeley WW. (2010). Network-level structural covariance in the developing brain. *Proc Natl Acad Sci U S A* 107(42):18191–18196.

3

Etiology and Neurological Effects of Perinatal Stroke

OUR STUDY OF the effects of early focal lesions on cognitive and behavioral development and on what these findings would reveal about plasticity began 30 years ago with a small group of about 15 children of various ages diagnosed with hemiplegic cerebral palsy (CP).[1] We have now seen and carefully evaluated in one or more cognitive or behavioral domains at least 250 children. Typical of hemiplegic CP cohorts, the majority of children we studied have had an arterial stroke (Golomb et al., 2007a; Kirton & de Veber, 2006; Krageloh-Mann & Horber, 2007; Wu et al., 2006), although some children have had other pathology, including intracranial hemorrhage[2] (which can occur in any location), grade 4 intraventricular hemorrhage (IVH) with associated white matter hemorrhage[3], focal periventricular leukomalacia (focal PVL)[4], and venous stroke or cerebral venous sinus thrombosis with stroke[5]. Our focus has been on infants born at term (>37 weeks) whose

[1] Hemiplegic CP is a clinical phenotype that, by definition, is the result of a focal injury that occurred in the pre-perinatal period and produces weakness on one side of the body. Hemiplegic CP is an umbrella term; there are many causes (e.g., brain malformation, focal periventricular leukomalacia, stroke).

[2] Intracranial hemorrhages in the newborn can occur after trauma or when a blood vessel malformation ruptures (arteriovenous malformation). Hemorrhage can affect any part of the brain. It does not occur in a particular vascular territory, unless it is a stroke with secondary hemorrhage.

[3] Technically, grade 4 IVH is not a hemorrhage in the ventricle with extension into the adjoining white matter; rather, it is a hemorrhagic stroke in the white matter itself. Small blood vessels (perforators) deep in the brain near the ventricle are involved (Goevart et al., 2000, 2009a). It typically occurs in small preterm infants (de Vries et al., 1997, 2001; Volpe, 2008). Fortunately, over the past 20 years, grade 4 IVH has become less common, due to advances in medical technology. IVH is sometimes seen in term infants (Volpe, 2008).

[4] Focal PVL is an ischemic (low blood flow and low tissue oxygen) injury in the white matter abutting the ventricle. Focal PVL generally occurs in the early third trimester. Thus, it is seen in preterm infants born around 34 weeks' gestation (Staudt, 2010) and in term infants, in whom it presumably occurred in utero.

[5] Veins as well as arteries can become occluded. CVST can be defined as the presence of a thrombus in a cranial venous sinus, a large deep brain vein, or a smaller cortical or deep vein, with partial or complete occlusion, with associated hemorrhagic stroke in most (Fitzgerald et al., 2006). Venous as opposed to arterial strokes generally occur early in the third trimester—periventricular venous stroke (Kirton & deVeber, 2009) (see Fig. 3.2).

neurological insult occurred during the perinatal period—towards the end of the third trimester through the 28th postnatal day[6]. In our studies we have excluded infants with birth asphyxia or an etiology (e.g., infection) that might be associated with a bilateral insult. We have generally excluded infants born preterm, especially those who had medical complications in the nursery. Given the plasticity of the immature nervous system, children with early focal lesions due to stroke are generally assumed to have an excellent outcome. However, many do have residual deficits of varying degrees (generally mild and often changing with age), as discussed in this volume. Our understanding of brain reorganization after early focal injury is still incomplete. However, children with early focal lesions provide the best available in vivo model for examining the response of the developing brain to localized injury, as well as the mechanisms of reorganization and plasticity.

EPIDEMIOLOGY

Stroke is more likely to occur in the term infant during the perinatal period than at any other time in childhood. The current estimated incidence of arterial stroke is about 1 in 4,000 births (Chalmers, 2005; de Veber et al., 2001; Golomb et al., 2001; Lee et al., 2005a; Lynch & Nelson, 2001; Lynch et al., 2002). The prevalence of focal injury, when hemorrhage is included as well, is as high as 1 in 2,700 births (Agrawal et al., 2009; Armstrong-Wells et al 2009; Kirkham & Cowan, 2011). The frequency of stroke may be even higher when both early (during the neonatal period) and late presenters (during the first year) are included; in one such cohort the incidence was 63 per 100,000 live births (Laugesaar et al., 2007). Cerebral venous sinus thrombosis (CVST) occurs in 2.6 per 100,000 newborns a year, and 50% to 80% have an associated stroke (Berfelo et al., 2010). One in 2,300 infants with neurological symptoms (e.g., seizures) in the nursery is estimated to have had a stroke (Schulzke et al., 2005).

Differences in the reported frequency of perinatal stroke reflect the method of ascertainment (e.g., prospective vs. retrospective chart review), inclusion criteria (e.g., solely arterial stroke, as opposed to including venous sinus thrombosis with stroke and hemorrhage as well), and whether children with both early and late presentations are included (Agrawal et al., 2009; Cowan & Mercuri 2011; de Veber et al., 2001; Estan & Hope, 1997; Golomb et al., 2001; Govaert et al., 2000; Laugesaar et al., 2007; Lee et al., 2005a; Lynch & Nelson, 2001;Nelson and Lynch 2004; Nelson, 2007; Perlman et al., 1994; Schulzke et al., 2005; Wu et al., 2004).

Children diagnosed with either hemiplegic CP and/or stroke are more often male (Golomb et al., 2009). Ethnicity and race (higher incidence in black infants compared with non-Hispanic white infants) may also play a role in stroke. Stroke rarely recurs (approximately 3% to 5%) (Kurnik et al., 2003), unless there is a clear risk factor like congenital heart disease or a thrombophilic (abnormal blood clotting) disorder (Herak et al., 2009). However, the fatality rate of perinatal stroke may be higher than in older children with stroke (Lynch and Nelson, 2001; Nelson and Lynch 2004).

---

[6] We have focused on the term infant whose neurological insult occurred towards the end of the third trimester through labor and delivery, maximizing the chance that we are including only children with single unilateral lesions.

CLASSIFICATION

In adults, arterial strokes in the left and right hemisphere affect different cognitive domains (e.g., language left hemisphere, spatial skills right hemisphere). Within each hemisphere three main arteries (the anterior [ACA], the middle [MCA], and the posterior cerebral arteries [PCA])[7] supply the cerebral cortex, and strokes within each of their territories produce specific cognitive and behavioral deficits (Fig. 3.1). Thus, strokes are typically described in terms of the particular brain artery that is involved; for example, MCA territory stroke. Furthermore, each of the three main arteries has multiple smaller branches (anterior, posterior, deep, superficial) that further determine what part of the brain territory it supplies will be affected by stroke (e.g., cortex and/or subcortex).

Perinatal strokes are left-sided in about two thirds of neonates. The strong bias towards the left is not well understood but probably reflects differences in blood flow patterns to the two sides of the brain, with emboli preferentially going leftward (Volpe, 2008). Term infants generally have large strokes involving the trunk of the MCA, damaging both cortical and subcortical regions (Bax et al., 2006; Wu et al., 2006). ACA and PCA infarcts occur in about 10% (Govaert et al 2009a; Husson et al., 2010; Kirton et al., 2008; Sreenan et al., 2000).

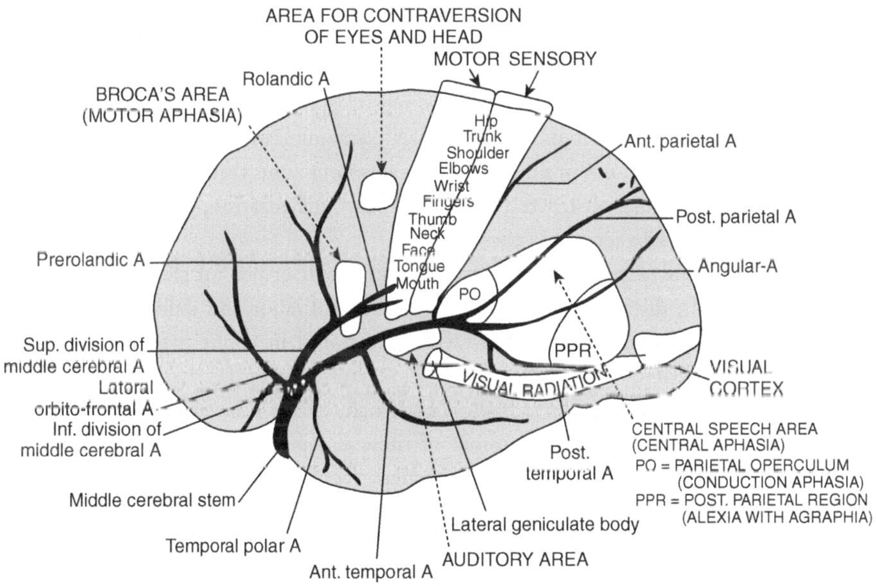

FIGURE 3.1 Vascular supply of the brain via the middle cerebral artery of the left hemisphere. The vascular distribution is the same in the right hemisphere but different cognitive functions are affected.

[7] The ACA and the MCA form the anterior circulation and originate from the internal carotid artery; the PCA is part of the posterior circulation supplied by the vertebral basilar system.

Some term infants (in some series as many as 15% to 30%) have multifocal arterial strokes involving multiple small branches of one or more of the three main arteries (Abels et al., 2006; Bax et al., 2006; de Vries et al., 1997; Raine et al., 1989; Wu et al., 2006). Rarely the internal carotid artery (ICA) (from which both the ACA and MCA originate) is occluded. In a small percent (often the late presenters, see below) a stroke occurs when a vein is occluded; these are generally veins deep within the brain near the ventricles (periventricular venous stroke) (de Vries et al., 2001; Kirton et al 2010; Kirton & de Veber 2009; Takanashi et al., 2003). In a recent prospectively studied cohort of 80 children presenting in the neonatal period, 50 strokes involved the left hemisphere (63%), 24 involved the right hemisphere (30%), and 6 were bilateral (8%). Seventy-three strokes (91%) involved the territory of the MCA, with extension to another territory in five patients. Seven neonates had strokes in another cerebral artery territory (ACA or PCA). Among the 73 children with stroke due to MCA territory strokes, 50 (68%) had only cortical involvement, 5 (7%) had only deep subcortical involvement, and 18 (25%) had both cortical and subcortical involvement (Husson et al., 2010).

ETIOLOGY, RISK FACTORS, AND ASSOCIATED FACTORS

A number of investigators have looked at the specific causes of stroke, as well as the risk and associated factors (Mineyko & Kirton 2011). A retrospective cohort study of 134 newborns with perinatal arterial stroke identified a range of clinical causes: embolism (blood clots) (25%); trauma (10%); infection/meningitis (8%); arterial venous malformation, arteriopathy, primary thrombosis—including blood loss, sepsis, asphyxia and prothrombotic conditions (e.g., polycythemia, inherited thrombophilias[8]), and unclassifiable (<5% in each group) (Govaert et al., 2009b). Causes of perinatal cerebral venous sinus thrombosis in this cohort included infection, trauma, obstructed venous outflow[9], dehydration, prothrombotic conditions, and asphyxia (Govaert et al., 2009b).

Risks for stroke and factors associated with stroke are described for the prenatal period (maternal and fetal), during the perinatal period around labor and delivery, and in the neonatal period. Risk and/or associated factors are found in about two thirds of cases of stroke (Cowan & Mercuri, 2011; Golomb et al., 2001; Kirton et al., 2011; Lee et al., 2005a; Mercuri et al., 2001; Nelson, 2007; Nelson & Lynch, 2004; Raju et al., 2007; Sreenan et al., 2000; 2005). Increasing the number of these independent risk/associated factors increases the likelihood of stroke. The role of genetic factors in both mother and newborn is under active investigation (Gibson et al., 2008; Mineyko & Kirton, 2011; Nelson, 2008). It should be emphasized, however, that a risk or association factor is not the same as a cause.

[8] Genetic disorders that result in abnormal blood clotting.

[9] The cerebral venous circulation is very vulnerable to interruption as the head is molded during delivery in both normal and instrumented deliveries and flow in the sinuses may vary hugely with inevitable swings in venous pressure. Changes in cranial venous pressure may alter inflow, especially if the infant is hypotensive (Cowan & Mercuri, 2011).

Prenatal Period—Maternal/Fetal Risk Factors

Pregnant women as well as their newborns are at increased risk for stroke (Jaigobin & Silver, 2000; Nelson & Lynch, 2004; Nelson, 2007). The placenta, itself, is a risk factor for stroke. It is a highly vascular organ with low blood flow, which makes it ripe for the formation of blood clots (Cowan & Mercuri, 2011). Abnormal placental blood vessels are not uncommon in stroke (Curry et al., 2007; Elbers et al., 2011; Kraus & Acheen, 1999; Redline, 2006), and emboli from the placenta may be the most common cause of neonatal stroke (Rutherford et al., 2011). Furthermore, placental abnormalities are associated with conditions that can also increase the risk of stroke, such as small-for-gestational-age (infants weighing less than expected for their gestational age), preterm birth, and preeclampsia (complications of pregnancy, including high blood pressure and swelling/edema) (Cheong & Cowan, 2009).

A number of additional risk factors with varying degrees of specificity have been identified on the maternal side, including infertility and infertility treatment, irregular menstrual cycles and polycystic ovary syndrome, primiparity (first pregnancy), preeclampsia, infection during pregnancy, prolonged rupture of membranes (>24 hours between rupture and delivery), chorioamnionitis (infection of the placenta), fever during labor, thrombophilias, autoimmune disorders, diabetes, hypothyroidism, and migraine (Nelson, 2008, 2009a; 2009b).

Risk factors on the fetal side include in utero cocaine exposure, thrombophilias, polycythemia (high red cell count), small for gestational age, and large for gestational age (Mineyko & Kirton, 2011; Raju et al., 2007; Rutherford et al., 2011). Being a twin (primarily monozygous/identical) with or without twin-to-twin transfusion syndrome (one twin gets more blood and the other gets less/too little) is associated with a higher risk of stroke.

Neonatal Risk Factors

Birth asphyxia, cardiac disorder, infection, polycythemia (increased red blood cells), dehydration, trauma, congenital heart disease, hypoglycemia (low sugar), and serious complications requiring procedures in the nursery all can increase the risk of stroke. Thrombophilias (genetic disorders with abnormal blood clotting) are a major risk factor (Herak et al., 2009; Kenet et al., 2010; Mercuri et al., 2001). About half of the infants with stroke investigated for thrombophilias are observed to have one or more abnormalities. In one study, 62 of 91 infants with stroke (68.1%) had at least one prothrombotic risk factor compared with 44 control subjects (24.2%) (Günther et al., 2000). Risk factors for hemorrhage (Armstrong-Wells et al., 2009; Jhawar et al., 2003; Kirkham & Cowan, 2011) include fetal distress, forceps delivery, Apgar score[10] at 1 minute less than 8, resuscitation in the delivery room, and low platelet count.

[10] The Apgar score was developed by Virginia Apgar in order to determine which newborns required special attention in the delivery room. A score of 0, 1, or 2 is given for heart rate, respiratory effort, tone, color, and reflex irritability at 1, 5, and 10 minutes. A score over 7 is generally considered normal. Newborns with scores below 3 need to be promptly resuscitated.

CLINICAL PRESENTATION

Left hemisphere strokes are much more common than right hemisphere strokes, occurring in about two thirds of neonates (Rutherford et al., 2011). About two thirds of children with perinatal stroke present acutely as newborns (early presenters) and the other third presumed to have had perinatal strokes present later—generally in the middle to the end of the first year (late presenters) (Kirton et al., 2008; Kirton & de Veber, 2009).

Early Presenters

When stroke presents acutely in the neonatal period (early presenters), seizures, starting on the first or second day of life, are the most common symptom, occurring in at least 75% or more (Estan & Hope, 1997; Perlman et al., 1994; Ramaswamy et al., 2004; Trauner & Mannino, 1986; Volpe, 2008). Unless these infants have suffered birth asphyxia (which would exclude them from our study), they are generally not encephalopathic (e.g., lethargy, floppy, poor feeders) between seizures (Govaert et al., 2000; Hajnal et al., 1999; Mercuri et al., 1999; Rafay et al., 2005; Sreenan et al., 2000; Trauner et al., 1993), although they can be (Kirton et al., 2011). The neurological examination is usually normal, although one recent multicenter prospective study reported that 30% had focal findings (Kirton et al., 2011). Clear signs of a hemiparesis, however, are very uncommon until 4 to 6 months of age (see Chapter 4).

Late Presenters

The other one third of children with perinatal stroke are not identified as newborns. Rather, they are retrospectively recognized on the basis of imaging findings to have had a stroke in the perinatal period (Kirton & de Veber, 2006; 2009). These late presenters, also referred to as presumed perinatal stroke, generally had a benign neonatal period. They typically present with signs of early handedness, hemiparesis, or seizures between 4 and 8 months or very rarely as toddlers with headache (Kirton & de Veber, 2009; Kirton et al., 2010; 2011). (While most have had an arterial stroke, about 10% are now recognized based on imaging to have had an in utero periventricular venous infarction[4] around 34 weeks' gestation (de Vries et al., 2001; Kirton et al., 2010; Takanashi et al., 2003). Hence, there are now three clinical and radiographic types of perinatal stroke: arterial strokes, usually in the MCA territory, that present acutely in the newborn; arterial strokes in the MCA territory that occurred in the perinatal period but present later with a hemiparesis; and prenatal (34 weeks' gestation) venous strokes that present later with hemiparesis (Fig. 3.2)(Kirton & deVeber, 2009)

DIAGNOSIS: IMAGING

Both cranial ultrasound and computed tomography (CT) scans are used in the nursery to diagnose stroke, but the rate of false negatives is high. The diagnosis of arterial stroke is made acutely and most accurately by magnetic resonance imaging (MRI) using a technique called diffusion-weighted imaging (DWI), which measures brain water content. Edema/swelling, reflecting tissue damage, occurs within minutes of a stroke and shows up on MRI as

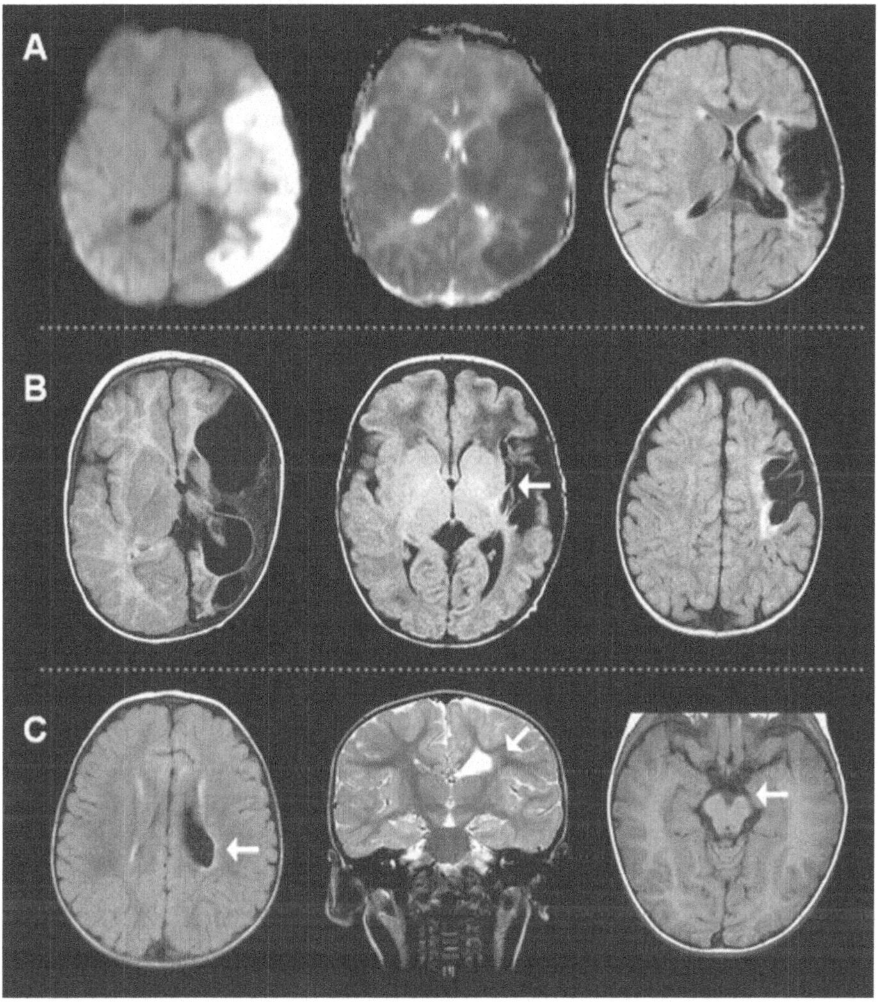

FIGURE 3.2 Perinatal stroke syndromes. (A) Acute symptomatic neonatal arterial ischemic stroke (PAS). A term neonate seized at 12 hours of age and magnetic resonance imaging revealed restricted diffusion in the middle cerebral artery (MCA) territory on diffusion-weighted imaging (left) and apparent diffusion coefficient analysis (center). Follow-up imaging demonstrates cystic encephalomalacia (right). (B) Presumed perinatal arterial ischemic stroke. Arterial MCA infarctions that are asymptomatic in neonates present later and can involve the entire MCA territory (left), occlusion of the distal M1 with sparing of basal ganglia (center), or divisions of the MCA (right). (C) Periventricular venous infarction also presents as presumed perinatal ischemic stroke, with focal lesions of the periventricular white matter (left and center) and atrophy of the ipsilateral cerebral peduncle (right). (Reprinted with permission from Kirton & deVeber, 2009.)

high signal intensity (SI) on DWI sequences. The quantitative measure of DWI, the apparent diffusion coefficient (ADC) map, can help determine the age of a stroke (Lequin et al., 2009).

Changes in the MRI after stroke continue for days, weeks, and months (Dudink et al., 2009; Lequin et al., 2009). The involved cortex shows low SI on T1-weighted images and high SI on T2-weighted images until day 6, when SIs reverse.[11] The white matter shows high SI on T1 images for the first 8 or 9 days and on T2 images for more than 2 weeks before converting to low SI. A checkerboard pattern of mixed high and low SI in the area of the stroke is often present at about 2 to 3 weeks after the stroke. Cystic tissue loss and atrophy appear as early as 3 to 4 weeks after the stroke and occur in most infants in 1 to 2 months. The optimal time for initial imaging is between days 3 and 10 after the stroke (Dudink et al., 2009; Husson et al., 2010; Lequin et al., 2009; Mercuri et al., 1995; Obernaus & Ashwal, 2008; Ramaswamy et al., 2004). During this timeframe the DWI is positive and other imaging sequences provide additional information about the timing and extent of the lesion (Fig. 3.3). MR angiography (MRA) confirms the location of an arterial occlusion in only about 20% to 30% of neonates with arterial stroke (Lequin et al., 2009). MR venography is useful for evaluating cerebral venous sinus thrombosis.

Imaging studies also document the occurrence of abnormalities remote from the lesion. Network injuries remote from the stroke itself could play a role in outcome. Secondary changes are seen in the thalamus and brain stem in the first week (Dudink et al., 2009). Later, thalamic atrophy ipsilateral to a stroke is often seen. Pulvinar (a nucleus that is part of the complex deep basal ganglia system) abnormalities along with its interconnections have been documented (Govert et al., 2008), as have abnormalities in internal capsule circuitry (Cowan & de Vries, 2005). Cerebellar atrophy, both ipsilateral and contralateral, is reported after large focal hemispheric stroke (Le et al., 2004; Niimura et al., 1999). Pre-Wallerian degeneration (secondary degeneration of cell axons and their myelin sheath/covering) in the corticospinal tract is another acute network injury (de Vries et al., 2005; Groenendaal et al., 2006; Kirton et al., 2007; Lequin et al., 2009). Pre-Wallerian degeneration in the brain stem has been reported as a persisting abnormal signal intensity occurring within a few days of stroke, with atrophy appearing over 5 to 8 weeks (Domi et al., 2009). These imaging findings can predict later motor outcome. Abnormalities of other networks are theoretically possible (Lequin et al., 2009).

MEDICAL EVALUATION

The medical workup includes an assessment of the heart, thrombophilia (blood coagulation) studies, and studies evaluating for metabolic and genetic problems that can cause stroke (Table 3.1).

OVERALL OUTCOME

Statistics about outcome are variable. Our cohort probably has a better overall outcome than the hemiplegic CP cohorts, since we have excluded children with multiple or bilateral lesions, infection, and neonates with hypoxic ischemic encephalopathy. Clinical risk factors

---

[11] MR imaging uses a range of techniques like T1 and T2 weighting to highlight different structures, to determine underlying etiology, and to date neurological events. High SI on T1 is thought to reflect an increase in the number of microglia cells and high protein content and accumulation of manganese in reactive astrocytic cells. The low cortical SI seen on T2 is thought to be related to petechial hemorrhages, release of myelin lipids, and/or calcifications.

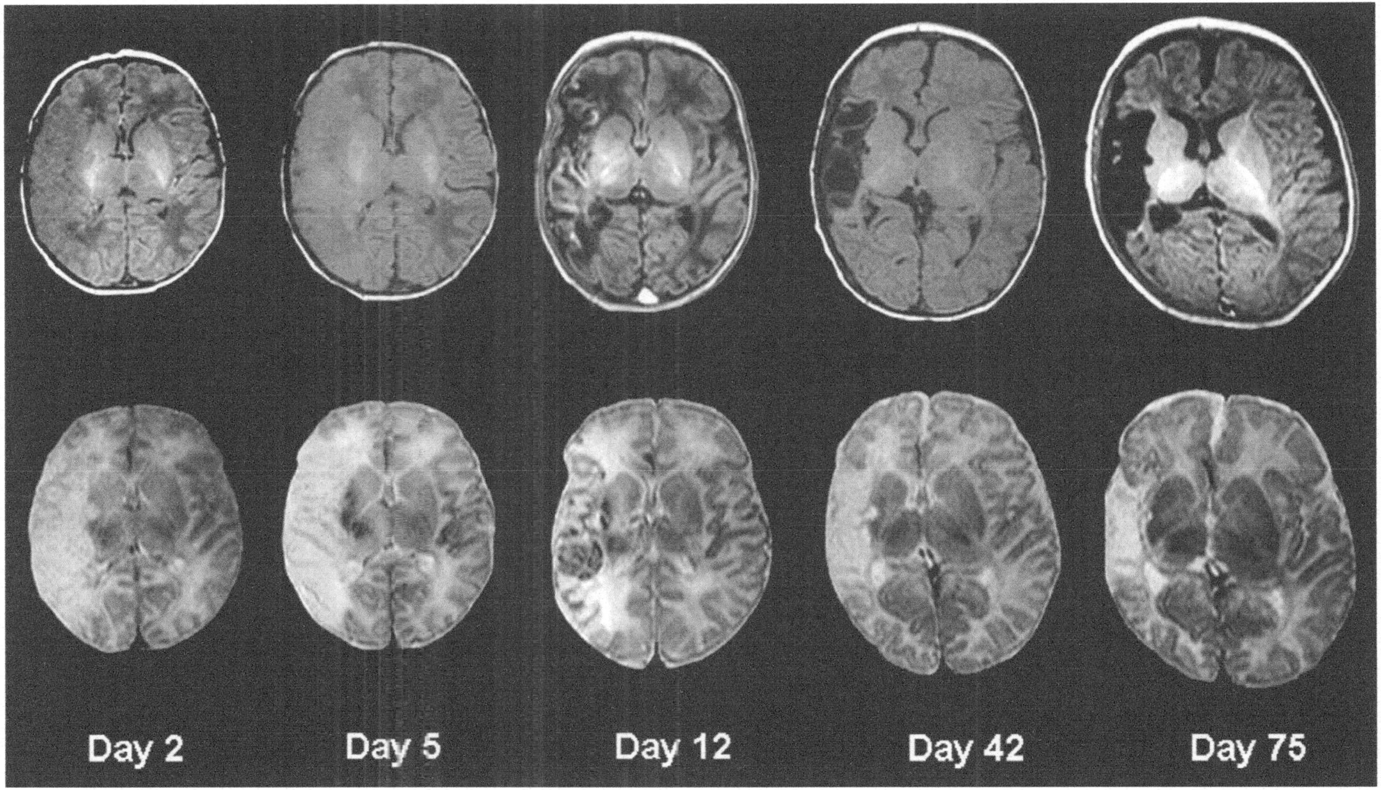

FIGURE 3.3 T1- and T2-weighted imaging of neonatal stroke. Serial T1-weighted (upper row) and T2-weighted (lower row) sequences within the first 3 months following perinatal stroke at term, involving the right middle cerebral artery in its cortical area, sparing deep gray matter. The pattern of changes over time is discussed in the text. (Reprinted with permission from Lequin et al., 2009.)

TABLE 3.1 DIAGNOSTIC EVALUATION OF PERINATAL STROKE

Neuroimaging
Symptomatic Neonatal Arterial Ischemic Stroke
Diffusion-weighted MRI to confirm or exclude acute arterial ischemic stroke, MR angiography (MRA) to assess for arterial occlusion
Symptomatic Neonatal Cerebral Sinovenous Thrombosis
Diffusion-weighted MRI to confirm or exclude venous edema or infarction, MR venography (MRV) to diagnose location and extent of venous thrombosis
Presumed Perinatal Arterial Ischemic Stroke or Periventricular Venous Infarction
T1-weighted MRI to confirm remote focal infarction, including FLAIR (fluid-attenuated inversion recovery) imaging for gliosis and features of periventricular venous infarction, gradient echo imaging looking for old blood (periventricular venous infarction)
History
Prenatal: Infertility, recurrent early pregnancy loss, fetal growth/movement, infections, bleeding, trauma, diabetes, hypertension, drug abuse (cocaine), smoking, alternative medications
Perinatal: Maternal fever, placental abnormality, umbilical cord abnormality, fetal status (heart rate, decelerations on fetal monitoring strips), mode of delivery, prolonged rupture of membranes, Apgar scores, umbilical cord gas (to determine acid–base balance, where acidosis is a marker of distress), resuscitation
Past medical history: Cardiac disease, systemic thrombosis, feeding and growth, hydration, infection, interventions
Maternal or family history: Thrombosis (deep vein thrombosis), recurrent early pregnancy loss, myocardial infarction or stroke at a young age
Physical Examination
Vital signs, growth parameters, fluid status, fontanel (bulging, pulsatile), dilated head and neck veins (CSVT), papilledema, asymmetrical movements or primitive reflexes, other neurological deficits (lethargy, low tone), seizures
Laboratory
Cardiac: Echocardiogram, electrocardiogram
Infectious: Blood cultures, TORCH (toxoplasmosis, rubella, cytomegalovirus, herpes simplex, human immunodeficiency virus) screen for congenital infection, cerebrospinal fluid evaluation for cells, protein, glucose, cultures
Prothrombotic Initial: Hemogram, C-reactive protein, protein C, protein S, fibrinogen, antithrombin, lipoprotein (a), anticardiolipin antibodies, lupus anticoagulant, partial thromboplastin time Follow-up (3–6 months): Activated protein C resistance, factor V Leiden, prothrombin gene mutation, methylene tetrahydrofolate reductase (MTHFR), lipoprotein (a), homocysteine, factors VIII/IX/XI. Consider evaluating parents if positive maternal or family history.
EEG: For any suspected seizures, consider repeat electroencephalography or video EEG monitoring.
Placental pathological exam if available

(Modified from Kirton and DeVeber, 2009 with permission)

for poor outcome in neonates with stroke include abnormal exam at discharge from the nursery, neonatal seizures, and an abnormal EEG (both epileptiform abnormalities [seizure potential] and focal slowing) (Bax et al., 2006; Mercuri et al., 1999; 2001; Sreenan et al., 2000; Wu et al., 2004). Notably, in our cohort, neonatal seizures did not predict an adverse outcome; in fact, the group with neonatal seizures did better than other groups (Trauner et al., 1993; Trauner & Mannino, 1986). Between 30% and 50% of children who had an arterial stroke are reported to be grossly neurologically normal (do not have a significant hemiplegia and have generally normal development) (Ballantyne et al., 2008; Golomb et al., 2008; Kirton et al., 2008; Lee et al., 2005b; Nelson & Lynch, 2004; Nelson, 2007; Trauner et al, 1993; Wu et al., 2005). Motor deficits are prominent in perinatal stroke syndromes, occurring in 30% to 60% of early presenters (Cowan & Mercuri, 2011; Lee et al., 2005b; Mercuri et al., 1999; 2004) and in more than 80% with presumed perinatal arterial stroke and periventricular venous infarction (which is biased by the fact that the presenting symptom is almost always motor) (Golomb et al., 2001; Kirton et al., 2008; 2010; Laugesaar et al., 2007; Mercuri et al., 1999). Recurrent seizures or epilepsy occurs in 20% to 50% of children in stroke and hemiplegic CP cohorts (Cowan & Mercuri, 2011; Fitzgerald et al., 2007; Mercuri et al., 1999; 2004; Trauner et al., 1993). Clear cognitive, language, and/or behavioral problems are reported in about 30%, and visual problems occur in about 20% to 30% (Golomb et al., 2001; 2007a; Ricci et al., 2008; Sreenan et al., 2000; Trauner et al., 1993; Westmacott et al., 2007, 2009). Somewhere between 60% and 80% have an abnormality in at least one domain, which varies from mild to severe (Cowan & Mercuri, 2011; Rutherford et al., 2011). Long-term neuropsychological studies like ours are leading to better definition of the evolution and spectrum of complex and generally mild cognitive and behavioral deficits.

Lesion size (Cioni et al., 1999; Lee et al., 2005b; Mecuri et al., 1999; 2001; 2004) and location (Boardman et al., 2005; Ganesan et al., 1999; Lee et al., 2005b; Mercuri et al., 1999; 2004) correlate modestly with general outcome. Those with lesions sparing the cortex appear to have a lower risk of cognitive, behavioral, language, or seizure disorders (Cowan & Mercuri, 2011; Kirton et al., 2008). In many but not all studies (Ballantyne et al., 2008), cognitive outcome correlates with size of lesion. Site and side of lesion are even less reliable predictors. The left MCA is the most common vessel involved in arterial stroke. Outcome may be affected by what part of the MCA is involved: main trunk, cortical- or lenticulostriate branches, anterior and posterior branches. Involvement of Broca's area, the internal capsule, Wernicke's area, or the basal ganglia predicted poorer overall outcome in some studies, but not in others (Ballantyne et al., 2007; Humphreys et al., 2000) (see Fig. 3.1).

Early findings on MRI (DWI sequences) of pre-Wallerian degeneration and corticospinal tract (CST) involvement are strongly predictive of later motor deficit, as are lesions involving cerebral cortex, basal ganglia, and the posterior limb of the internal capsule (Boardman et al., 2005; de Vries et al., 1997; Domi et al., 2009; Mercuri et al., 1999). In a recent large prospective study of 80 children with arterial stroke, assessed at age 2 years, 26% of those with MCA infarcts (three quarters of those with complete MCA territory involvement) had a hemiplegia. CST involvement was an even better predictor of motor outcome. Involvement of the CST was associated with hemiplegia in two thirds, whereas its absence was associated with normal motor development in 94% of cases (Husson et al., 2010) (see Chapter 4 for further discussion).

SEIZURES AND EPILEPSY

Neonatal seizures, occurring at the same time as the stroke, are generally few in number and easy to control. An abnormal neonatal EEG (both epileptiform abnormalities and focal slowing) predicts poorer outcome at 15 months (Bouza et al., 1994; Cowan & Mercuri, 2011; Golomb et al., 2008; Mercuri et al., 1999; 2004; Selton et al., 2003; Sreenan et al., 2000). The temporal lobe and hippocampus are often damaged in both MCA and PCA strokes and presumably serve as the substrate for acute and chronic seizures (Remillard et al., 1974; Squire et al., 2003). In arterial stroke cortical as opposed to subcortical lesions may increase the risk for later epilepsy (Kirton et al., 2008).

The reported frequency of seizures and epilepsy[12] is quite variable. Most children who have seizures as newborns never have them again (Wanigasinghe et al., 2010; Wusthoff et al., 2011). Epilepsy, ranging from mild to severe (Bruck et al., 2001; Carlsson et al., 2003; Humphreys et al., 2000; Oskoui & Shevell 2005; Uvebrant 1988), is reported in anywhere from one quarter to one third to even one half of the patients in generic hemiplegic CP cohorts. Epilepsy is reported in anywhere from 20% to 50% of children in series that are limited to children with arterial stroke (Estan & Hope, 1997; Fitzgerald et al., 2007; Golomb et al., 2001; 2007b; Kirton et al., 2008; Koelfen et al., 1995; Lee et al., 2005b; Mercuri et al., 2001; Sreenan et al., 2000; Trauner et al., 1993). Seizures can recur/occur at any age. Evidence of stroke on prenatal ultrasound and family history of epilepsy may be associated with earlier onset of later epilepsy. In Golomb et al.'s (2007b) retrospective review of 64 children with stroke (both early and late presenters) 75% presented with seizures (mostly neonatal), and 65% continued to have or developed epilepsy after 6 months of age. The median age at time of seizure development was 16 months (range 7 months to 10 years).

Generally seizures are easily controlled with medication, but some children have persistent seizures and some develop intractable epilepsy (Table 3.2). In a cohort of 110 children with infantile spasms[13] 10 had had a stroke (Golomb et al., 2006). In Golomb et al.'s (2007b)

TABLE 3.2 ASSOCIATED WITH EPILEPSY AT FOLLOW-UP

Presentation with neonatal seizures	+
Presentation with infantile spasms	+
Cognitive impairment at the last follow-up	+
Middle cerebral artery infarction	–
Large-branch middle cerebral artery infarction	+/–
Initial abnormal EEG	–

(Modified from Fitzgerald et al., 2007)

[12] Epilepsy is defined as having two or more seizures, but a neonatal seizure and a single seizure later in childhood would not be considered epilepsy.

[13] Infantile spasms represent an age-dependent seizure type that starts between ages 6 months and 3 years and is often associated with cognitive impairments and later epilepsy of other types.

cohort epilepsy resolved in 25%; 45% had epilepsy as of last follow-up (median age at follow-up 3.5 years). Two thirds were eventually seizure-free with treatment and 25% of the children with epilepsy had severe epilepsy at last follow-up, with one or more seizures per month. Rarely, surgery is required to control the seizures. Both children and adults with perinatal stroke, who come to hemispherectomy because of intractable seizures, show improvement of both motor and cognitive function postoperatively (Carreno et al., 2002; Cukiert et al., 2009; Guzzetta et al., 2006). Hemispherectomy can diminish spasticity, especially in the contralateral lower limb, resulting in improved gait. The absence of seizures and epileptic discharge on EEG after surgery is associated with overall cognitive improvement.

Children in generic hemiplegic CP cohorts, as well as those with well-documented stroke, who have epilepsy have a poorer cognitive outcome and may have significant cognitive declines (Ballantyne et al., 2008; Carlsson et al., 2003; Chilosi et al., 2001; Cohen & Duffner, 1981; Dall'Oglio et al., 1994; Vargha-Khadem et al., 1992). In a sense, epilepsy may transform focal pathology into generalized pathology and thus interferes with plasticity. Our patients with epilepsy acquired language more slowly (Ballantyne et al., 2008; Rowe et al., 2009). Ballantyne et al. (2008) also documented that full-scale IQ declined over time in those who had seizures, but not in those who did not (Fig. 3.4) (see Chapter 9 for further discussion of changes of IQ over time).

OUTCOME: EARLY AND LATE PRESENTERS

The outcome in this population may differ to some degree according to the timing of presentation (early vs. late), as well as between late presenters with arterial versus venous stroke (Kirton et al., 2010). The latter not only have different lesion locations, but the insults occur at different times, term versus about 34 weeks' gestation (Staudt et al 2010). Lesion location may differ as well for the two arterial stroke groups. Late presenters are more likely to have involvement of the entire MCA territory, leading to both cortical and subcortical

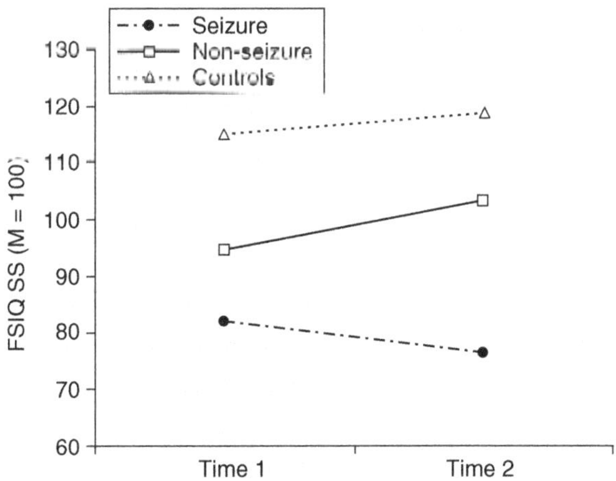

FIGURE 3.4 Mean for IQ measures (WPPSI/WPPSI-R) at Time 1 and for IQ measures (WISC-R/WISC-3) at Time 2. Full-scale IQ for the seizure and non-seizure subgroups, and control group. (Reprinted with permission from Ballantyne et al., 2008.)

involvements, while early presenters tend to have one or the other (Abels et al., 2006; de Vries et al., 1997; Golomb et al., 2001; Govaert et al., 2000).

Early presenters have more adverse events during pregnancy and delivery and placental pathology is more common. In those with late presentation–presumed perinatal stroke, the neonatal period was generally uncomplicated even when examined in retrospect. In Laugesaar et al.'s (2007) cohort of 26 cases of presumed perinatal arterial stroke (late presenters), only one quarter had any symptoms in the neonatal period (Table 3.3). On the other hand, thrombophilias are more common among the late presenters, suggesting that inherited disorders, rather than adverse events around the time of delivery, play a more important role in the etiology of stroke in the late presenters than in the early presenters.

Motor outcome differs in the two groups. Among children with late presentation, the rate of hemiplegia of more than 80% is consistent with the motor deficit being by far the most common presenting symptom. However, the degree varies from mild to severe. Some children declare handedness early; some children have a clear hemiparesis. The rate of motor disability is lower in children who presented in the neonatal period—about 25% to 30%

TABLE 3.3 COMPARISON BETWEEN EARLY AND LATE PRESENTERS

	Early Presenters
Sex*	More boys, fewer girls
Side of damage	No difference
Prematurity	No difference
Protein C deficiency**	No difference
Homocysteinemia**	No difference
Preeclampsia	No difference
Intrauterine growth restriction (IUGR)	No difference
Chorioamnionitis	No difference
First delivery*	More primiparas
Mean birth weight*	Heavier
Cardiac disorders	No difference
Thrombophilia	No difference
Infection	No difference
Maternal disorders	No difference
Placenta disorders*	More frequent
Birth asphyxia*	More frequent
Hemiparesis*	More with severe, less with mild to moderate
Epilepsy	No difference

* Significant differences in frequency between the two groups. Early presenters (n = 12), late presenters (n = 26).

** Protein C deficiency and homocysteinemia are also types of thrombophilias. Note that birth asphyxia was an exclusionary criteria in our study; hence, our subjects may have less severe deficits.

(Boardman et al., 2005; Curry et al., 2007; Golomb et al., 2001; Husson et al., 2010; Kirton et al., 2008; Laugesaar et al., 2007; Lee et al., 2005b; Mercuri et al., 1999; 2004; Sreenan et al., 2000). The data suggest, however, that when early presenters have a hemiparesis, it is generally more severe than in the late presenters (Laugesaar et al., 2007).

Epilepsy in childhood occurs at a similar rate in early presenters and late presenters (Estan & Hope, 1997; Fitzgerald et al., 2007; Fujimoto et al., 1992; Golomb et al., 2001; 2007a; Kirton et al., 2008; Koelfen et al., 1995; Laugesaar et al., 2007; Lee et al., 2005b; Sreenan et al., 2000; Wu et al., 2004). However, since age of seizure onset/recurrence is extremely variable, duration of follow-up affects this statistic.

Overall, it appears that late presenters may have a worse outcome, but this difference may be limited to the occurrence of hemiparesis. Further investigation of possible differences in etiology and pathology in the early versus late presenters, as well as longer follow-up, is warranted.

Late Presentation: Arterial Versus Periventricular Venous Stroke

Recent evidence suggests that periventricular venous stroke (de Vries et al., 2001; Takanashi et al., 2003) is the second most common type of presumed perinatal stroke in late presenters and explains most isolated subcortical presumed perinatal strokes in the periventricular white matter (see Fig. 3.2) (Kirton et al., 2010). The clinical presentations and risk factor profiles in late presenters with periventricular venous stroke and presumed perinatal arterial stroke differ to some degree. Studying 12 children (20%) with venous stroke and 47 (80%) with arterial stroke, Kirton et al. (2010) found that delays in diagnosis were common. The median time to parental concern was 5 months, with delays in physician concern (7 months) and diagnosis (12 months); delays were somewhat longer in the venous stroke group. Most children presented with asymmetrical motor development, but children with arterial stroke were more likely to present with seizures or nonmotor, developmental delays. Perinatal, obstetrical, and neonatal factors were common (76%), with acute perinatal factors present in more than half. One or more occurred more frequently in arterial (31 of 47 cases; 66%) compared with venous stroke (2 of 12 cases; 17%). Delivery by cesarean section occurred at a similar rate in the two groups (although at a higher rate than usual—42%). Neonatal risk factors occurred in 14 cases (24%), all in the presumed perinatal arterial stroke cases. Thrombophilia occurred in almost half the children. The frequency may have been slightly higher in venous stroke, but the sample size of the venous stroke group was too small to be sure. The greater association of acute perinatal risk factors with arterial stroke suggests that arterial strokes occur perinatally, while venous stroke occurs earlier in the third trimester, and by a different mechanism.

PREVENTION AND TREATMENT

Perinatal stroke rarely repeats, suggesting that environmental factors play an important role (Nelson, 2009b). Nelson speculates that maternal fever, thyroid disorder, family history of neurological problems or seizures, low socioeconomic status, and placental abnormalities may be causal factors that have not been given enough consideration. Understanding these better may enhance prevention.

Given the greater plasticity of the developing brain, the early timing of perinatal stroke is often assumed to confer an advantage and a more favorable outcome (Nelson & Lynch, 2004). Nonetheless, most children with perinatal stroke suffer some morbidity, perhaps even at greater rates than older infants and children (Anderson et al., 2010, 2011; Lansing et al., 2004), which suggest that our understanding of brain reorganization after perinatal stroke is incomplete. Perinatal strokes provide the ideal in vivo model for examining the response of the developing brain to focal injury. There is more work to be done.

REFERENCES

Abels L, Lequin M, Govaert P (2006). Sonographic templates of newborn perforator stroke. *Pediatr Radiol* 36:663–669.

Agrawal N, Johnston SC, Wu YW, Sidney S, Fullerton HJ (2009). Imaging data reveal a higher pediatric stroke incidence than prior US estimates. *Stroke* 40:3415–3421.

Anderson V, Jacobs R, Spencer-Smith M, Coleman L, Anderson P, Williams J, Greenham M, Leventer R (2010). Does early age at brain insult predict worse outcome? Neuropsychological implications. *J Pediatr Psychol* 35(7):716–727.

Anderson V, Spencer-Smith M, Wood A. (2011). Do children really recover better? Neurobehavioural plasticity after early brain insult. *Brain* 134; 2197–2221.

Armstrong-Wells J, Johnston SC, Wu YW, Sidney S, Fullerton HJ (2009). Prevalence and predictors of perinatal hemorrhagic strokes: results from the Kaiser pediatric stroke study. *Pediatrics* 123:823–828.

Ballantyne AO, Spilkin AM, Hesselink J, Trauner DA (2008). Plasticity in the developing brain: intellectual, language and academic functions in children with ischaemic perinatal stroke. *Brain* 131:2975–2985.

Ballantyne AO, Spilkin AM, Trauner DA. (2007). Language outcome after perinatal stroke: does side matter? *Child Neuropsychol* 13: 494–509.

Bax M, Tydeman C, Flodmark O (2006). MRI pattern in the European hemiplegic CP by age. *JAMA* 296:1602–1608.

Berfelo FJ, Kersbergen KJ, van Ommen CH, Govaert P, van Straaten HLM, Poll-The BT, van Wezel-Meijler G, Vermeulen RJ, Groenendaal F, de Vries LS, de Haan TR (2010). Neonatal cerebral sinovenous thrombosis from symptom to outcome. *Stroke* 41:1382–1388.

Boardman JP, Ganesan V, Rutherford MA, Saunders DE, Mercuri E, Cowan F (2005). Magnetic resonance image correlates of hemiparesis after neonatal and childhood middle cerebral artery stroke. *Pediatrics* 115(2):321–327.

Bouza H, Rutherford M, Acolet D, Pennock JM, Dubowitz LM (1994). Evolution of early hemiplegic signs in full-term infants with unilateral brain lesions in the neonatal period: a prospective study. *Neuropediatrics* 25:201–207.

Bruck I, Antoniuk SA, Spessatto A, Bem RS, Hausberger R, Pacheco CG (2001). Epilepsy in children with cerebral palsy. *Arq Neuropsiquiatr* 59:35–39.

Carlsson M, Hagberg G, Olsson I (2003). Clinical and aetiological aspects of epilepsy in children with cerebral palsy. *Dev Med Child Neurol* 45:371–376.

Carreno M, Kotagal P, Perez Jiminez A, Mesa T, Bingaman W, Wyllie E (2002). Intractable epilepsy in vascular congenital hemiparesis: clinical features and surgical options. *Neurology* 59:129–131.

Chalmers EA (2005). Perinatal stroke: risk factors and management. *Br J Haematol* 130:333–343.

Cheong JL, Cowan FM. (2009). Neonatal arterial ischaemic stroke: obstetric issues. *Semin Fetal Neonatal Med* 14:267–271.

Chilosi AM, Cipriani P, Bertuccelli B, Pfanner PL, Cioni G (2001). Early cognitive and communication development in children with focal brain lesions. *J Child Neurol* 16:309–316.

Cioni G, Sales B, Paolicelli PB, Petacchi E, Scusa MF, Canapicchi R (1999). MRI and clinical characteristics of children with hemiplegic cerebral palsy. *Neuropediatrics* 30:249–255.

Cohen ME, Dufner PK (1981). Prognostic indicators in hemiparetic cerebral palsy. *Ann Neurol* 9:353–357.

Cowan F, Mercuri E (2011). Neonatal stroke. In: Ganesan V, Krikham F. Strokes in Childhood (pp. 189–194). London: MacKeith Press.

Cowan FM, de Vries LS (2005). The internal capsule in neonatal imaging. *Semin Fetal Neonatal Med* 10:461–474.

Cukiert A, Cukiert CM, Argentoni M, Baise-Zung C, Forster CR, Mello VA, Burattini JA, Mariani PP (2009). Outcome after hemispherectomy in hemiplegic adult patients with refractory epilepsy associated with early middle cerebral artery infarcts. *Epilepsia* 50:1381–1384.

Curry CJ, Bhullar S, Holmes J, Delozier CD, Roeder ER, Hutchison HT (2007). Risk factors for perinatal arterial stroke: a study of 60 mother–child pairs. *Pediatr Neurol* 37:99–107.

Dall'Oglio AM, Bates E, Volterra V, Di Capua M, Pezzini G (1994). Early cognition, communication and language in children with focal brain injury. *Dev Med Child Neurol* 36: 1076–1098.

de Veber G, Andrew M, Adams C, Bjornson B, Booth F, Buckley DJ, Camfield CS, David M, Humphreys P, Langevin P, MacDonald EA, Meaney B, Shevell M, Sinclair DB, Yager, J, Gillett, J (2001). Cerebral sinovenous thrombosis in children. *N Engl J Med* 345:417–423.

de Vries LS, Groenendaal F, Eken P, van Haastert IC, Rademaker KJ, Meiners LC (1997). Infarcts in the vascular distribution of the middle cerebral artery in preterm and full-term infants. *Neuropediatrics* 28:88–96.

de Vries LS, Roelants-van Rijn AM, Rademaker KJ, Van Haastert IC, Beek FJ, Groenendaal F (2001). Unilateral parenchymal haemorrhagic infarction in the preterm infant. *Eur J Paediatr Neurol* 5:139–149.

de Vries LS, Van der Grond J, Van Haastert IC, Groenendaal F (2005):Prediction of outcome in new-born infants with arterial ischaemic stroke using diffusion-weighted magnetic resonance imaging. *Neuropediatrics* 36:12–20.

Domi T, deVeber G, Shroff M, Kouzmitcheva E, MacGregor DL, Kirton A (2009). Corticospinal tract pre-wallerian degeneration: A novel outcome predictor for pediatric stroke on acute MRI. *Stroke* 40:780–787.

Dudink J, Mercuri E, Al-Nakib L, Govaert P, Counsell SJ, Rutherford MA, Cowan FM (2009). Evolution of unilateral perinatal arterial ischemic stroke on conventional and diffusion-weighted MR imaging. *AJNR Am J Neuroradiol* 30:998–1004.

Elbers J, Viero S, MacGregor D, deVeber G, Moore AM (2011). Placental pathology in neonatal stroke. *Pediatrics* 127:e722–e729.

Estan J, Hope P (1997). Unilateral neonatal cerebral infarction in full term infants. *Arch Dis Child Fetal Neonatal* 76:88–93.

Fitzgerald KC, Williams LS, Garg BP, Carvalho KS, Golomb MR (2006). Cerebral sinovenous thrombosis in the neonate. *Arch Neurol* 63:405–409.

Fitzgerald KC, Williams LS, Garg BP, Golomb MR (2007). Epilepsy in children with delayed presentation of perinatal stroke. *J Child Neurol* 22:1274–1280.

Fujimoto S, Yokochi K, Togari H, Nishimura Y, Inukai K, Futamura M, Sobajima H, Suzuki S, Wada Y (1992). Neonatal cerebral infarction: symptoms, CT findings and prognosis. *Brain & Development* 14:48–52.

Ganesan, V., Ng, V., Chong, W.K., Kirkham, F.J., Connelly, A. (1999). Lesion volume, lesion location, and outcome following middle cerebral artery territory stroke. *Archives of Disease in Childhood* 81: 295–300.

Gibson CS, Maclennan AH, Dekker GA, Goldwater PN, Sullivan TR, Munroe DJ, Tsang S, Stewart C, Nelson KB (2008). Candidate genes and cerebral palsy: a population-based study. *Pediatrics* 122:1079–1085.

Golomb MR, Fullerton HJ, Nowak-Gottl U, deVeber G (2009). Male predominance in childhood ischemic stroke: findings from the International Pediatric Stroke Study. *Stroke* 40:52–57.

Golomb MR, Garg BP, Carvalho KS, Johnson CS, Williams LS (2007b). Perinatal stroke and the risk of developing childhood epilepsy. *J Pediatr* 151:409–413.

Golomb MR, Garg BP, Saha C, Azzouz F, Williams LS (2008). Cerebral palsy after perinatal arterial ischemic stroke. *J Child Neurol* 23:279–286.

Golomb MR, Garg BP, Williams LS (2006). Outcomes of children with infantile spasms after perinatal stroke. *Pediatr Neurol* 34:291–295.

Golomb MR, MacGregor DL, Domi T, Armstrong DC, McCrindle B, Mayank S, deVeber GA (2001). Presumed pre- and perinatal stroke: risk factors and outcomes. *Ann Neurol* 50:163–168.

Golomb MR, Saha C, Garg BP, Azzouz F, Williams LS (2007a). Association of cerebral palsy with other disabilities in children with perinatal arterial ischemic stroke. *Pediatr Neurol* 37:245–249.

Govaert P, Matthys E, Zecic A, Roelens F, Oostra A, Vanzieleghem B (2000). Perinatal cortical infarction within middle cerebral artery trunks. *Arch Dis Child Fetal Neonatal* 82:59–63.

Govaert P, Ramenghi L, Taal R, De Vries L, deVeber G (2009a). Diagnosis of perinatal stroke I: definitions, differential diagnosis and registration. *Acta Paediatr* 98:1556–1567.

Govaert P, Ramenghi L, Taal R, Dudink J, Lequin M (2009b). Diagnosis of perinatal stroke II: mechanisms and clinical phenotypes. *Acta Paediatr* 98:1720–1726.

Govaert P, Zingman A, Jung YH, Dudink J, Swarte R, Zecic A, Meersschaut V, van Engelen S, Lequin M (2008). Network injury to pulvinar with neonatal arterial ischemic stroke. *NeuroImage* 39:1850–1857.

Groenendaal F, Benders MJ, de Vries LS (2006). Pre-Wallerian degeneration in the neonatal brain folloing perinatal cerebral hypoxia-ischemia demonstrated with MRI. *Semin Perinatol* 30(3):146–150.

Günther G, Junker R, Starter R, Schobess R, Kurnik K, Kosch A, Nowak-Gottl U (2000). Symptomatic ischemic stroke in full-term neonates: role of acquired and genetic prothrombotic risk factors. *Stroke* 31:2437–2441.

Guzzetta F, Battaglia D, Di Rocco C, Caldarelli M (2006). Symptomatic epilepsy in children with porencephalic cysts secondary to perinatal middle cerebral artery occlusion. *Childs Nerv Syst* 22:922–930.

Hajnal BL, Sahebkar-Moghaddam F, Barnwell AJ, Barkovich AJ, Ferriero DM (1999). Early prediction of neurologic outcome after perinatal depression. *Pediatr Neurol* 21:788–793.

Herak DC, Antolic MR, Krleza JL, Pavic M, Dodig S, Duranovic V, Brkic AB, Zadro R (2009). Inherited prothrombotic risk factors in children with stroke, transient ischemic attack, or migraine. *Pediatrics* 123:e653–660.

Humphreys P, Whiting S, Pham B (2000). Hemiparetic cerebral palsy: clinical pattern and imaging in prediction of outcome. *Can J Neurol Sci* 27:210–219.

Husson B, Hertz-Pannier L, Renaud C, Allard D, Presles E, Landrieu P, Chabrier S (2010). Motor outcomes after neonatal arterial ischemic stroke related to early MRI data in a prospective study. *Pediatrics* 126:912–918.

Jaigobin C, Silver FL (2000). Stroke and pregnancy. *Stroke* 31:2948–2295.

Jhawar BS, Ranger A, Steven D, Del Maestro RF (2003). Risk factors for intracranial hemorrhage among full-term infants: a case-control study. *Neurosurgery* 52:581–590.

Kenet G, Lutkhoff LK, Albisetti M, Bernard T, Bonduel M, Brandao L, Chabrier S, Chan A, deVeber G, Fiedler B, Fullerton J, Goldenberg N, Grabowski E, Gunther G, Heller C, Holzhauer S, Iorio A, Journeycake J, Junker R, Kirkham F, Kurnik K, Lynch J, Male C, Manco-Johnson M, Mesters R, Monagle P, van Ommen H, Raffini L, Rostasy K, Simioni P, Strater R, Young G, Nowak-Gottl U (2010). Impact of thrombophilia on risk of arterial ischemic stroke or cerebral sinovenous thrombosis in neonates and children: a systematic review and meta-analysis of observational studies. *Circulation* 121:1838–1847.

Kirkham F, Cowan F. (2011). Intracranial hemorrhage in the newborn. In: Ganesan V, Kirkham F. Strokes in Childhood. London: MacKeith Press, pp. 194–198.

Kirton A, Armstrong-Wells J, Chang T, deVeber G, Rivkin MJ, Hernandez M, Carpenter J, Yager JY, Lynch JK, Ferriero DM, Members of the IPSS (2011). Symptomatic neonatal arterial ischemic stroke. The International Pediatric Stroke Study. *Pediatrics* 128:1–9.

Kirton A, deVeber G (2006). Cerebral palsy secondary to perinatal ischemic stroke. *Clin Perinatol* 33:367–386.

Kirton A, deVeber G (2009). Advances in perinatal ischemic stroke. *Pediatr Neurol* 40: 205–214.

Kirton A, deVeber G, Pontigon A-M, Macgregor D, Shroff M (2008). Presumed perinatal ischemic stroke: vascular classification predicts outcomes. *Ann Neurol* 63:436–443.

Kirton A, Shroff M, Pontigon AM, deVeber G (2010). Risk factors and presentations of periventricular venous infarction vs arterial presumed perinatal ischemic stroke. *Arch Neurol* 67:842–848.

Kirton A, Shroff M, Pontigon AM, deVeber G (2010): Risk factors and presentations of periventricular venous infarction versus arterial presumed perinatal ischemic stroke. *Archives Neurology* 67:842–848.

Kirton A, Shroff M, Visvanathan T, deVeber G (2007). Quantified corticospinal tract diffusion restriction predicts neonatal stroke outcome. *Stroke* 38:974–980.

Koelfen W, Freund M, Varnholt V (1995). Neonatal stroke involving the middle cerebral artery in term infants: clinical presentation, EEG and imaging studies, and outcome. *Dev Med Child Neurol* 37:204–212.

Krageloh-Mann I, Horber V (2007). The role of magnetic resonance imaging in elucidating the pathogenesis of cerebral palsy: a systematic review. *Dev Med Child Neurol* 49:144–156.

Kraus FT, Acheen VI (1999). Fetal thrombotic vasculopathy in the placenta: cerebral thrombi and infarcts, coagulopathies, and cerebral palsy. *Hum Pathol* 30:759–769.

Kurnik K, Kosch A, Sträter R, Schobess R, Heller C, Nowak-Gottl U (2003). Recurrent thromboembolism in infants and children suffering from symptomatic neonatal arterial stroke: a prospective follow-up study. *Stroke* 34:2887–2892.

Lansing A, Max J, Delis D, Fox P, Lancaster J, Manes F, Schatz A (2004). Verbal learning and memory after childhood stroke. *J Intl Neuropsychol Soc* 10:742–752.

Laugesaar R, Kolk A, Tomberg T, Metsvaht T, Lintrop M, Varendi H, Talvik T (2007). Acutely and retrospectively diagnosed perinatal stroke: a population-based study. *Stroke* 38:2234–2240.

Le SE, Saeed N, Cowan FM (2004). MRI imaging quantification of cerebellar growth following hypoxic injury to the neonatal brain. *AJNR Am J Neuroradiol* 25:463–468.

Lee J, Croen LA, Backstrand KH, Yoshida CK, Henning LH, Lindan C, Ferriero DM, Fullerton HJ, Barkovich AJ, Wu YW (2005a). Maternal and infant characteristics associated with perinatal arterial stroke in the infant. *JAMA* 293:723–729.

Lee J, Croen LA, Lindan C, Nash KB, Yoshida CK, Ferriero DM, Barkovich AJ, Wu YW (2005b). Predictors of outcome in perinatal arterial stroke: a population-based study. *Ann Neurol* 58:303–308.

Lequin MH, Dudink J, Tong KA, Obenaus A (2009). Magnetic resonance imaging in neonatal stroke. *Semin Fetal Neonatal Med* 14:299–310.

Lynch JK, Hirtz DG, DeVeber G, Nelson KB (2002). Report of the National Institute of Neurological Disorders and Stroke workshop on perinatal and childhood stroke. *Pediatrics* 109:116–123.

Lynch JK, Nelson KB (2001). Epidemiology of perinatal stroke. *Curr Opinion Pediatr* 13: 499–505.

Mercuri E, Barnett A, Rutherford M, Guzzetta A, Haataja L, Cioni G, Cowan F, Dubowitz L (2004). Neonatal cerebral infarction and neuromotor outcome at school age. *Pediatrics* 113:95–100.

Mercuri E, Cowan F, Gupte G, Manning R, Laffan M, Rutherford M, Edwards AD, Dubowitz L, Roberts I (2001). Prothrombotic disorders and abnormal developmental outcome in infants with neonatal cerebral infarction. *Pediatrics* 107(6):1400–1404.

Mercuri E, Cowan F, Rutherford M, Acolet D, Pennock J, Dubowitz L (1995). Ischaemic and haemorrhagic brain lesions in newborns with seizures and normal Apgar scores. *Arch Dis Child Fetal Neonatal Ed* 73:F67–74.

Mercuri E, Rutherford M, Cowan F, Pennock J, Counsell S, Papadimitriou M, Azzopardi D, Bydder G, Dubowitz L (1999). Early prognostic indicators of outcome in infants with neonatal cerebral infarction: a clinical, electroencephalogram, and magnetic resonance imaging study. *Pediatrics* 103:39–46.

Mineyko A, Kirton A (2011). The black box of perinatal ischemic stroke pathogenesis. *J Child Neurol* 26: 1154–1160.

Nelson KB (2007). Perinatal ischemic stroke. *Stroke* 38:742–745.

Nelson KB (2008). Causative factors in cerebral palsy. *Clin Obstet Gynecol* 51:749–762.

Nelson KB (2009a). Infection in pregnancy and cerebral palsy. *Dev Med Child Neurol* 51(4): 253–254.

Nelson KB (2009b). Preventing cerebral palsy: paths not (yet) taken. *Dev Med Child Neurol* 51(10):765–766.

Nelson KB, Lynch JK (2004). Stroke in newborn infants. *Lancet Neurol* 3:150–158.

Niimura K, Chugani, D, Muzik O, Chugani H (1999):Cerebellar reorganization following cortical injury in humans. *Effects of lesion size and age. Neurology* 52:792–798.

Obenaus A, Ashwal S (2008). Magnetic resonance imaging in cerebral ischemia: focus on neonates. *Neuropharmacology* 55:271–280.

Oskoui M, Shevell MI (2005). Profile of pediatric hemiparesis. *J Child Neurol* 20:471–476.

Perlman JM, Rollins NK, Evans D. (1994). Neonatal stroke: clinical characteristics and cerebral blood flow velocity measurements. *Pediatr Neurol* 11:281–284.

Rafay MF, Cortez MA, deVeber GA, Tan-Dy C, Al-Futaisi A, Yoon W, Fallah S, Moore A (2009). Predictive value of clinical and EEG features in the diagnosis of stroke and hypoxic ischemic encephalopathy in neonates with seizures. *Stroke* 40:2402–2407.

Raine J, Davies H, Gamsu HR (1989). Multiple idiopathic emboli in a full term neonate. *Acta Paediatr Scand* 78:644–646.

Raju TN, Nelson KB, Ferriero D, Lynch JK, the NICHD-NINDS Perinatal Stroke Workshop Participants (2007). Ischemic perinatal stroke: summary of a workshop sponsored by the National Institute of Child Health and Human Development and the National Institute of Neurological Disorders and Stroke. *Pediatrics* 120:609–616.

Ramaswamy V, Miller SP, Barkovich AJ, Partridge JC, Ferriero DM (2004). Perinatal stroke in term infants with neonatal encephalopathy. *Neurology* 62:2088–2091.

Redline RW (2006). Placental pathology and cerebral palsy. *Clin Perinatol* 33:503–516.

Remillard GM, Ethier R, Andermann F (1974). Temporal lobe epilepsy and perinatal occlusion of the posterior cerebral artery. *Neurology* 24:1001–1009.

Ricci D, Mercuri E, Barnett A, Rathbone R, Cota F, Haataja L, Rutherford M, Dubowitz L, Cowan F (2008). Cognitive outcome at early school age in term-born children with perinatally acquired middle cerebral artery territory infarction. *Stroke* 39:403–410.

Rowe ML, Levine SC, Fisher J, Goldin-Meadow S (2009). The joint effects of biology and input on the language development of brain-injured children. *Dev Psychol* 45:90–102.

Rutherford RA, Ramenghi LA, Cowan FM (2011). Neonatal stroke. Arch Dis Child Fetal Neonatal Ed [August online version].

Schulzke S, Weber P, Luetschg J, Fahnenstich H (2005). Incidence and diagnosis of unilateral arterial cerebral infarction in newborn infants. *J Perinat Med* 33:170–175.

Selton D, Andre M, Hascoet JM (2003). EEG and ischemic stroke in full-term newborns. *Neurophysiol Clin* 33:120–129.

Squier W, Salisbury H, Sisodiya S (2003). Stroke in the developing brain and intractable epilepsy: effect of timing on hippocampal sclerosis. *Dev Med Child Neurol* 49:580–585.

Sreenan C, Bhargava R, Robertson CM (2000). Cerebral infarction in the term newborn: clinical presentation and long- term outcome. *J Pediatr* 137:351–355.

Staudt M. (2010). Reorganization after pre- and perinatal brain lesions. *J Anat* 217:469–474.

Takanashi J, Barkovich AJ, Ferriero DM, Suzuki H, Kohno Y (2003). Widening spectrum of congenital hemiplegia: periventricular venous infarction in term neonates. *Neurology* 61:531–533.

Trauner DA, Chase C, Walker P, Wulfeck B (1993). Neurologic profiles of infants and children after perinatal stroke. *Pediatr Neurol* 9:383–386.

Trauner DA, Mannino FL (1986). Stroke in neonates [response to letter to the editor]. *J Pediatr* 109:400.

Uvebrant P (1988). Hemiplegic cerebral palsy aetiology and outcome. *Acta Paediatr Scand Suppl* 1345:1–100.

Vargha-Khadem F, Isaacs E, Van der Werf S, Robb S, Wilson J (1992). Development of intelligence and memory in children with hemiplegic cerebral palsy. The deleterious effect of seizures. *Brain* 115: 315–329.

Volpe JJ (2008). Neurology of the Newborn (5th ed.). Philadelphia: Elsevier.

Wanigasinghe J, Reid SM, Mackay MT, Reddihough DS, Harvey AS, Freeman JL (2010). Epilepsy in hemiplegic cerebral palsy due to perinatal arterial ischaemic stroke. *Dev Med Child Neurol* 52:1021–1026.

Westmacott R, Barry V, MacGregor D, deVeber G (2007). Intellectual function in preschool and school-aged children with a history of acute neonatal stroke. *Stroke* 38:581.

Westmacott R, MacGregor D, Askalan R, deVeber G (2009). Late emergence of cognitive deficits after unilateral neonatal stroke. *Stroke* 40:2012–2019.

Wu YW, Lindan CE, Henning LH, Yoshida CK, Fullerton HJ, Ferriero DM, Barkovich AJ, Croen LA (2006). Neuroimaging abnormalities in infants with congenital hemiparesis. *Pediatr Neurol* 35:191–196.

Wu YW, Lynch JK, Nelson KB (2005). Perinatal arterial stroke: understanding mechanisms and outcomes. *Semin Neurol* 25:424–434.

Wu YW, March WM, Croen LA, Grether JK, Escobar GJ, Newman TB (2004). Perinatal stroke in children with motor impairment: a population-based study. *Pediatrics* 114:612–619.

Wusthoff CJ, Kessler SK, Vossough A, Ichord R, Zelonis S, Halperin A, Gordon D, Vargas G, Licht DJ, Smith SE (2011). Risk of later seizure after perinatal arterial ischemic stroke: a prospective cohort study. *Pediatrics* 127:e1550–1557.

PART TWO
Behavioral Studies

4

Somatosensory and Motor Processes

KENNARD'S (1940) SEMINAL WORK on animal recovery after brain damage introduced the concept that motor recovery was better after early brain injury than after late brain injury. Goldman's studies (1974) indicated that the same lesion might cause a deficit in an adult, but not in an infant. However, she also showed that deficits change over time, as progressive encephalization of function occurs with maturation. A specific motor function may initially depend on subcortical structures and later on cortical structures that have matured and more efficiently mediate the task. Thus, in the case of early focal brain injury deficits that were not apparent at a younger age can actually appear. Furthermore, task demands change with maturation. Simple proximal arm movements sufficient for early motor tasks may be mediated by ipsilateral corticospinal tracts (CSTs), which branch bilaterally onto spinal motor neurons (Carr et al., 1994), while dexterous hand movements depend on contralateral CSTs. The greater plasticity of the immature nervous system has been touted as the explanation for the better outcome after neonatal than adult stroke. But plasticity has limits, and some byproducts of plasticity, like mirror movements, may actually impair function. Furthermore, plasticity appears to be modality specific: the sensory and motor systems are not as plastic as the cognitive systems.

Studies of motor and sensory outcome after early focal lesions have focused on the type and degree of deficits, how to predict deficits clinically and radiologically, and patterns of motor and sensory reorganization. Hemiplegic cerebral palsy (CP) is a clinical phenotype that, by definition, is the result of a focal injury that occurred in the pre-perinatal period and produces weakness on one side of the body. Hemiplegic CP is an umbrella term; there are many causes, such as brain malformation and focal periventricular leukomalacia. Pre-perinatal stroke is the etiology in 20% to 40% or more of children with "generic" (cause not specified) hemiplegic CP (Golomb et al., 2007; Humphreys et al., 2000; Kirton & deVeber, 2006; Krageloh-Mann & Horber, 2007; Uvebrant, 1988; Wu, 2004; 2005; 2006). This chapter will discuss studies focusing on children with hemiplegic CP of any etiology. The causative lesion (e.g., stroke, focal periventricular leukomalacia) will be indicated whenever it is known. Over the past two decades, with the increased availability of brain imaging, many hemiplegic CP studies include only children with stroke. The terms "hemiparesis" and "hemiplegia" will be used somewhat interchangeably throughout to describe the phenotype (since many studies do not specify degree of deficit) but will be modified by mild, moderate, and severe whenever possible.

MOTOR DEVELOPMENT AFTER EARLY FOCAL LESIONS AND THE EMERGENCE OF HEMIPARESIS

Because of limited motor demands/activities, neonates do not place much demand on the contralateral CSTs, and hemiparesis, despite an apparent lesion on CT or MRI, is rarely apparent at birth (Bouza et al., 1994). Severity of neonatal seizures, EEG abnormalities, and abnormalities on the neurological examination at discharge from the nursery often predict later motor disability (Golomb et al., 2008; Guzzetta et al., 2007; Kato et al., 2004; Mercuri et al., 1999; 2004; Sreenan et al., 2000). Although late presenters (infants noted to have a hemiparesis in the middle to late first year of life and found on imaging studies to have had a pre- or perinatal injury, usually due to stroke [see Chapter 3]) almost always have a hemiparesis, early presenters (who are diagnosed in the newborn nursery and who generally have neonatal seizures around the time a stroke occurs) are likely to have a more severe hemiparesis in the long run (Laugesaar et al., 2007).

Various motor signs during infancy have been used to predict later hemiparesis. Generalized body movements emerge as early as 6 to 12 weeks post term. Infants with stroke or focal periventricular lesions destined to have a hemiparesis have abnormal generalized movements from the outset. In those with the most unfavorable outcomes, fidgety movements are absent on the involved body side. Asymmetries in segmental movements also predict later hemiparesis (Cioni et al., 2007; 2010).[1] Three- to 6-month-old infants who have abnormal motor activity like unilateral lack of kicking and asymmetric independent finger movements are at increased risk for developing a hemiparesis (Guzzetta et al., 2003; 2010; Janneke et al., 2009; Yokochi et al., 1995). By about 4 months of age, a paucity of movement on the hemiparetic side becomes clinically apparent, and infants who will eventually have a hemiparesis fail to reach for and hold objects with that hand at 5 months. Early declaration of handedness is a strong predictor of hemiparesis, and the earlier handedness is declared the more severe the ultimate motor deficit is likely to be (Cohen & Duffner, 1981). Among late presenters the median age of parental concern about hemiparesis is 5 months, with delays in physician concern until 7 months, and diagnosis at around 12 months (Boardman et al., 2005; Curry et al., 2007; Golomb et al., 2001; 2003; Husson et al., 2010; Kirton et al., 2008, 2010; Laugesaar et al., 2007; Lee et al., 2005; Mercuri et al., 1999; 2004; Sreenan et al., 2000;

[1] Among the generalized body movements, writhing movements occur first. They are characterized by small to moderate amplitude, slow to moderate speed, and an ellipsoid shape. Writhing movements gradually disappear and are replaced with fidgety movements. Fidgety movements are continuous (except during fussing, crying, and focused attention), small movements of moderate speed and variable acceleration involving the neck, trunk, and limbs, which occur in all directions. They do not involve all body parts simultaneously, but typically migrate from one to another. Fidgety movements gradually disappear from 15 weeks post term but may still be present up to 6 months of age. Voluntary and anti-gravity movements appear at 15 to 20 weeks post term (Cioni et al., 2007; Ferrari & Cioni, 2010).

Uvebrant, 1988). One explanation for delayed presentation, particularly in milder cases, is that fine finger dexterity, the province of the contralateral CST, is not expected until late in the first year and this skill continues to evolve throughout the toddler period. From a physiologic vantage the progressive displacement at the spinal cord level of surviving contralateral corticospinal projections from the damaged hemisphere by ipsilateral corticospinal projections from the intact hemisphere continues over the first 2 years (Martin et al., 2007; 2009; Eyre et al.,2001; 2007) (see below). This also factors into the delay in clinical presentation of hemiparesis.

Long-term motor development has been monitored in children with "generic" hemiplegic CP. When evaluated longitudinally from 16 to 70 months, these children acquire some early fine motor skills (Peabody Developmental Motor Scales, Folio & Fewell, 1983) but then appear to decline (in reality they are not improving in keeping with their age), unless their impairment is very mild (Hanna et al., 2003). By age 5 years, even moderately affected children perform significantly less well than normal children. In this same cohort the quality of upper extremity function (QUEST,[2] DeMatteo et al., 1992, 1993) peaked at 3.5 years and declined thereafter. Levels of hand and arm function in an individual child do not necessarily parallel each other (Hanna et al., 2003). At a projected age of 18 months, low bimanual performance score, measured with the Assisting Hand Assessment (AHA[3]; Krumlinde-Sundholm et al., 2007), predicts future hand impairment. Children with low 18-month scores rarely perform bimanual play tasks independently, while children with high 18-month scores use the hemiparetic hand at least as a fairly useful assisting hand by age 3 years. Children with better initial unimanual skills (Manual Abilities Classification System (MACS)[4] scores, Eliasson et al., 2006a) do better and continue to improve longer than those with lower initial MACS scores (Holmefur et al., 2010). Some, but not all, motor functions in the hemiparetic arm can continue to improve into adolescence. Spontaneous hand use improves slightly, but hand grip improves considerably more and until a later age (Fedrizzi et al., 2003; Pagliano et al., 2001). Over a 13-year follow-up period spanning adolescence, some continuing improvement in the bimanual skills needed for everyday life and in grip-lift synergy (see below) occurs (Eliasson et al., 2006b). Consistent with Goldman's animal model, the differing trajectories of motor development/recovery suggest that different brain regions may mediate the same motor functions at different ages.

Disuse is another marker of level of impairment and predictor of outcome. Many children with hemiparesis ignore their affected limb (Trauner, 2003) and even cross the midline with their intact hand to perform tasks that they are quite capable of doing with the

[2] Quality of Upper Extremity Function (QUEST) (DeMatteo et al., 1992; 1993) is an impairment-based measure that includes items specifically related to hand function and also assesses movements of the adjacent joints. It mainly tests for impairments in reaching and grasping, assessing activities like picking up a piece of cereal, a pencil, and a cube. The test consists of four domains: disassociated movements, grasp, weight bearing, and protective extension. Everyday activities are used to elicit the required movement—for example, rock a doll for eliciting elbow supination, push a wall for wrist dorsiflexion, and hit a balloon for elevation and abduction of the shoulder (Hega et al., 2007).

[3] Assisting Hand Assessment (AHA) tasks include unimanual skills like put down, manipulate, move forearm, grasp, readjust grip, vary grasp, reach, calibrate and bimanual skills like release, stabilize by grip, orient object, move fingers, move upper arm, initiate use, coordinate, change strategies, hold, approach object (Krumlinde-Sundholm et al., 2007).

affected hand. They avoid bimanual activities. While many hemiparetic children also have sensory deficits, the magnitude is not sufficient to explain disuse. Developmental disuse and neglect can exacerbate the magnitude of the motor problem (Taub, 1976; Taub & Wolf, 1997) because reorganization of the motor system, which is activity dependent, is not optimized (Eyre et al., 2001; 2007; Martin, 2005; Martin et al., 2007; 2009) (see below).

THE RANGE OF MOTOR IMPAIRMENTS

Hemiplegic CP can affect both arm and leg—often to different degrees, reflecting the location of the lesion. Since most strokes are in the middle cerebral artery (MCA) territory (see Chapter 3), the arm is generally more affected than the leg. By contrast, periventricular lesions may affect the leg more than the arm. Motor deficits manifest as weakness, spasticity, slowness and impaired dexterity/individual finger movements, and apraxia (Ferrari & Cioni, 2010).

The Leg

The typical resting posture in hemiplegic CP consists of posterior elevation and retraction of the pelvis, internal rotation and adduction at the hip, extension at the knee, plantar flexion and inversion at the ankle, and flexion of the toes. Most children with "generic" hemiplegic CP walk eventually, and almost all those with stroke walk on time (Golomb et al., 2001, 2003; Koelfen et al., 1993; Trauner & Mannino, 1986; Trauner et al., 1993) and function at the highest levels as measured by the Gross Motor Function Classification System (GMFCS) (Rosenbaum et al., 2002).[4] Although parents of children with stroke tend to rate their children's gait as normal (Golomb et al., 2003), gait abnormalities are common (Fonseca et al., 2004; Ounpun et al., 2001, 2009; Scrutton 2000; Wren et al., 2005) . Interestingly, a circumducting gait[5], typical in adult stroke, is relatively infrequent in children with hemiplegic CP. In addition, arm posture is abnormal and arm swing is decreased (Riad et al., 2011).

The Arm

Corticospinal tract lesions secondary to MCA stroke cause distal weakness in the face of relatively preserved proximal power, because the proximal arm has some ipsilateral CST innervation (Jankowska & Edgley, 2006). Arm abnormalities in children with hemiplegic CP nevertheless occur, including weakness, spasticity, decreased range of movement (ROM), stiffness, abnormal compensatory postures, and apraxia (e.g., less fluid and generally slower movements). After stroke, weakness is maximal at the elbow and wrist and in the hand (Brown et al., 1987; Brown & Walsh, 2001; Mackey et al., 2006; Yokochi et al., 1992). Spasticity, a rate-dependent increase in tone attributed to hyperactivity of the spinal stretch reflex, is notable (Bax et al., 2005; Peacock, 2009). Range of motion (the ability to move, for

---

[4] Gross Motor Function Classification System (GMFCS)—Level I (limitations only in more advanced gross motor skills); Level II (limitations walking outdoors and in the community) (Beckang et al., 2007; Rosenbaum et al., 2002).

[5] In a circumducting gait the leg is stiff and the foot is in extension so the leg is "too long". Therefore, to step forward the leg swings around/is rotated away from the body, then towards it, forming a semicircle.

example, the wrist completely in all directions) is decreased (Brown & Walsh, 2001). The hemiplegic upper limb is usually maintained in a flexed posture at the elbow, wrist, and fingers and is internally rotated (Brown & Walsh, 2001; Colebatch & Gandevia, 1989; Ponten et al., 2005). The typical posture of the child with hemiplegic CP is shown in Figure 4.1.

The Hand

Children with hemiplegic CP have more problems with fine motor than with gross motor function. Impairments of the hand include slowness, weakness, spasticity, stiffness, decreased dexterity (uncoordinated movements, incomplete finger individualization), apraxia, and mirror movements. These difficulties co-occur to varying degrees in the same child. Both unimanual and bimanual functions are affected.

Weakness is mild in about 60%, moderate in about 35%, and severe in about 5% with "generic" hemiplegic CP (Bax et al., 2006). Children with relatively mild impairment have grip strength that is only 50% of normal (Eliasson et al., 1995a; 1995b). Functional use of the hand is strongly correlated with strength, as are speed (Brown & Walsh, 2001) and finger pinch and fingertip pinch force (Duque et al., 2003). Spasticity, hyperactive deep tendon reflexes, ankle clonus[6], and a Babinski sign are generally present on the neurological examination. Based on voluntary grasp and release patterns of the hand, wrist, and fingers, most

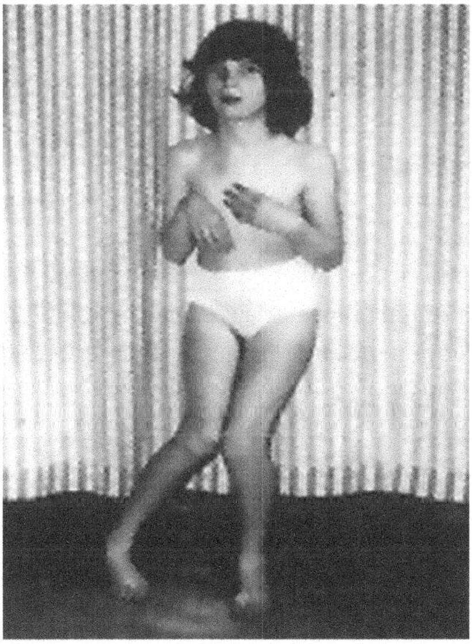

FIGURE 4.1 Typical posture of child with hemiplegic CP. In children with hemiplegic CP the head and trunk are flexed toward the involved side. In the upper extremity the scapula is depressed and retracted, the shoulder is adducted and internally rotated, the elbow is flexed, the forearm is pronated, the wrist is flexed and turned toward the fifth finger, and the fingers are flexed. (With permission from Brown & Walsh, 2001).

[6] Ankle clonus is tested for by rapidly flexing the foot upward. Clonus is an alternating involuntary muscular contraction and relaxation in rapid succession.

school-age children with "generic" hemiplegic CP function at level 1 or 2 on the Zancolli spasticity classification scale[7] (Arner et al., 2008; Zancolli et al., 1983).

Speed and strength are strongly correlated (Brown & Walsh, 2001), and level of hand function correlates with both. Dexterity/motor execution in both the hand and fingers is generally compromised even in a seemingly mildly affected hand (Brown et al., 1987; Duff & Gordon, 2003; Duque et al., 2003; Eliasson & Gordon, 2000; Eliasson et al., 1991, 1992, 1995a; 1995b;Forssberg et al., 1999; Gordon et al., 1999; Gordon & Duff, 1999;Gordon et al., 2003; Krumlinde-Sundholm & Eliasson, 2002; Steenbergen et al., 2000). Finger tapping, finger sequencing, and peg placement into holes on a board are performed slowly; a simple block pick-up task takes about three times longer with the affected hand than the unaffected hand (Brown et al., 1987; Krumlinde-Sundholm et al., 1998), and even putting blocks in a box can be a problem (Duque et al., 2003). Dexterity is inversely correlated with sensory function; sensory impairments have a strong negative effect on dexterity.

Difficulties with motor planning/apraxia are common. Dexterity correlates with the developmental level of the grip-lift synergy, indicating that good motor execution also requires good motor planning (Forssberg et al., 1999; Zancolli et al., 1983). Apraxia, defined as the inability to perform learned skilled movements despite the motor and sensory ability to do so, occurs in many children with hemiplegic CP. In "generic" CP cohorts (which probably included some children with bilateral brain abnormalities) about 40% of children had a mild deficit (75% of the function of the good hand), 20% had a moderate deficit, (50% to 75% function), 20% had a severe deficit (25% to 50% function), and 20% had very severe dysfunction (less than 25% ability in the affected compared to the unaffected hand) when performing activities of daily living (Bax et al., 2005; Fedrizzi et al., 1994; Neville & Goodman, 2006). Step-by-step anticipatory motor planning, which is needed, for example, to properly pick up a cup, or throw and catch a ball, is impaired (Steenbergen & Gordon, 2006). Children with CP often get stuck in the initial step of a movement and do not develop the synergy required for smooth coordinated reaching (Steenbergen et al., 2000). Timing, fluidity, speed, and velocity are atypical (Chang et al., 2005; Mackey et al., 2006; Steenbergen et al., 2000; Trombly 1993; Utley & Sugden, 1998; Van Roon et al., 2005; Van Thiel et al., 2002). Arm movements are slow (Van Thiel & Steenbergen, 2001) and more submovements occur (Chang et al., 2005; Utley & Sugden, 1998). Alteration of the stereotypical shoulder/elbow recruitment order (Steenburgen et al., 2000), more variable hand trajectories (Van Thiel et al., 2002), and increased trunk involvement during reaching (Van Roon et al., 2005) are also notable. Ten-year-olds, particularly those with right hemisphere lesions, have difficulty imitating arm positions (Gobel and Brown, 2009). Despite the apparent simplicity, this task requires planning, as well as the ability to use proprioceptive feedback. Subtle deficits are often present in the unaffected arm (Dellatolas et al., 2005; Steenbergen & Meulenbroek, 2006; Steenbergen & Van der Kamp, 2004), which may affect the ability to compensate during complex motor tasks.

Anticipatory motor planning has been studied in small groups of carefully characterized hemiparetic children using experimental measures of force control during grasping and

[7] Zancolli classification: Level 1, can completely extend the fingers with a neutral position of the wrist or with less than 20° of flexion; Level 2, fingers can be actively extended, but only with more than 20° of wrist flexion (Zancolli et al., 1983).

lifting objects (Eliasson et al., 1991; 1992; 1995a;1995b; Forssberg et al., 1999; Gordon et al., 1999; Gordon & Duff, 1999, Steenbergen et al., 1998; Steenbergen & Gordon, 2006) as well as by detailed assessments of object release skills (Eliasson & Gordon, 2000; Gordon et al., 2003). Abnormal movement planning underlies grip-lift synergy problems in hemiplegic CP (plan and scale the rate of grip and load forces according to features of the object being grasped) (Duff & Gordon, 2003; Duque et al., 2003; Eliasson et al., 1991; 1992; 1995a; 1995b; Forssberg et al., 1999; Gordon & Duff, 1999; Gordon et al., 1999; Steenbergen et al., 1998, 2000; 2004; 2008; Steenbergen & Gordon, 2006). Normally, grip and load forces are initiated simultaneously and increase in parallel, but children with hemiplegic CP have immature or pathological patterns of grip-lift synergy (Eliasson & Gordon 2000; Eliasson et al., 1991; 1992; 1995a; Gordon & Duff, 1999). When children with hemiplegic CP grasp an object they often press too hard (Eliasson et al., 1992; 1995b; Gordon & Duff, 1999; Gordon et al., 1999). To lift objects smoothly, planning both grasp and manipulation is necessary as the object's weight and center of mass can be determined only after an object has been lifted. Sensory deficits have a negative impact on performance (Eliasson et al., 1995a; 1995b; Forssberg et al., 1995; Gordon et al., 1991; Gordon & Duff, 1999). Performance is better with familiar objects and with practice (Duff & Gordon, 2003). Children with hemiplegic CP also have difficulty with the "time in contact" and "replace and release" of objects (Steenbergen et al., 2000). They replace objects faster and more abruptly after a prolonged and uncoordinated release of the grasp. Increasing task difficulty, for example by speeding it up or destabilizing the surface on which the object is placed (Eliasson & Gordon, 2000; Gordon et al., 2003), increases the degree of deficit.

Motor imagery deficits may also contribute to apraxia (Craje et al., 2010; Mutsaarts et al., 2007; Steenbergen & Gordon, 2006; Steenbergen et al., 2007. Practice effects and transfer of information from the good to the impaired hand suggest that anticipatory planning may be based on internal models of an object's physical properties, acquired during previous experience (Gordon et al., 1999; Mutsaarts et al., 2006). Furthermore, fingertip force modulation is best when the objects to be lifted are varied by size, suggesting that visual input can enhance performance (Crajé et al., 2009; Duff & Gordon, 2003; Steenbergen et al., 2007). Thus, the ability to form and retain internal representations of both familiar and novel objects facilitates anticipatory control (Johansson & Westling, 1990). Sensory deficits may interfere with the generation of internal representation (Gordon & Duff, 1999). Poor anticipatory control may also reflect a limited ability to integrate sensory and motor information via motor imagery (Mutsaarts et al., 2005; 2006; Steenbergen & Bekkering, 2006). The sensory–motor dissociation (see below) that often results from brain reorganization after early focal injury may also contribute. The left hemisphere may dominate the use of motor imagery; deficits are greater after left hemisphere damage than after right (Craje et al., 2010; Fadiga et al., 1999; Mutsaarts et al., 2007; Stinear et al., 2007; Van Elk et al., 2010). The posterior parietal cortex, in particular, appears to be active during both end posture motor planning and use of motor imagery (Mutsaarts et al., 2005; 2006; 2007).

The Good Hand

Some studies show minimally impaired strength even in the "unimpaired" hand (Kuhtz-Buschbeck et al., 2000). Task-dependent minor dexterity and motor planning impairments have also been found in the presumed unaffected hand (Brown et al., 1989; Duque et al., 2003; Gordon et al., 1999; Mercuri et al., 1999; Mutsaarts et al., 2005; Steenbergen et al., 2008; Steenbergen & Van der Kamp, 2004; Steenbergen & Meulenbroek, 2006). Handwriting difficulties are common (Tükel Kavak & Eliasson, 2011). Mild deficits are documented on grip-lift synergy and replace and release tasks, especially when task difficulty is increased (Duque et al., 2003; Gordon et al., 1999; 2003). Two- to 4-year-old children with stroke can reach through apertures of varying sizes to get a toy with both the affected and the unaffected hand, but they overestimate their ability to fit their hand into small holes even with the unaffected limb (Dimitropoulou et al., 2007). Adolescents with hemiplegic CP work in a step-by-step fashion (Mutsaarts et al., 2005; 2006) and do not plan ahead. For example, when they complete a sequential task, they do not achieve the typical "end posture comfort"[8] even with the "unimpaired hand" (Rosenbaum et al., 2001; Steenbergen & Gordon, 2006; Steenbergen et al., 2004; Steenbergen & Bekkering, 2006).

Mild abnormalities of the "unaffected" hand, particularly in the older studies, could result from subtle bilateral injury. In children with well-documented stroke the severity of the impairment on the unaffected side does not parallel the severity of impairment in the hemiparetic hand (Mercuri et al., 1999). Subtle deficits in the unaffected hand could reflect the absence of a contribution from the damaged hemisphere's ipsilateral CST tract to normal hand function at the cortical or spinal level (Duque et al., 2003) and/or the fact that the intact hemisphere generally carries the burden of controlling both hands. Left hemisphere lesions in adults cause bilateral apraxia and this appears to be true in hemiplegic CP as well; the good hand in children with left lesions shows more impairment than the good hand of those with right hemisphere lesions (Steenbergen et al., 2004; Steenbergen & Gordon, 2006; Van Elk et al., 2010).

Bimanual Coordination

Bimanual coordination is impaired in children with hemiplegic CP. Indeed, it may be their greatest motor deficit (Gordon & Steenbergen, 2008a; Sakzewski et al., 2010). Difficulties are due to both poor dexterity in the impaired hand and apraxia (Duque et al., 2003; Greaves et al., 2010; Utley & Steenbergen, 2006). Bimanual coordination has been measured simply by rating impaired hand assist skills on everyday bimanual activities like opening a bottle or holding and cutting paper. Even when the impaired hand appears to have good function, grip position is atypical during bimanual tasks (Krumlinde Sundholm et al., 1998) and "end posture comfort is often sacrificed" (Mutsaarts et al., 2006; Steenbergen et al., 2004; Steenbergen & Bekkering, 2006) just as it is in unimanual tasks. Bimanual motor planning is affected by a range of task constraints that have clear analogues in everyday life (Utley et al., 2004). For example, Gordon et al. studied bimanual coordination using an experimental

[8] End posture comfort means that the hand is in a comfortable position at the target location even when this necessitated an uncomfortable posture at the home location (Rosenbaum et al., 2001). When eating with a knife and fork, anticipatory planning is evidenced by the macroscopic variation in grip type. The knife is picked up with a full grip with the thumb pointing towards the blade of the knife. However, if you pick up a knife to pass it to someone else, you probably adopt another grip type, with the thumb pointing towards the handle so that another person can take the knife without any danger (Janssen et al., 2009).

drawer-opening task while varying speed and difficulty. Children aged 8 to 16 years had to open a drawer with one hand and flick a light switch with the other. Under the standard condition, performance was slower than controls and sequential rather than simultaneous. Interestingly, performing the task under time constraints (as fast as possible) facilitated bimanual coordination. The intact hand can influence the impaired hand (Hung et al., 2004). The task took longer when accuracy constraints were increased, and the effect was the same regardless of which hand (affected or unaffected) was used to open the drawer (Hung et al., 2010).

The degree of unimanual dexterity and the extent of spasticity of the impaired hand affect performance on bimanual tasks. During bimanual activities the demands on the impaired, assisting hand are not the same as for the intact hand. The intact hand executes actions where dexterity and manipulation as well as high-quality sensibility are crucial (Krumlinde-Sundholm & Eliasson, 2002; Steenbergen et al., 2008). Bimanual coordination is affected even if the impaired hand is relatively dexterous; furthermore, deficits are reciprocal—the impaired hand affects the intact hand and vice versa (Hung et al., 2004, 2010; Punt et al., 2005; Utley et al., 2004). The fact that the affected hand can interfere with normal hand function suggests that some aspects of motor reorganization/plasticity can have negative ramifications. Mirror movements, a byproduct of reorganization (see below), can also hamper bimanual performance. Two interacting control processes may be involved in bimanual tasks (Utley & Steenbergen, 2006): a common control process that coordinates both hands, and a hand-specific control process that controls each hand independently. Different task constraints may have different effects on the two systems (Aramaki et al., 2006). Sometimes "more is not better" (Hung et al., 2010).

ANATOMICAL CORRELATES OF HEMIPARESIS AND MOTOR REORGANIZATION

Overall, there is less potential for reorganization/plasticity of the motor and sensory systems than for the cognitive systems (Anderson et al., 2011; Muller et al., 1998a; 1998b) after early focal lesions, be it early-third-trimester periventricular lesions or late-third-trimester stroke. This plasticity differential may be a manifestation of the fact that the motor and sensory systems are more primitive and mature earlier, while cognitive systems develop later and continue to evolve long after birth. The motor and sensory systems are also more localized and dependent on specific pathways, while cognitive systems are distributed and interconnected, potentially permitting more extensive intra- and interhemispheric reorganization. Both intra- and interhemispheric motor reorganization is relatively limited or utilized inefficiently, possibly counterproductively (e.g., mirror movements). Plasticity or lack thereof is paralleled by the apparent, rather than subtle, deficits in motor and sensory function as compared with cognitive systems.

ANATOMICAL CORRELATES

Size and Location of Lesions

Recent studies of perinatal stroke populations (in contrast to the "generic" hemiplegic CP populations) document that the presence of motor and other neurological deficits often, but not always, correlates with size of lesion (Cioni et al., 1999; Lee et al., 2005; Mercuri et al., 1999, 2004; Westmacott et al., 2009). Lesion topography, specifically the combined involvement of cortex, basal ganglia, and posterior limb of the internal capsule, almost invariably predicts a moderate hemiparesis after stroke (Boardman et al., 2005; Cowan & de Vries 2005; de Vries et al., 1997; Ganesan et al., 1999; Humphreys et al., 2000; Lee et al., 2005; Mercuri et al., 1999, 2004; Westmacott et al., 2009). About 50% of children with stroke have severe involvement of the hand with loss of individuated finger movements (Cowan & de Vries, 2005). In a chart review study that identified 40 children (from among about 200,000) with late presentation of stroke (perinatal stroke presenting with hemiparesis in the first year), large lesion size and injury to Broca's area, internal capsule, Wernicke's area, or basal ganglia increased the risk for hemiparesis (Lee et al., 2005). In children with presumed prenatal venous stroke, motor outcomes were predicted by basal ganglia involvement including leg hemiparesis, spasticity, and need for assistive devices (Kirton et al., 2008). The periventricular subcortical focus of the injury explains the greater leg involvement since CSTs supplying the legs abut the ventricles. Regardless of lesion type, lesions involving any part the CST almost always cause a motor deficit. When the CST is spared, motor development is almost always normal (Duque et al., 2003; Husson et al., 2010).

Motor deficits associated with some lesions change over time. Following a cohort longitudinally from 15 months to school age, Mercuri et al. (1999; 2004) found that children with isolated internal capsule lesions often had only minor motor signs by school age; they generally did not have a clear hemiparesis (Barnett et al., 2002; Cowen & de Vries, 2005; Mercuri et al., 1999; 2004). While some children in their cohort improved, some had a greater motor deficit at school age than they had had as a preschooler (Mercuri et al., 1999; 2004). Although MRI abnormalities are generally present in children with motor deficits at age 3 to 11 years, some children with abnormal MRIs have only transient motor dysfunction and some children with normal MRIs have permanent motor abnormalities (Bax et al., 2006; Candy et al., 1993; Feldman et al., 1990; Krageloh-Mann & Horber, 2007; Ludeman et al., 2008; Wu et al., 2004; 2005). By and large, children with hemiparesis who have a normal MRI are likely to outgrow the hemiparesis by age 3 years, a phenomenon that has been termed "disappearing CP" (Nelson & Ellenberg, 1982; Wu et al., 2006).

Imaging Correlates of Hemiparesis

With respect to vascular anatomy, complete occlusion of the MCA is highly likely to result in a hemiparesis (Husson et al., 2010), but distal branch occlusions are less reliable predictors of motor outcome. There is more individual variability in terms of the structures affected after distal branch occlusions (Govaert et al., 2000). For example, in a cohort of 18 children (presenting with neonatal seizures) with unilateral stroke limited to branches of the MCA, only 4 had a hemiparesis; 3 children had a main trunk occlusion and 1 child had a cortical plus lenticulostriate lesion from distal branch occlusion(s). Other children with cortical plus lenticulostriate territory lesions did not have hemiparesis, nor did children with only cortical or lenticulostriate branch occlusions (de Vries et al., 1997). The specific territory supplied by MCA branches and the extent of the resulting lesion can be quite variable.

The degree of Wallerian degeneration (degeneration of a nerve fiber distal to the injury, characterized by loss of the myelin that covers the nerve and resulting in atrophy and destruction of the nerve axon) of the descending CSTs also predicts the occurrence and degree of hemiparesis (Bouza et al., 1994). In a group of children with stroke, deficits in manual and digital dexterity and apraxia correlated with the extent of cerebral peduncle asymmetry (Duque et al., 2003). (The difference in size of the two cerebral peduncles reflects the difference in size of the descending contralateral CSTs; a large asymmetry is usually, but not always, an indicator of motor reorganization via ipsilateral CSTs). Regardless of lesion type (congenital malformations, periventricular lesions, stroke usually in the MCA territory), an MRI signal abnormality (T2-weighted sequence) in the CST pathway predicts a later hemiparesis (Staudt et al., 2000, 2005). Special MRI sequences that can directly assess CST axon projections (diffusion tensor imaging [DTI]) have also been used to try to predict motor outcome in infants. Specific abnormalities (lower fractional anisotropy and higher transverse diffusivity) and particular locations are associated with worse motor outcome (Holmstrom et al., 2011; Ludeman et al., 2008). Evidence of pre-Wallerian degeneration of the CST (demonstrated on diffusion weighted image [DWI] sequences) immediately after stroke (particularly in the cerebral peduncle [de Vries et al., 2005], midbrain, and pons [Domi et al., 2009]) is another effective predictor of poor motor outcome (Kirton et al., 2007) (Fig. 4.2). Imaging (DWI) has recently been used to look not only at primary lesions,

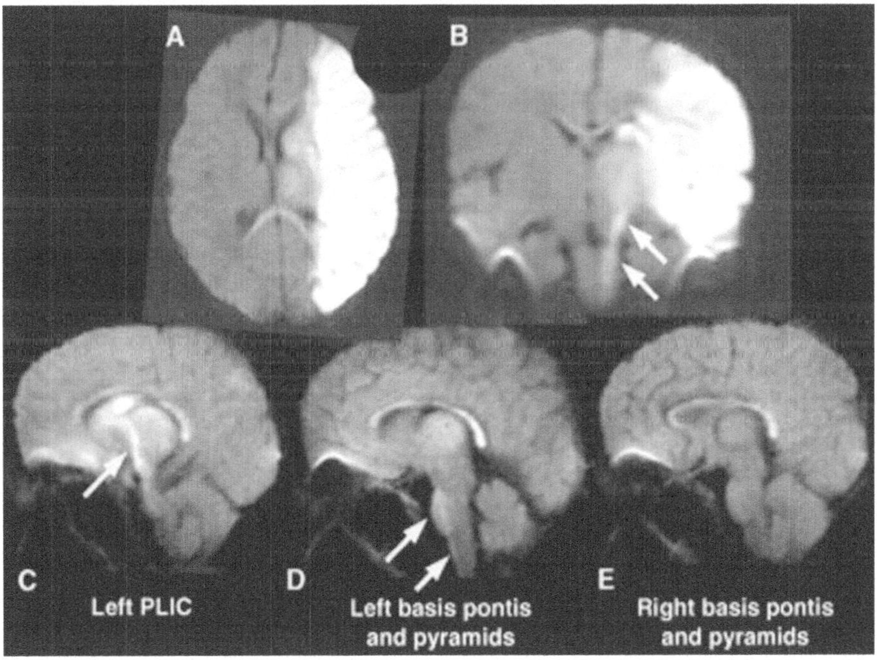

FIGURE 4.2 (A) Large left MCA infarction in a term neonate. Coronal (B) and sagittal (C, D, E) images demonstrate restricted diffusion of ipsilateral descending CSTs remote from the area of infarct (*arrows*). This probably represents pre-Wallerian degeneration, and its extent is predictive of motor outcome. PLIC, posterior limb of internal capsule. (From Kirton et al., 2007, with permission.)

but also at secondary lesions (i.e., the effects of a primary lesion on remote networks). Secondary injury to the pulvinar, presumably caused by damage to its cortical targets and connecting axons, has been described in children with stroke (Govaert et al., 2008). Excitotoxicity or deafferentation is the proposed mechanism. Pulvinar changes after neonatal stroke in term infants may be analogous to thalamic changes, remote from the periventricular lesions in preterm infants (see below). Such findings highlight the importance of imaging, and the fact that both primary and secondary measures of injury need to be investigated to better understand and potentially treat those at high risk for poor motor outcome.

Imaging Correlates of Motor Reorganization

The presence of ipsilateral CSTs can in some instances be predicted based only on routine MRI (Staudt et al., 2000, 2005). Functional imaging (fMRI) provides additional information about motor reorganization patterns. fMRI in subjects with ipsilateral CST reorganization generally reveals significant activation of the intact hemisphere during movement of both the contralateral intact hand and the ipsilateral hemiparetic hand. Activation occurs in the ipsilateral "hand knob" area, indicating that intrahemispheric hand representation is the same regardless of the hemisphere mediating it (Cao et al., 1994; Staudt et al., 2002). Activation during movement of the paretic hand can also occur in secondary motor areas and in the cerebellum, bilaterally (Muller et al., 1998a; 1998b). In a cohort limited to subjects with MCA strokes, fMRI during paretic hand movement in those with preserved contralateral CSTs documented strong activation in the contralateral central sensorimotor region (affected hemisphere), including the "hand knob" area of the precentral gyrus and the central sulcus. In subjects with periventricular lesions and reorganization via ipsilateral CST, fMRI indicates that the basal ganglia reorganizes ipsilaterally, much like the motor cortex (Juenger et al., 2008).

REORGANIZATION OF THE MOTOR SYSTEM

The Normal CST

Contralateral CSTs are required for fractionation of movements and the control of small groups of muscles in a highly selective manner, both crucial to skilled voluntary movement and the acquisition of new motor skills (Lemon, 2008). The normal CST originates from neurons in the frontal and parietal cortex. (Note that only 60% of the axons actually originate in the primary motor cortex.) The tract travels through the anterior half of the posterior limb of the internal capsule and then forms the cerebral peduncles before reaching the brain stem (Fig. 4.3). In the lower medulla the CST crosses the midline to the contralateral side, forming the medullary pyramid/decussation. The lateral contralateral CST travels down the spinal cord, synapsing directly onto motor neurons that control fine finger movements (Armand, 1982). Some fibers (ranging from 10% to 25% in different individuals) do not cross the midline, remain ipsilateral, and form the ventral ipsilateral CST (Davidoff, 1990). The ventral CST, as it travels down the spinal cord, branches extensively, innervating motor neurons on both sides of the spinal cord (hence proximal motor sparing and mirror movements, see below) (Vulliemoz et al., 2005).

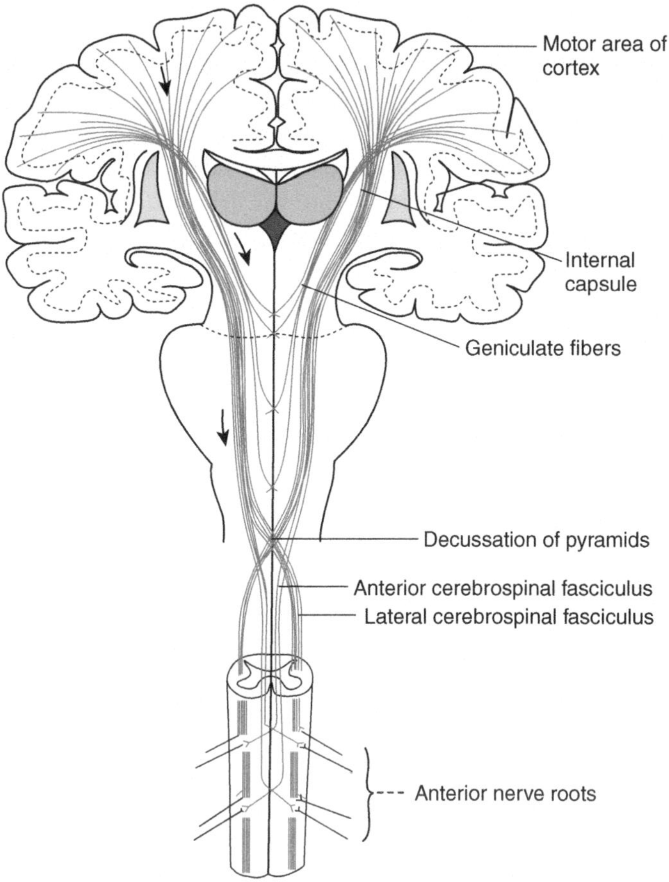

FIGURE 4.3 Normal anatomical organization of the somatosensory system. (With permission, http://deltabiology.com/wp-content/uploads/2012/02/674-2-iline-bp_default.gif.)

Maturation of the Normal CST

Typical of the areal specification process in efferent pathways, CST neurons initially exhibit "exuberant distribution" (O'Leary & Kroll, 2009). Both ipsilateral and contralateral CST projections from each hemisphere to the spinal cord are present by the middle of the second trimester and are detectable for the first 3 months of postnatal life. Thereafter, progressive withdrawal of the ipsilateral projections occurs, resulting in a clear contralateral dominance by 18 months. Maturation of the CST is activity dependent. It is driven by activity in the motor cortex, which depends in turn on the motor activity of the limbs, which is mediated by the CSTs. This affects the balance between projection and withdrawal of contralaterally and ipsilaterally projecting CST axons (Eyre et al., 2001; 2007; Martin 2005; Martin et al., 2007; 2009).

Maturation of the Corticospinal Tract after Early Focal Injury

Inactivity of the hemiparetic side after stroke alters the typical activity-dependent competition between the ipsi- and contralaterally projecting CSTs, with the result that ipsilateral projections from the intact hemisphere generally take over the space that contralateral projections from the damaged hemisphere ordinarily would have filled (Eyre et al., 2007) (Fig. 4.4); compounding the problem, motor cortex excitability is abnormal (Berweck et al., 2008). Because of disuse, organization of the CSTs becomes progressively more abnormal over time. Since the primary motor cortex (and adjoining premotor and somatosensory cortices) is the principal origin of the CSTs, early-third-trimester periventricular lesions have less effect on this maturation process (Staudt, 2007a; 2007b; 2010a), which is driven by cortical activation. In addition, the hemiparesis associated with periventricular lesions tends to be milder and the disuse less prominent; hence, the normal development of contralateral CST efferents from the damaged hemisphere is less affected and contralateral CSTs are the rule.

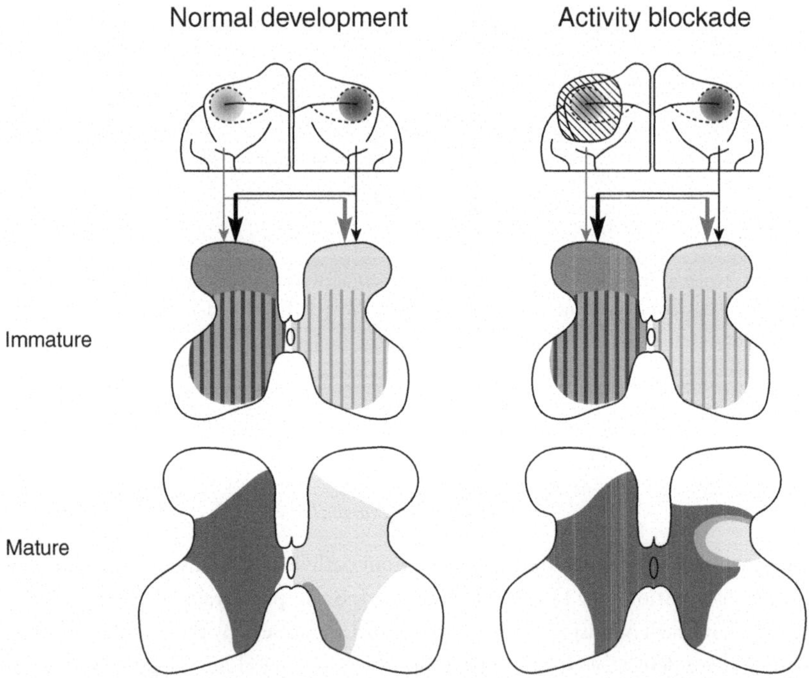

FIGURE 4.4 Early in development, the CST projections to the spinal cord are bilateral. With maturation the connections are pruned back to become strongly contralateral and unilateral. This process is due to activity-dependent competition between the two halves of the CST. If activity is blocked in one half, for example after a perinatal arterial ischemic stroke, the projections from that half are highly restricted and ineffective. On the other hand, the bilateral projections from the other side, which are normally pruned back, persist into maturity. (Adapted from Martin et al., 2007, with permission.)

Imaging studies document abnormal hypertrophy of ipsilateral CST projections from the contralesional hemisphere that parallel loss of physiological function of the contralateral CSTs (Staudt et al., 2005). Transcranial magnetic stimulation (TMS) documents that the absence of motor evoked potentials from the contralateral CST at 2 years is associated with failure to develop a grasp. The presence of ipsilateral central motor conduction delays from the normal hemisphere after TMS predicts the failure to develop manipulation skills. Erye et al. (2007b) argue that the predominance of an ipsilateral CST projection is maladaptive and actually interferes with function. Rather than reflecting "reparative plasticity," ipsilateral CST efferents from the intact hemisphere to the hemiparetic side compound the hemiparesis by competitively displacing surviving contralateral CST projections from the damaged hemisphere and preventing normal pruning (Martin, 2005; Martin et al., 2007; 2009). The scenario may be similar to disuse amblyopia, which occurs in the visual cortex when strabismus goes untreated and one eye goes unused (Eyre et al., 2007). "Developmental disuse" worsens ultimate function. Early stimulation of use of the impaired hand could theoretically facilitate activity-dependent plasticity, as it has in animal models, and enhance primary motor cortex representation and CST connectivity (Chakrabarty et al., 2009) (see Chapter 10, Clinical Implications).

Motor Reorganization Patterns[9]

Three reorganization patterns of the CST are described based on a combination of radiographic and physiological evidence (in order of frequency): (1) ipsilateral CST control of the impaired hand by the intact hemisphere (reflecting the persistence of ipsilateral CST projections from the intact motor cortex to spinal cord motor neurons controlling the affected hand, which would normally have been withdrawn during development in an activity-dependent fashion [Martin, 2005; Martin et al., 2007; 2009]); (2) contralateral CST control of the impaired hand by the damaged hemisphere; and (3) combined ipsilateral and contralateral CST control of the impaired hand (rare) (Carr et al., 1993, Carr 1996; Cincotta et al., 2000; Holmström et al., 2010; Maegaki et al., 1997; Nezu et al., 1999; Staudt et al., 2004; Thickbroom et al., 2001; Uvebrant, 1988). The type of reorganization of the CST after early injury is affected by the timing of the injury during the pre-perinatal period, the type of injury, and the plasticity potential of the CST itself at the time of injury, all of which are strongly interrelated (Staudt et al., 2004). Size of lesion and location of lesion also affect reorganization (Staudt et al., 2002).

[9] The motor reorganization pattern is determined using transcranial magnetic stimulation (TMS) (Staudt, 2010b). Stimulation of the motor cortex produces activity in the hand controlled by the stimulated area. Thus, determinations about ipsi- and contralateral CST innervation can be made. Note that fMRI is not as reliable for determining the motor reorganization pattern. Bilateral fMRI activation can be a false localizer. Bilateral fMRI activation can occur even when there is no physiologic evidence of an active CST. For example, ipsilesional activation could be associated with mirror movements, or with increased task complexity. Disinhibition of the intact motor cortex because of reduced transcallosal input by the damaged hemisphere can result in bilateral fMRI activation that does not reflect the active CST. Thus, TMS is the only accurate way to demonstrate the CST representation of the paretic hand, be it ipsilateral or contralateral.

Type of Reorganization and Outcome

Regardless of time of lesion and type of lesion, motor function is best preserved in children whose impaired hand is controlled by contralateral CST efferents from the damaged hemisphere (along with sensory afferents to the same damaged hemisphere resulting in a sensory–motor association) (Benecke et al., 1991; Carr et al., 1993, Carr 1996; Eyre, 2007; Farmer et al., 1991; Holmström et al., 2010; Macdonell et al., 1999; Maegaki et al., 1997; Nezu et al., 1999; Nirkko et al., 1997; Staudt, 2007a; 2007b; 2010a;, 2004; Thickbroom et al., 2001; Vandermeeren et al., 2002). (Ipsilateral CSTs [from intact hemisphere to impaired hand] may play a role in fine-tuning motor function even when contralateral CSTs have primary control of the impaired hand [Lotze et al., 2009].)

Although ipsilateral CSTs are not optimal for motor control, a range of residual hand functions associated with this reorganization pattern and good motor function has been reported (Cao et al., 1994; Holmström et al., 2010). Recovery in adults is much less common and much more limited after large MCA strokes that involve both its cortical and subcortical territory. Adult recovery is almost always mediated by contralateral CSTs (Krakauer, 2005). Reorganization with ipsilateral CST control of the impaired hand does not occur in adults. Although ipsilateral CSTs are less optimal for mediating recovery after pre-perinatal focal damage, the availability/plasticity underlying their occurrence permits considerably better motor recovery than is accessible to the adult nervous system. Interestingly, recovery of fine coordinated finger movements is reported in adults after subcortical strokes if the ipsilesional/contralateral CST mediates the recovered function (Lemon, 2008). This is similar to the pattern of motor reorganization and outcome after early-third-trimester periventricular injury (Staudt, 2007b; 2010a).

Time of Lesion

The earlier the lesion within the pre-perinatal period, the greater the likelihood that motor reorganization will occur via contralateral CSTs. Thus, contralateral CSTs are generally found after periventricular lesions, which typically occur early in the third trimester (Staudt et al., 2007b; 2010a). Although disrupted by the lesion, both the ipsi- and contralateral CST projections have already reached their spinal cord targets at the time of the injury. Contralateral CST efferent projections persist (Staudt, 2010a; Staudt et al., 2002; Eyre, 2007) and ipsilateral CST projections are withdrawn in a more typical fashion over time. Furthermore, periventricular lesions occur while thalamocortical somatosensory afferents are plastic and can "bypass" periventricular lesions before reaching the somatosensory cortex in the damaged hemisphere (Staudt, 2007b; 2010a; Staudt et al., 2006a; 2006b). Thus, somatosensory representation of the paretic hand is contralateral, remaining in the affected hemisphere, and the sensory and motor systems are associated in the same hemisphere and presumably work in parallel (Staudt et al., 2006a; 2006b; Thickbroom et al., 2001). Clinically, these patients have good arm function, and mild to moderate impairments of hand and finger control, with finger sequencing the most impaired skill. Sensory function is frequently intact for two-point discrimination and proprioception, although not necessarily for complex cortical sensory functions like stereognosis and graphesthesia (see below). Better motor outcome with contralateral CST could reflect the sensory–motor association (versus dissociation), the better sensory function (perhaps reflecting the fact the sensory cortex, reached albeit by a circuitous route, is intact), and/or greater use in the first year of an initially better hand, which allows for activity-dependent pruning and the normal maintenance of a contralateral CST.

By contrast, children with late-third-trimester lesions (usually stroke) generally have ipsilateral CSTs (ipsilateral CST projects to the affected hand from the intact hemisphere) and usually do not have useful hand function (Guzzetta et al., 2007; Staudt, 2010a; Staudt et al., 2004; Thickbroom et al., 2001) (Fig. 4.5). Afferent sensory projections are still directed to the damaged hemisphere, resulting in a sensory–motor dissociation. Clinically, these patients have good arm function, moderately impaired hand function, and markedly impaired finger function. Despite crossed sensory pathways, most have sensory deficits for two-point discrimination as well as complex cortical sensory functions. Presumably, sensory function that is not mediated by primary sensory cortex is abnormal (see below). Damage to the primary motor cortex, the sensory–motor dissociation inevitably associated with ipsilateral CSTs, and the presence of significant sensory deficits, given the importance of sensory function in motor control, may all contribute to the relative severity of motor dysfunction associated with the reorganization pattern seen after late-third-trimester lesions.

Interactions of Type and Time of Lesion: Effect on Motor Reorganization and Outcome

As indicated, time of lesion and type of lesion interact; periventricular lesions occur early in the third trimester, while stroke occurs late in the third trimester. Earlier lesions tend to result in contralateral CST reorganization and later lesions in ipsilateral CST reorganization. Not only does time of lesion generally determine reorganization pattern, but the later the lesion in the third trimester, the less effective the ipsilateral CST is for producing good hand function. In other words, the efficacy of ipsilateral CSTs decreases significantly toward the end of the third trimester (Staudt et al., 2004). The structural properties of the lesion could be relevant to the correlation between the time of the lesion and the reorganizational potential at the time of the insult (Staudt et al., 2004). Patients with the "latest" lesions (MCA stroke) also tend to have the most extensive lesions. If true, hand function should largely depend on the contralesional hemisphere, making the size and topography of the lesion less relevant in those patients whose paretic hand is controlled by the contralesional hemisphere via ipsilateral corticospinal projections (solid circles in Fig. 4.6). However, a significant correlation between the time of lesion (within the third trimester) and hand function is still present—the earlier the lesion, the better the hand function. Thus, gestational age at the time of the insult and the effectiveness of reorganization via ipsilateral CSTs are correlated. The persisting correlation between time of lesion and type of lesion in terms of ipsilateral CST efficacy could also reflect differences in "nonprimary" motor contributions from the ipsilesional hemisphere (Staudt et al., 2004). In other words, the poorer outcome in patients with MCA strokes (vs. those with periventricular white matter lesions (and perhaps those with venous strokes earlier in the third trimester; see Chapter 3) may be due in part to the larger lesion size of the former. This argument is countered by a case study. The patient reported had a unilateral brain malformation and a contralesional/ipsilateral CST reorganization pattern. A hemispherectomy for refractory seizures did not affect motor function. The patient had satisfactory hand function, showing that this can occur with

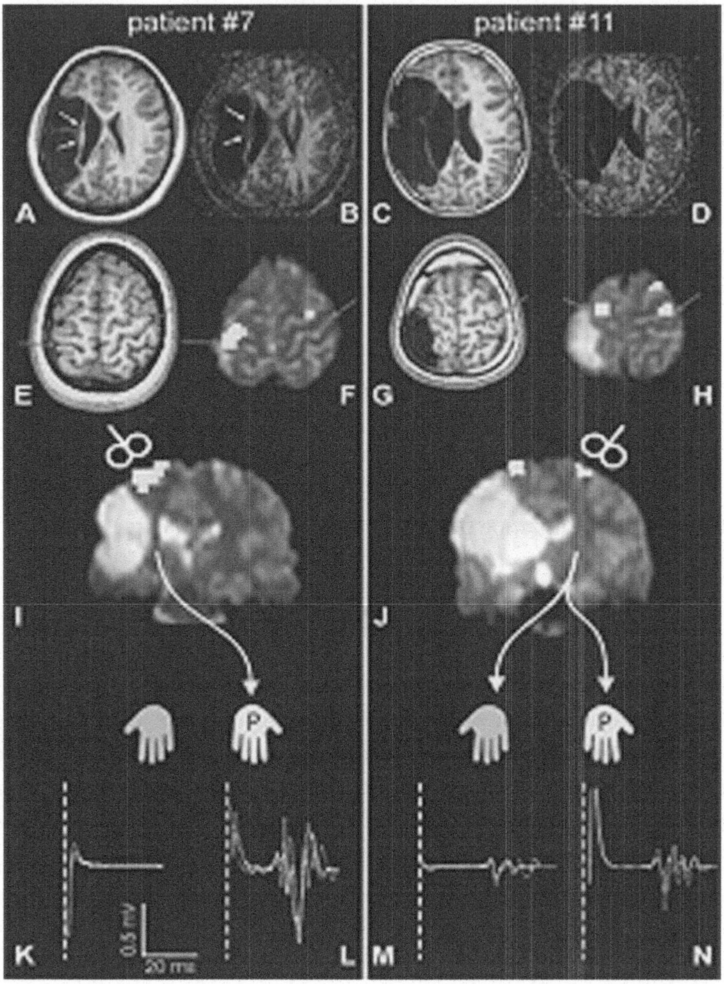

FIGURE 4.5 fMRI and TMS findings for two hemiplegic patients with MCA lesions. In Patient 7 (left column), both TMS and DTI indicated preserved crossed corticospinal projections in a small "bridge" of intact white matter in the affected hemisphere (white arrows in A, B). In Patient 11, in whom the lesion abolished the CST projections from the affected hemisphere, TMS revealed ipsilateral fast-conducting projections from the intact hemisphere to the impaired hand. fMRI showed bilateral activation in both subjects. In Patient 7, the "hand knob" area of the central sulcus was activated in affected hemisphere, whereas in the contralesional hemisphere, activation was located in the precentral sulcus (premotor cortex). In Patient 11, activation was observed in the "hand knobs" of both hemispheres and, in addition, in the precentral sulcus of the contralesional hemisphere. Note that most patients with MCA infarctions and ipsilateral corticospinal pathways showed severe motor impairments, so that an fMRI assessment of active hand function is not possible. Hence, Patient 11 is not typical for this subgroup of patients. (B, D) Axial diffusion tensor imaging at the level of the maximum extent of the lesion. (F, H, I, J). fMRI activation during paretic hand movement at the level of the "hand knob," superimposed on axial (F, H) and coronal (I, J) reconstructions from the averaged (functional) echo planar imaging. On these, a white "figure-eight coil" symbol indicates the hemisphere from which motor evoked potentials (MEP) in the paretic hand (P) could be elicited. These MEP curves are shown in K to N for both the nonparetic hand (K, M) and the paretic hand (L, N). Corresponding anatomical images are shown in A, C, E, and G. Red arrows mark the position of the central sulcus. (Reprinted with permission from Staudt et al., 2004.) (See color insert.)

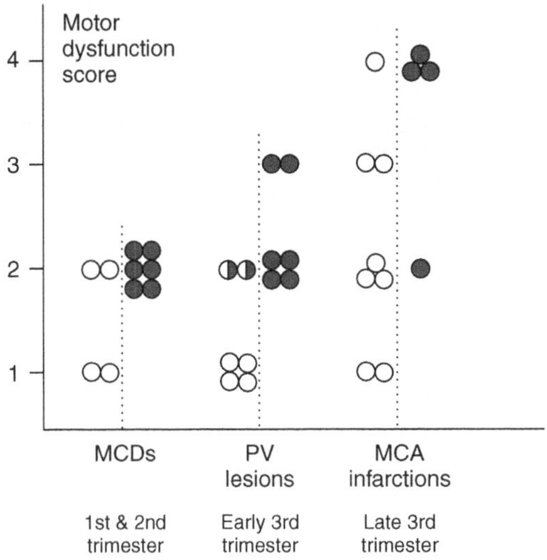

FIGURE 4.6 Comparison of hand function scores among patients with congenital lesions acquired during the three major time periods (malformations of cortical development [MCDs]—first and second trimester of pregnancy; periventricular [PV] lesions—early third trimester of pregnancy; MCA infarctions—late third trimester of pregnancy). Open circles represent patients with preserved crossed corticospinal projections from the affected hemispheres, solid circles, patients with reorganized ipsilateral projections from the contralesional hemispheres; and half-solid circles, patients with both preserved contralateral and reorganized ipsilateral corticospinal projections to the paretic hand. Because of the lower efficacy, shifting the motor representation of the paretic hand to the contralesional hemisphere might not have been a better alternative for these patients, in contrast with patients with malformations of cortical development and periventricular lesions, in whom reorganization with ipsilateral corticospinal tracts could always "offer" a satisfactory hand function (scores 2 and 3). (Reprinted with permission from Staudt et al., 2004.)

purely ipsilateral control without any contribution from the affected hemisphere (Staudt et al., 2001). Thus, the poor hand function of many patients with MCA strokes and ipsilateral CSTs cannot simply be explained by a lack of any "nonprimary" motor contributions from the affected hemisphere due to the size of the brain lesion. More likely, the potential for plasticity/reorganization of the intact hemisphere is already diminished by the late third trimester. Less efficient overall reorganization of ipsilateral CSTs among patients with late-third-trimester MCA strokes results in an even less effective hand. (Recent imaging data suggest that fiber tracking may elucidate different outcomes in patients with similar structural lesions [Holmström et al., 2011; Hoon et al., 2002; 2009; Murakami et al., 2008; Nagae et al., 2007; Staudt et al., 2001 case study].) Even among those subjects with preserved contralateral CSTs from the affected hemisphere (open circles in Fig. 4.6), there was a functional difference between patients with MCA strokes and patients with malformations and periventricular lesions. All of the latter had either good hand function or only moderate impairment, whereas about half of those with MCA strokes were severely impaired. Thus, even when reorganization occurs via contralateral CSTs, time of lesion during the pre-perinatal period affects motor outcome.

Motor Reorganization: Size of Periventricular Lesions

The effect of extent of lesion on motor reorganization has been best delineated for periventricular lesions (Staudt, 2007b, 2010a; Staudt et al., 2002). Ultimately, type of CST reorganization still appears to be the primary factor affecting outcome (Carr et al., 1993; Maegaki et al., 1997; Nezu et al., 1999; Staudt 2010a; Staudt et al., 2002). Patients with small lesions and minor hand impairment (unless the lesion is "strategically placed") have intact contralateral CST projections from the damaged hemisphere to the paretic hand, whereas those with large lesions and more severe hand deficits (impaired individual finger movements) have ipsilateral CST projections from the intact hemisphere to the paretic hand.

Disadvantages of Reorganization: Mirror Movements

Overt mirror movements (MM) are common in normal children and can persist until age 10 years; the intensity decreases with age (Connolly & Stratton, 1968). Mirror movements in young children are thought to reflect intrahemispheric activation during voluntary movements of both the ipsilateral and contralateral CSTs, with the former suppressed towards the end of the first decade by transcallosal inhibition via a more completely myelinated corpus callosum (Nass 1985; Yakolev & LeCours, 1967). In adults transcallosal interhemispheric inhibition of ipsilateral CSTs has been shown to play a significant role in suppressing MM during complex unimanual motor activities (Hubers et al., 2008). Note also that contralateral CSTs are monosynaptic, while ipsilateral CSTs are polysynaptic and branch bilaterally to motor neurons on both sides of the spinal cord (Martin et al., 2007; 2009). Thus, activation of the ipsilateral CST is particularly likely to result in MM. Alternatively, or in addition, the activation of M1 primary motor cortex (contralateral CSTs) in both hemispheres that occurs during unimanual tasks (Mayston et al., 1999) may play a role in MM. Imaging studies show that both unilateral mental motor imagery and actual finger-to-thumb opposition activate the motor cortex of both hemispheres (Cincotta et al., 2003; Gemignani et al., 2004). Pure unimanual motor activity requires that motor output be restricted to the M1 primary motor cortex contralateral to the voluntary movement (Carson, 2005). In this setting the corpus callosum presumably suppresses MM by inhibiting activation of the motor cortex in the non-voluntarily active hemisphere (Hubers et al., 2008). In addition, a number of other neural pathways mediate bilateral interactions between the upper limbs, including primary motor cortex, premotor cortex, supplementary motor area, basal ganglia, and cerebellum (Carson, 2005). Some of these pathways may also play a role in promoting normal mirroring.

In children with hemiplegic CP, MM are prominent and persistent (Nass, 1985; Woods & Teuber, 1978). Mirror movements can be elicited with a wide range of tasks. Complex tasks and tasks requiring strength tend to elicit more MM. The relationship between presence and extent of MM and degree of motor deficit is debated. The degree of MM correlates in some studies, but not in others, with the extent of the motor deficit, whether it is measured by unimanual dexterity, spasticity, and/or strength or bimanual adeptness (Carr et al., 1993; Holmström et al., 2010; Kuhtz-Buschbeck et al., 2000; Staudt et al., 2004; Woods & Teuber, 1978). However, MM may not occur at all in either hand, when the impaired hand is completely plegic (Woods & Teuber, 1978). The reported laterality of MM has also varied from study to study, probably reflecting an interaction among a number of factors, including task used, age of subjects, and degree of motor deficit. Most studies document more mirroring in the good hand when the impaired hand voluntarily performs the task (Kuhtz-Buschbeck et al., 2000; Staudt et al., 2004; Wood & Teuber, 1978). Some report more mirroring in the impaired hand when the good hand voluntarily performs the task (Cernacek, 1961; Green, 1967). Changes in the laterality pattern of mirroring with age may reflect the maturation of the corpus callosum and the emergence of transcallosal inhibition (Nass, 1985).

The exaggerated and persistent MM in hemiplegic CP have generally been attributed to activation of a compensatory ipsilateral CSTs from the intact hemisphere to the impaired hand, which projects from primary motor cortex of the unaffected hemisphere to ipsilateral or both ipsilateral and contralateral spinal motoneurons (Carr et al., 1993; Cincotta et al., 2000; Farmer et al., 1991; Forssberg et al., 1999; Macdonell et al., 1999; Maegaki et al., 1997; Nezu et al., 1999; Nirkko et al., 1997; Norton et al., 2008; Staudt et al., 2002; 2004; Thickbroom et al., 2001). Based on neurophysiological studies, Carr et al. (1993) identified two subgroups with ipsilateral reorganization and different clinical deficit patterns. Those with projections to bilateral spinal motor neurons had marked mirroring (also Farmer et al., 1991) and a mild to moderately impaired hand capable of independent finger movements, while those with only ipsilateral spinal motor neuron projections had minimal mirroring and a moderately impaired hand with few independent finger movements. A third group with a contralateral CST had no mirroring, and a mildly impaired hand with good independent finger movements.

Not all investigators find a correlation between the presence or degree of MM and ipsilateral versus contralateral CST reorganization; that is, the presence of MM does not always indicate ipsilateral CST reorganization (Staudt, 2010a; Staudt et al., 2004; Holmström et al., 2010). When MM were evaluated in the context of the degree of paresis of the affected hand in a group of patients with stroke, subjects with MM in the intact hand during voluntary movements of the paretic hand had contralateral CST projections (Staudt et al., 2004). Thus, MM in the intact hand may not be specific for reorganization with ipsilateral CSTs, but may represent a nonspecific motor "overflow" phenomenon in patients with significant motor impairment (Staudt et al., 2004). On the other hand, some laterality patterns of MM may be predictive of the reorganization pattern. MM in the paretic hand, while moving the intact hand voluntarily, were documented by Staudt et al. (2004) only in patients with ipsilateral CST projections to the paretic hand. Only patients with ipsilateral CSTs showed marked involuntary MM not only in the nonparetic hand while moving the paretic hand voluntarily, but also in the paretic hand while moving the nonparetic hand voluntarily (Holmström et al., 2010; Staudt, 2010). These data suggest that only MM in the paretic hand can be used as a clinical sign of reorganization with ipsilateral CSTs.

Motor reorganization via ipsilateral CSTs from the intact hemisphere to the impaired hand has functional consequences. The normal and impaired hands do not function independently (Hong et al., 2004; 2010). MM may be the "tip of the iceberg" indicative of qualitative differences in motor performance between patients with ipsilateral and contralateral CSTs (Staudt, 2010a). An abnormal ipsilateral CST in the intact hemisphere may be responsible for subtle abnormalities of motor control in that intact hemisphere. MM can interfere with bimanual activities (Kuhtz-Buschbeck et al., 2000; Holmström et al., 2010). Thus, MM are an example of maladaptive plasticity and represent a potential drawback of motor reorganization via an ipsilateral CST.

SOMATOSENSORY SYSTEM

As discussed, there is less potential for reorganization/plasticity of the somatosensory and motor systems than for the cognitive systems (Anderson et al., 2011; Muller et al., 1998a; 1998b) after early focal lesions. The motor and sensory systems are more localized and dependent on specific pathways as well as on each other (sensorimotor integration), while cognitive systems are distributed and interconnected, potentially permitting more extensive intra- and interhemispheric reorganization. Although reorganization of the sensory system pathways maintains a typical contralateral pattern, the sensory system may be even less plastic than the motor system. Little reorganization of the somatosensory cortex is possible. The frequency and severity of sensory deficits, as well as their relatively high rate of bilaterality, suggest this. Furthermore, because of the different reorganization patterns of the somatosensory and motor systems, hemispheric dissociation of the sensory and motor systems is common, potentially exacerbating the deficit in both domains.

THE RANGE OF SENSORY IMPAIRMENTS

Sensory Deficits

Sensory deficits in the affected hand are reported in anywhere from 40% to over 90% of children with generic hemiplegic CP (Bolanos et al., 1989; Clayton et al., 2003; Himmelmann et al., 2007; McLaughlin et al., 2005; Riquelmea & Montoya, 2010; Van Heest et al., 1993; Yekutiel et al., 1994). Sensory deficits are also sometimes found in the unaffected hand (Cooper et al., 1995; Lesny et al., 1993; Wingert et al., 2009). Differences in the features of the cohorts studied (type of lesion and possible bilateral lesions in older studies), age at testing, as well as differences in the tests used and even the manner in which the same task is administered, all contribute to the wide variation in findings. Sensory functions tested in this population include touch, pain, temperature, position sense/proprioception (determining the direction of movement—up or down for finger or toe)/kinesthesia, vibration, two-point discrimination (determining whether one or two points are applied to the fingertip, usually done with a paper clip opened to 3 mm and if necessary on account of poor performance 7 mm), graphesthesia (determining with eyes closed what number or shape is traced on the palm of the hand), and stereognosis (determining what has been placed in the hand) for objects, textures, and two- and three-dimensional shapes. Deficits are most frequently reported for cortical sensory functions (graphesthesia and stereognosis and two-point discrimination), while touch, pain, temperature, and vibration are generally better preserved (Gordon & Duff, 1999; Krumlinde-Sundholm & Eliasson, 2002; Lesny, 1993; Tachdjian & Minear, 1958; Uvebrant, 1988; Wilson & Wilson, 1967a; 1967b; Wilke et al., 2009). Stereognosis requires a blend of tactile, kinesthetic, and proprioceptive sensations, as well as requiring active manipulation of the stimulus (Krumlinde-Sundholm & Eliasson, 2002). The impairment is not surprising given that deficits in each component are described. Proprioceptive and kinesthetic deficits have been variably reported (Tachdjian & Minear 1958; Tizard et al., 1954; Uvebrantm 1988; Wingert et al., 2009). Failure to compare the affected with the unaffected hand and failure to use controls may explain why deficits in proprioception and kinesthesia are inconsistently reported. Kinesthetic testing, unless performed with specialized equipment, does not control for movement velocity or degree of displacement (e.g., standard neurological testing of joint position sense). Wingert et al. (2009) raise the question of whether decreased or abnormal limb use could also secondarily contribute to proprioceptive deficits, such as stiffer muscle spindles secondary to spasticity (Gobel & Brown, 2009). Stereognosis and graphesthesia are more complex in terms of the cognitive requirements for performing the task than are those involved in measuring the primary sensory modalities (Bolanos et al., 1989; Cooper et al., 1995; Dahlin et al., 1998; Gordon & Duff, 1999; Krumlinde-Sundholm & Eliasson, 2002; Mihran & Tachdjian, 1958; Van Heest et al., 1993; Wingert et al., 2008; Wilson and Wilson 1967a, 1967b; Yekutiel et al., 1994). An association and sometimes an interaction between performance on various sensory tests is well described (Krumlinde-Sundholm & Eliasson, 2002; Wilke et al., 2009).

A comprehensive evaluation of sensory function in 25 children aged 5 to 18 years with mild (n = 21) (pincer grip and/or fractionated finger movements possible) or moderate (n = 4) (whole hand grip possible) hemiplegic CP assessed a range of sensory tasks (Fig. 4.7). While performance on all the sensory tasks correlated significantly with each other, indicating that they all measured some shared skills, tests of two-point discrimination with a separation of 3 mm and 7 mm (the size of the fingertip) (Bolanos et al., 1989; Yekutiel et al., 1994), stereognosis for familiar objects (Cooper et al., 1995; Uvebrant, 1988; Yekutiel et al., 1994), and functional sensibility assessed with the pick-up test (comparing performance with and without visual input) were the most useful measures of sensibility (Krumlinde-Sundholm & Eliasson, 2002).

SENSORY–MOTOR INTERACTION

There is a strong correlation between sensibility and motor dexterity (Gordon & Duff, 1999; Krumlinde-Sundholm & Eliasson, 2002; Van Heest et al., 1993; per contra Cooper et al., 1995). Sensory impairments can compound motor deficits. The negative effects of sensory deficits on motor function are not surprising since sensory feedback is fundamental to the execution of voluntary movement of the hand (Gandevia et al., 1992; McCloskey & Prochazka, 1993) and a prerequisite for fine manual dexterity and precision finger movements (Krumlinde-Sundholm & Eliasson, 2002; Tachdjian & Minear, 1958; Taub, 1976; Taub & Wolf, 1997). Impaired sensory function has wide-ranging ramifications for motor function, both at the planning and execution stages (Clayton et al., 2003). Visual information is used to guide the hand in space and in preparation for grasping an object, and tactile input regulates the force of the grasp, provides the control to keep an object from slipping, and helps the hand manipulate objects (Eliasson et al., 1995a;1995b; Gordon & Duff, 1999; Jeannerod 1984; Johansson & Westling 1990). Sensory information from the fingertips is needed when lifting objects with a precision grip to adjust grip force amplitude (Herrmsdoerfer & Nowak, 2009; Johansson & Westling, 1990). This keeps objects, particularly small ones, from slipping, enhances the smoothness of the lift, and facilitates anticipatory control (Eliasson et al., 1995a;1995b; Forssberg et al., 1995).

Lack of sensory input has been shown to delay motor learning (Asanuma & Arissian, 1984). Inadequate sensory information about the tactile or proprioceptive characteristics of an object (e.g., weight, texture) interferes with the development of a plan for grasping and manipulating objects with the fingertips (Gordon & Duff, 1999; Hermsdoerfer & Nowak, 2009). The excessive grip force found in children with hemiplegic CP could be related to impaired tactile

HEMIPLEGIC CHILDREN		DOMINANT HAND					HEMIPLEGIC HAND					
SIDE AFFECTED	AGE	2 PD 3 mm	Pick-up test	STER objects	MONOF	STER forms	2 PD 3 mm	2 PD 7 mm	Pick-up test	STER objects	MONOF	STER forms
R	6	10	1	6	4	5	0	0	0	3	0	0
L	6	10	1	6	4	5	0	0	0	3	2	1
L	13	10	1	6	4	6	0	0	0	3	2	1
R	11	10	1	6	4	6	0	4	0	3	2	0
R	9	10	1	6	4	4	0	0	1	3	4	0
R	6	10	1	6	4	5	0	0	1	3	4	2
R	16	10	1	6	4	6	0	0	2	3	4	0
R	12	10	1	6	4	5	0	0	4	2	4	1
L	14	10	1	6	4	6	0	0	4	1	4	1
L	12	10	1	6	4	5	0	0	4	1	4	1
R	5	10	1	6	4	2	0	0	4	1	3	1
L	13	10	1	6	4	4	0	6	6	1	4	4
R	16	10	1	6	4	6	0	10	6	2	4	1
L	5	10	1	6	4	4	2	10	6	2	4	3
R	8	10	1	6	4	6	3	8	6	1	4	2
R	12	10	1	6	4	6	5	10	6	1	4	6
L	16	10	1	6	4	6	6	10	6	1	4	3
L	18	10	1	6	4	5	6	10	6	1	4	4
R	8	10	1	6	4	4	10	10	6	1	4	5
L	8	10	1	6	4	4	10	10	6	1	4	4
L	10	10	1	6	4	4	10	10	6	1	4	4
R	11	10	1	6	4	5	10	10	6	1	4	4
L	11	10	1	6	4	6	10	10	6	1	4	4
R	15	10	1	6	4	6	10	10	6	1	4	3
R	11	10	1	6	4	4	10	10	6	1	4	3

Fairly Capable/ Capable | Modestly Capable | Minimally Capable | Incapable

FIGURE 4.7 Sensory function in hemiplegic CP. Distribution of results from 25 participants with hemiplegic CP. Left panel shows results from dominant hand and right panel shows results from hemiplegic hand. Shading indicates grades of ability capable to incapable and numbers in boxes are scores achieved. Stereognosis (STER) of objects was assessed by the tactile identification of six familiar objects: Lego brick, eraser, a wooden bead, a paper pellet, a coin, and a shirt button. The objects were first presented to the children when they could see them and they were asked to examine them by touch and name them. The children then indicated from a visual array which item they were feeling. Stereognosis of forms was assessed with 10 flat plastic geometric forms about 45 mm in diameter and 6 mm thick (Ayres, 1972). Functional sensibility was determined by comparing performance on the pick-up test with and without visual feedback (Krumlinde-Sundholm et al., 1998). The pick-up test required that ten wooden cubes, sized 10 mm per side, were picked out of a box (120 × 120 × 40mm), one at a time, as quickly as possible. It was used as a measure of dexterity when performed with visual feedback and as a measure of functional sensibility when performed without visual feedback. (A cutoff value of 2.5 times the speed of the performance when able to see was chosen to be indicative of abnormality, as none of the control children took longer to perform the test than 2.3 times the speed of the test performed when looking.) Some hemiplegic CP children could not perform at all without looking, although they could pick up the cubes when they could see them. Two-point discrimination (2 PD) was assessed using a bent wire paper clip (Moberg, 1991). First a distance of 3 mm, which is considered normal (Cope & Anthony, 1992; Moberg, 1990), was tested; if the child could not discriminate the two points, a distance of 7 mm was tried. The Semmes–Weinstein monofilaments (MONOF) (Weinstein, 1993) were used to evaluate threshold values for touch. (Reprinted with permission from Krumlinde-Sundholm & Eliasson, 2002.)

regulation. Ultimately, they are able to adjust grip force and develop anticipatory control for different textures given enough practice (Eliasson et al., 1995a; Forssberg et al., 1995). Increasing the amount of sensory information available can improve motor function. For example, sensory information about an object can be transferred from the uninvolved to the involved hand, resulting in improved motor performance (Gordon et al., 1999).

Bimanual Functions

Bimanual activities are not affected by sensibility level to the same extent as unimanual function. Although there is a strong correlation between deficient sensibility and dexterity even in children with mild hemiparesis, the relationship between sensory functions like two-point discrimination and the impaired hand's contribution during bimanual tasks like cutting with scissors, carrying a tray, opening a bottle of soda, and using a knife and fork to cut "food" (a "sausage" made of plastic putty) is weak (Krumlinde-Sundholm et al., 1998). Functional sensibility, assessed on the pick-up test (see Fig. 4.7 for description) performed without visual input, does correlate with dexterity and the quality of the hemiplegic hand function in bimanual performance. The functional sensibility score here, though, is really a combined measure of both motor and sensory function, and so is not ideal for assessing the effect of sensibility level (Krumlinde-Sundholm & Eliasson, 2002). The lack of correlation is probably due to the fact that the impaired hand's role in bimanual coordination is really secondary; the bulk of the work is done by the unaffected hand.

ORGANIZATION AND REORGANIZATION OF THE SOMATOSENSORY SYSTEM

Organization of the Normal Somatosensory System

The mature somatosensory pathway projects from exteroceptive (sensitive to environmental factors) and proprioceptive (sensitive to factors within the body) receptors in the extremities to the dorsal root ganglion of the spinal cord. From there the fibers split into two groups, a lateral group (the anterolateral group) and a medial group (dorsal column-medial lemniscal group). The lateral group projects to the substantia gelatinosa and nucleus proprius, where it synapses onto second-order neurons. The pathway then crosses over to the contralateral side and forms the spinothalamic tract. The spinothalamic tract mediates pain, temperature, and global touch. The medial group fibers project to and synapse with cells of the dorsal column nucleus in the medulla. There the pathway crosses over to the contralateral side and forms the medial lemniscus. The medial lemniscus mediates position sense and fine discrimination touch. After crossing over, both the spinothalamic tract and the medial lemniscus project to the ventral posterior nucleus of the thalamus. The thalamocortical afferents then project via the posterior limb of the internal capsule to primary somatosensory cortex and the posterior parietal lobule.

The somatosensory cortex has a specific cytoarchitecture and chemoarchitecture, distribution of efferent and afferent pathways, and gene expression patterns. Two major forms of gene products influence the intrinsic generation of areal identity (morphogens and transcription factors). Genetic regulation of arealization includes the regulatory genes that control specification and patterning centers, and signaling molecules that establish the initial patterning of these genes. The specification and differentiation of the somatosensory cortex is determined by both intrinsic (e.g., genetic mechanisms that operate within the cortex) and by extrinsic factors (e.g., thalamocortical afferent input, brain damage) (O'Leary & Kroll, 2009).

Reorganization of the Somatosensory System after Early Focal Injury: Somatosensory Cortex

Regional specification of the postcentral gyrus as the primary somatosensory cortex occurs early in gestation, well before the thalamocortical afferents reach it and limit reorganization (Juenger et al., 2011). Therefore, cortical lesions (like MCA strokes) affect sensory function to a significantly greater degree than even large white matter periventricular lesions (Wilke et al., 2009). A careful analysis of the exact location of damage of somatosensory cortex in a group of patients with MCA strokes revealed that small regions in the somatosensory cortex (S1), secondary somatosensory cortex (S2), and the inferior parietal cortex were damaged significantly more frequently in those with marked sensory deficits versus those with mild sensory deficits. All the subjects in this study had contralateral CSTs as their motor reorganization pattern and mild to moderate motor deficits (Juenger et al., 2011). Thus, sensory cortex appears to be fixed very early in prenatal development and very specific cortical areas need to be intact if sensory function is not to be severely compromised after MCA strokes. Furthermore, sparing of these important regions is the exception. Here brain injury is an extrinsic factor that significantly alters areal specification.

In addition, evidence of interhemispheric cortical reorganization of the sensory system, as seen in the motor system, is equivocal at best (Wilke et al., 2009). Assessing functional connectivity in relation to sensory impairment, Dinomais et al. (2011) found that patients with MCA strokes displayed more sensory deficits, as well as significantly reduced functional connectivity in the secondary somatosensory cortex, but not in the primary somatosensory cortex, when compared with a group with periventricular lesions. However, when gray matter volume loss was taken into account, the difference between the groups disappeared. Although reduction in functional connectivity within the somatosensory network was associated with more sensory deficits, the deficits were better explained by the overall degree of cortical damage. Despite limited intra- and interhemispheric reorganization (Wilke et al., 2009), deficits after somatosensory cortex lesions do show some variance. Varying degrees and kinds of sensory impairment occur in "generic" hemiplegic CP for no clearly identifiable reason (Guzzetta et al., 2007; Thickbroom et al., 2001).

Reorganization of the Somatosensory System after Early Focal Injury: Thalamocortical Afferents

In contrast to the lack of cortical reorganization capacity, the somatosensory system appears to possess both axonal plasticity (Juenger et al., 2011) and spatial plasticity (Wilke et al., 2009). Unlike the CSTs, which already project "exuberantly" to ipsi- and contralateral spinal cord by gestational week 24 (and over time reorganize by pruning in an activity-dependent fashion postnatally) (Eyre et al., 2007), sensory afferents reach the contralesional cortex (layer IV) at the very beginning of the third trimester (gestational week 26) but still undergo considerable third-trimester and postnatal elaboration (Kostovic & Jovanov-Milosevic, 2006; Kostovic & Judas, 2010). In contrast to the lack of areal specificity in the early distribution of efferent motor projection neurons, the areal specificity of sensory afferent originating in the principal thalamic sensory nuclei is evident in the early stages of their development. Thalamocortical afferent targeting is primarily controlled intracortically by guidance molecules and influenced by neural activity. Thalamocortical afferent projections exhibit areal specificity throughout development (O'Leary & Kroll, 2009). Nonetheless, thalamocortical sensory afferent fibers can reorganize after early- and even late-third-trimester injury (axonal plasticity). Sensory afferents have the capacity to "bypass" even large periventricular lesions (spatial plasticity) by passing through undamaged tissue, presumably into intact somatosensory cortex in the postcentral gyrus (Staudt et al., 2006a) (Fig. 4.8). Imaging studies (DTI) confirm this by showing fibers actually curving around periventricular lesions (Staudt et al., 2002; 2006b). The same potential is present after late-third-trimester stroke/cortical insults, although the "bypass" capacity may not be as extensive (Guzzetta et al., 2007; Staudt 2010a; Staudt et al., 2006b) and the sensory cortex target is not completely intact. Thus, axonal plasticity mediates reorganization of the sensory system through spatial alterations of thalamocortical afferent pathways. Thalamocortical somatosensory projections can "bypass" a lesion and follow alternative routes to the

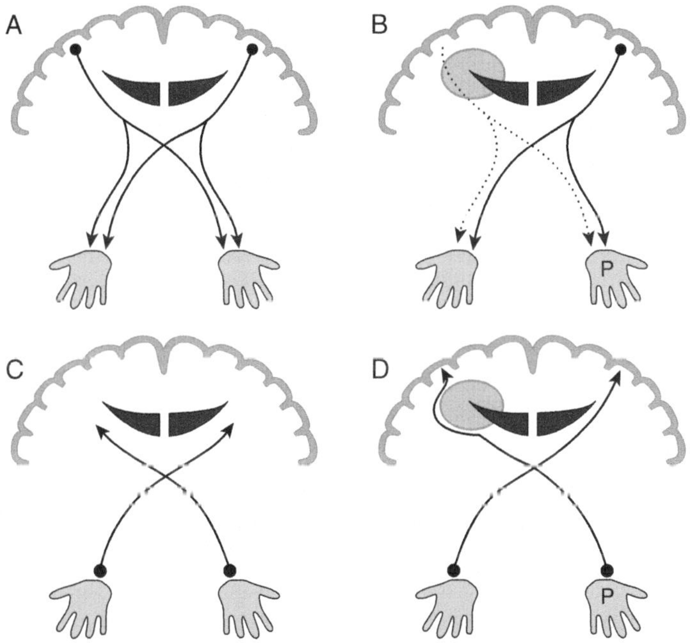

FIGURE 4.8 Schematic of the development of corticospinal motor pathways (top) and thalamocortical somatosensory projection (bottom). At the beginning of the third trimester (A, C), corticospinal motor projections have already arrived at their spinal target areas with still-bilateral projections from each motor cortex, whereas thalamocortical sensory axons have not yet reached their cortical destination. Hypothetically, a unilateral periventricular lesion (gray circle) will not affect thalamocortical somatosensory projections directly, so that the defective tissue can then be bypassed and the cortical target zone can be reached in its original topography (D). The lesion will, however, disrupt the corticospinal motor projections from the affected hemisphere. This will result in a lack of corticospinal input to spinal motor neurons of the paretic hand so that the withdrawal of the ipsilateral projections from the contralesional hemisphere will be inhibited (B). (Reprinted with permission from Staudt et al., 2006a.)

somatosensory cortex, which can differ significantly from predictions that would be made from "adult" anatomy (Staudt et al., 2006b).

Reorganization: Ipsilateral versus Contralateral Afferent Projections

Reorganization of the motor system is a prolonged, dynamic (activity-dependent) process that occurs either via ipsilateral or contralateral CST efferents (more often the former). Importantly, this process is modulated by factors such as the age at lesion and type of lesion. In striking contrast, sensory afferents virtually always remain contralateral (per contra, Maegaki et al., 1999; Ragazzoni et al., 2002) regardless of the time of the injury, be it an early-third-trimester periventricular injury or a late-third-trimester stroke. While motor activity itself plays a role in motor reorganization (Eyre et al., 2007; Martin et al., 2007, 2009), sensory impairments/feedback do not affect the reorganization of sensory afferents. Nor does the type of reorganization of sensory afferents appear to affect the type of CST motor reorganization. All degrees of sensory impairment are documented in children with both ipsilateral and contralateral CST motor reorganization (Guzzetta et al., 2007). The role of the sensory system in driving the type of CST motor reorganization, if present at all, is probably masked by other more critical factors, such as the location and extent of the lesion. This contrasts with the marked effect that sensory deficits have on motor function.

Reorganization: Imaging Data

Imaging studies corroborate the ipsilesional/contralateral reorganization of somatosensory function. fMRI studies demonstrate that the primary somatosensory representation of the hemiparetic hand is in the Rolandic cortex of the affected hemisphere, even with large periventricular brain lesions (Staudt, 2007b; 2010a; Staudt et al., 2006a; 2006b). Passive movement of both the unaffected and affected hands results in fMRI activation in the contralateral hemispheres (Thickbroom et al., 2001). Passive movement or tactile stimulation of the impaired hand can produce ipsilateral activation, but only in non-primary sensory cortex (Bernasconi et al., 2000; Bittar et al., 2000; Chu et al., 2000). There appears to be some correlation between extent of sensory impairment and extent of cortical activation in the contralateral perirolandic region after sensory stimulation (Cao et al., 1994; Chu et al., 2000; Guzzetta et al., 2007; Thickbroom et al., 2001), but individual variability is very common (Chu et al., 2000). Sensory stimulation does produce some activity in the ipsilateral hemisphere, but the degree of ipsilateral activation does not correlate with the quality of sensory function, consistent with the view that the unaffected hemisphere does not play a major role in restoring sensory function (Guzzetta et al., 2007).

Reorganization: Neurophysiologic Data

Somatosensory evoked potentials following peripheral nerve stimulation are generally absent or abnormal after stroke in the affected and unaffected hemispheres, respectively (Cooper et al., 1995; Ferri et al., 2001). In one case study somatosensory evoked potentials showed slow-conducting, probably non-lemniscal connections between the affected arm and ipsilateral non-primary somatosensory cortex (Ragazzoni et al., 2002).

Reorganization: Sensory-Motor Association and Dissociation[10]

Since reorganization of the motor system is primarily through ipsilateral CSTs, and reorganization of the sensory system is primarily contralateral, a dissociation between the hemisphere mediating motor function and the hemisphere mediating sensory function is common. The functional consequences of sensory–motor association versus sensory–motor dissociation are not yet well understood. However, data are accumulating to suggest that overall outcome is affected by the status of sensory–motor integration circuitry. Motor function and sensory function appear to be reciprocally related when they are represented in the same hemisphere, while they are only partially or even totally unrelated if sensory–motor dissociation occurs (Guzzetta et al., 2007) (Fig. 4.9). The advantage of sensory–motor association may be mediated partly by intrahemispheric interconnections between primary sensory and motor cortex, which are considered crucial for the quality of motor performance and for the degree of recovery following focal lesions (Asanuma & Arissian, 1984). This view is supported by the demonstration of severe metabolic depression in the thalamus (part of the sensory relay system) ipsilateral to the affected hemisphere in adults with poor or no improvement of hand function after stroke (Binkofski et al., 1996). The thalamus plays an important gating role. Recent DTI studies of preterm infants with periventricular lesions demonstrate that thalamocortical tract integrity, responsible for transmitting sensory information, correlates better with motor outcome than does CST integrity (Hoon et al., 2002; 2009; Nagae et al., 2007; Wilke et al., 2009),[11] supporting the importance of intrahemispheric sensorimotor integration. Both motor and sensory deficits found in hemiplegic CP due to periventricular lesions could be related to the severity of injury in the diffuse thalamocortical projections (posterior thalamic radiation) to the somatosensory and parietal cortex (Coq et al., 2008).

Not all investigators find sensory–motor association to be an advantage. Comparing a small group of patients with MCA strokes and contralateral CSTs to a group with periventricular lesions and ipsilateral CSTs (the reverse of the typical motor reorganization pattern seen after these two lesion types), all of whom had about equal mild to moderate motor deficits, Wilke et al. (2009) found that the periventricular lesion group with sensory–motor dissociation had fewer sensory deficits, particularly on two-point discrimination, and to a lesser degree for vibration. These investigators speculate that a damaged hemisphere may not

---

[10] Cajal, over a century ago, speculated that the motor system was crossed because the sensory system was crossed. Crossing at the optic chiasm was necessary for optimal vision; hence, crossing of the tactile pathways became necessary so that these two sensory inputs would be co-localize, generating a global sensory representation contralateral to the stimulus. Since manual skills mediated by the CST are dependent on adequate visual and tactile inputs, the motor system needs to be crossed in parallel with the crossed sensory representation to ensure that the correct limb is activated by sensory stimuli. Crossed output and input tracts facilitate multimodal function in association cortex (Vulliemoz et al., 2005). Assuming this scenario, reorganization that involves sensory–motor association (see below) would be more effective than reorganization in which the sensory and motor systems dissociate (i.e., are controlled in different hemispheres). The clinical correlation between motor and sensory deficits suggests that sensorimotor integration is important to best motor outcome (Thickbroom et al., 2001).

[11] Fiber tracking may turn out to be a better way of determining extent of injury and predicting degree of deficit than traditional imaging (Holmstrom et al., 2011; Murakami et al., 2008).

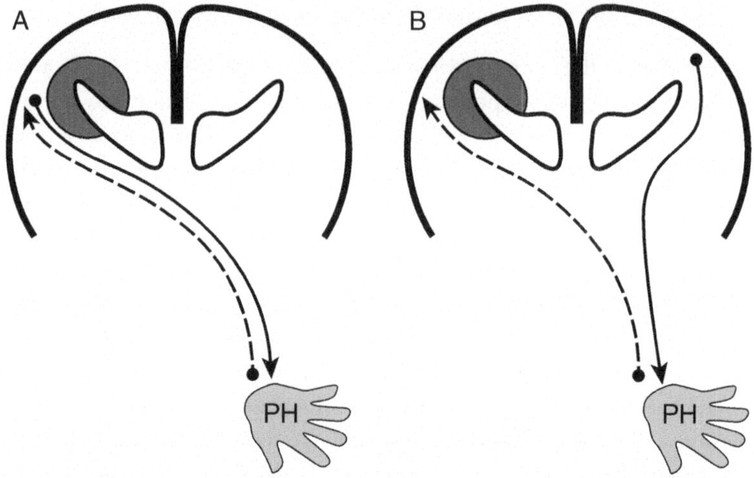

FIGURE 4.9 Schematic representation of the different types of sensory (S) and motor (M) reorganization following early brain lesion. (a) Both motor function and sensory function reorganize in the ipsilesional hemisphere. (b) A dissociation between motor and sensory function is observed: motor function is reorganized in the contralesional hemisphere and sensory function is reorganized in the ipsilesional hemisphere. (From Guzzetta et al., 2007, with permission.)

be able to support both motor and sensory function; hence, those with sensory–motor dissociation fare better from a sensory vantage than those with sensory–motor association. Sensory–motor integration may not be the only factor relevant to preserving sensory function. On the other hand, the damage to sensory cortex itself from the MCA stroke likely has a profound effect on sensory function. Consistent with this notion, some studies have shown a correlation between degree of sensory impairment and extent of cortical activation during fMRI (Guzzetta et al., 2007; Wilke et al., 2009).

Outcome: Plasticity Is Modality-Specific

Cognitive outcome after early-third-trimester periventricular injury and late-third-trimester stroke is significantly better than motor and sensory outcome. Obvious motor and sensory deficits are the rule, while cognitive deficits in a range of domains, while present, are considerably more subtle. Although the motor cortex is capable of reorganization, a less effective ipsilateral (vs. contralateral) CST is the most common reorganization pattern. Nevertheless, even an ipsilateral CST after perinatal injury allows for better motor function than occurs after stroke in adults. The clinical motor deficit itself may actually interfere further with recovery, since the activity-dependent maturation of the CST at the spinal level is disrupted and ipsilateral CST projection are not pruned and thus do not allow for the normal elaboration of a contralateral CST necessary for the development of normal dexterity. Thus, deficits emerge and evolve over time. The sensory system undergoes very early areal specification and thus lacks cortical plasticity; sensory pathways cannot move from a damaged to undamaged hemisphere. While axonal and spatial plasticity allow for continuing contralateral representation of sensory functions, the afferent pathways are anatomically atypical and clinical deficits are apparent. Furthermore, the commonly resulting sensory motor disassociation (motor function in the intact hemisphere and sensory function in the damaged one) may interfere with sensory motor integration necessary to optimize motor and sensory function. The evolutionarily old sensory and motor systems, with less capacity for reorganization than cognitive systems, also appear to be strongly interrelated: dysfunction in one has significant negative consequences for the other. This contrasts with newer cognitive systems that are both more adaptable and exhibit more widely distributed networks. Some of the treatments discussed in Chapter 10 have begun to make use of our knowledge of motor and somatosensory reorganization.

REFERENCES

Anderson V, Spencer-Smith M, Wood A (2011). Do children really recover better? Neurobehavioural plasticity after early brain insult. *Brain* 134:2197–2215.

Aramaki Y, Honda M, Sadato N (2006). Suppression of the nondominant motor cortex during bimanual symmetric finger movement: a functional magnetic resonance image study. *Neuroscience* 141:2147–2153.

Armand J (1982). The origin, course and terminations of corticospinal fibers in various mammals. *Prog Brain Res* 57:329–360.

Arner M, Eliasson AC, Nicklasson S, Sommerstein K, Hagglund G (2008). Hand function in cerebral palsy: Report of 367 children in a population-based longitudinal health care program. *J Hand Surg* 33:1337–1347.

Asanuma H, Arissian S (1984). Experiments on functional role of peripheral input to motor cortex during voluntary movement in the monkey. *J Neurophysiol* 52:212–227.

Ayres, A. J. (1972). *Sensory integration and learning disorders*. Los Angeles: Western Psychological Services.

Barnett A, Mercuri E, Rutherford M, Haataja L, Frisone MF, Henderson S, Cowan F, Dubowitz L (2002). Neurological and perceptual-motor outcome at 5–6 years of age in children with neonatal encephalopathy: relationship with neonatal brain MRI. *Neuropediatrics* 33: 242–248.

Bax M, Goldstein M, Rosenbaum P, Leviton A, Paneth N, Dan B, Jacobsson B, Damiano D (2005). Proposed definition and classification of cerebral palsy. *Dev Med Child Neurol* 47: 571–576.

Bax M, Tydeman C, Flodmark O (2006). Clinical and MRI correlates of cerebral palsy. The European Cerebral Palsy Study. *JAMA* 296:1602–1608.

Beckang E, Carlsson G, Carlsdotter S, Uvebrant P (2007). The natural history of gross motor development in children with cerebral palsy. *Dev Med Child Neurol* 49:751–756.

Benecke R, Meyer BU, Freund HJ (1991). Reorganisation of descending motor pathways in patients after hemispherectomy and severe hemispheric lesions demonstrated by magnetic brain stimulation. *Exp Brain Res* 83:419–426.

Bernasconi A, Bernasconi N, Lassonde M, Toussaint PJ, Meyer E,Reutens DC, Gotman J, Andermann F, Villemure JG (2000). Sensorimotor organization in patients who have undergone hemispherectomy:a study with (15)O-water PET and somatosensory evoked potentials. *Neuroreport* 11:3085–3090.

Berweck S, Walther M, Brodbeck V, Wagner N, Koerte I, Henschel V, Juenger H, Staudt M, Mall V (2008). Abnormal motor cortex excitability in congenital stroke. *Pediatr Res* 63: 84–88.

Binkofski F, Seitz R, Arnold S, Classen J, Benecke R, Freund H (1996). Thalamic metabolism and corticospinal tract integrity determine motor recovery in stroke. *Ann Neurol* 39:460–470.

Bittar RG, Olivier A, Sadikot AF, Andermann F, Reutens DC (2000). Cortical motor and somatosensory representation: effect of cerebral lesions. *J Neurosurg* 92:242–248.

Boardman JP, Ganesan V, Rutherford MA, Saunders DE, Mercuri E, Cowan F (2005). Magnetic resonance image correlates of hemiparesis after neonatal and childhood middle cerebral artery stroke. *Pediatrics* 115:321–326.

Bolanos AA, Bleck EE, Firestone P, Young L (1989). Comparison of stereognosis and two-point discrimination testing of the hands of children with cerebral palsy. *Dev Med Child Neurol* 31:371–376.

Bouza H, Dubowitz LM, Rutherford M, Pennock J (1994). Prediction of outcome in children with congenital hemiplegia: a magnetic resonance imaging study. *Neuropediatrics* 25:60–66.

Brown JV, Schumacher U, Rohlmann A, Ettlinger G, Schmidt RC, Skreczek W (1989). Aimed movements to visual targets in hemiplegic and normal children: is the "good" hand of children with infantile hemiplegia also normal? *Neuropsychologia* 27:283–302.

Brown JK, van Rensburg F, Walsh G, Lakie M, Wright GW (1987). A neurological study of hand function of hemiplegic children. *Dev Med Child Neurol* 29:287–304.

Brown JK, Walsh EG (2001). Neurology of the upper limb. In Neville B, Goodman R (eds), Congenital Hemiplegia. London: Mac Keith Press, pp. 113–149.

Candy EJ, Hoon AH, Capute AJ, Bryan RN (1993). MRI in motor delay: important adjunct to classification of cerebral palsy. *Pediatr Neurol* 9:421–429.

Cao Y, Vikingstadt EM, Huttenlocher PR, Towle VL, Levin DN (1994). Functional magnetic resonance studies of the reorganization of the human hand sensorimotor area after unilateral brain injury in the perinatal period. *Proc Natl Acad Sci USA* 91:9612–9616.

Carr LJ (1996). Development and reorganization of descending motor pathways in children with hemiplegic cerebral palsy. *Acta Paediatr* 416:53–57.

Carr LJ, Harrison LM, Evans AL, Stephens JA (1993). Patterns of central motor reorganization in hemiplegic cerebral palsy. *Brain* 116:1223–1247.

Carr LJ, Harrison LM, Stephens JA (1994). Evidence for bilateral innervation of certain homologous motoneurone pools in man. *J Physiol* 475:217–227.

Carson RG (2005). Neural pathways mediating bilateral interactions between the upper limbs. *Brain Res Rev* 49:641–662.

Cernacek J (1961). Contralateral motor irradiation—cerebral dominance. Its changes in hemiplegia. *Arch Neurol* 4:165–172.

Chakrabarty S, Shulman B, Martin JH (2009). Activity-dependent codevelopment of the corticospinal system and target interneurons in the cervical spinal cord. *J Neurosci* 29: 8816–8827.

Chang J, Wu T, Su F (2005). Kinematical measure for spastic reaching in children with cerebral palsy. *Clin Biomech* 20:381–388.

Chu D, Huttenlocher PR, Levin DN, Towle VL (2000). Reorganization of the hand somatosensory cortex following perinatal unilateral brain injury. *Neuropediatrics* 31:63–69.

Cincotta M, Borgheresi A, Liotta P, Montigiani A, Marin E, Zaccara G, Ziemann U (2000). Reorganization of the motor cortex in a patient with congenital hemiparesis and mirror movements. *Neurology* 55:129–131.

Cincotta M, Borgheresi A, Ragazzoni A, Vanni P, Balestrieri F, Benvenuti F, Zaccara G, Ziemann U (2003). Motor control in mirror movements: studies with transcranial magnetic stimulation. *Supp Clin Neurophysiol* 56:175–180.

Cioni G, Einspieler C, Paolicelli P (2007). Other approaches to neurological assessment. In: Cioni G (ed), Neurological Assessment in the First Two Years of Life. London: MacKeith Press, pp. 56–61.

Cioni G, Sales B, Paolicelli PB, Petacchi E, Scusa MF, Canapicchi R (1999). MRI and clinical characteristics of children with hemiplegic cerebral palsy. *Neuropediatrics* 30: 249–255.

Cioni G, Sgandurra G, Muzzini S, et al. (2010). Forms of hemiplegia. In: Ferrari A, Cioni G. (eds), The Spastic Forms of Cerebral Palsy: A Guide to the Assessment of Adaptive Functions. Springer Verlag Italia, pp. 331–356.

Clayton K, Fleming JM, Copley J. (2003) Behavioral responses to tactile stimuli in children with cerebral palsy. *Phys Occup Ther Pediatr*. 23(1):43–62.

Cohen ME, Dufner PK (1981). Prognostic indicators in hemiparetic cerebral palsy. *Ann Neurol* 9:353–357.

Colebatch JG, Gandevia SC (1989). The distribution of muscular weakness in upper motor neuron lesions affecting the arm. *Brain* 112:749–763.

Connolly K, Stratton P. (1968) Developmental changes in associated movements. *Dev Med Child Neurol*. 10(1):49–56

Cooper J, Majnemer A, Rosenblatt B, Birnbaum R (1995). The determination of sensory deficits in children with hemiplegic cerebral palsy. *J Child Neurol* 10:300–309.

Cope E, Anthony J. (1992) Normal values for the two-point discrimination test. *Pediatric Neurology* 8: 251–4.

Coq JO, Strata F, Russier M, Safadi FF, Merzenich MM, Byl NN (2008). Impact of neonatal asphyxia and hind limb immobilization on musculoskeletal tissues and S1 map organization: Implications for cerebral palsy. *Exp Neurol* 210: 95–108.

Cowan FM, de Vries LS (2005). The internal capsule in neonatal imaging. *Semin Fetal Neonatal Med* 10:461–474.

Crajé C, Van der Kamp J, Steenbergen B (2009). Visual information for action planning in left and right congenital hemiparesis. *Brain Res* 1261:54–64.

Craje C, van Elka M, Beerena M, van Schieb HT, Bekkeringa H, Steenbergenb B (2010). Compromised motor planning and motor imagery in right hemiparetic cerebral palsy. *Res Dev Disabilities* 31:1313–1322.

Curry CJ, Bhullar S, Holmes J, Delozier CD, Roeder ER, Hutchison HT (2007). Risk factors for perinatal arterial stroke: a study of 60 mother-child pairs. *Pediatr Neurol* 37:99–107.

Dahlin LB, Komoto-Tufvesson Y, Salgeback S (1998). Surgery of the spastic hand in cerebral palsy. Improvement in stereognosis and hand function after surgery. *J Hand Surg [Br]* 23: 334–339.

Davidoff RA (1990). The pyramidal tract. *Neurology* 40:332–339.

Dellatolas G, Filho GN, Souza L, Nunes LG, Braga LW (2005). Manual skill, hand skill asymmetry, and neuropsychological test performance in school children with spastic cerebral palsy. *Laterality* 10:161–182.

DeMatteo C, Law M, Russell D, Pollock N, Rosenbaum P, Walter S (1992). QUEST: Quality of Upper Extremity Skills Test. Quest Manual. Ontario: CanChild Press.

DeMatteo C, Law M, Russell D, Pollock N, Rosenbaum P, Walter S. (1993). The reliability and validity of Quality of Upper Extremity Skills Test. *Physical and Occupational Therapy in Pediatrics* 13:1–18.

de Vries LS, Groenendaal F, Eken P, Van Haastert IC, Rademaker KJ, Meiners LC (1997). Infarcts in the vascular distribution of the middle cerebral artery in preterm and full-term infants. *Neuropediatrics* 28:88–96.

de Vries LS, van der GJ, van Haastert IC, Groenendaal F (2005). Prediction of outcome in newborn infants with arterial ischaemic stroke using diffusion-weighted magnetic resonance imaging. *Neuropediatrics* 36:12–20.

Dimitropoulou K, Adolph K, Nass R (2007). Reaching in hemiplegic CP. Presented at American Academy of Neurology meeting, Boston, April 2007.

Dinomais M, Groeschel S, Staudt M, Krageloh-Mann I, Wilke M (2011). Relationship between functional connectivity and sensory impairment: Red flag or red herring? *Hum Brain Mapp* 33:628–638. *[e-pub March 9].*

Domi T, deVeber G, Shroff M, Kouzmitcheva E, MacGregor DL, Kirton A (2009). Corticospinal tract pre-wallerian degeneration: a novel outcome predictor for pediatric stroke on acute MRI. *Stroke* 40:780–787.

Duff SV, Gordon AM (2003). Learning of grasp control in children with hemiplegic cerebral palsy. *Dev Med Child Neurol* 45:746–757.

Duque J, Thonnard JL, Vandermeeren Y, Sébire G, Cosnard G, Olivier E (2003). Correlation between impaired dexterity and corticospinal tract dysgenesis in congenital hemiplegia. *Brain* 126:732–747.

Eliasson AC, Forssberg H, Hung Y-C, Gordon AM (2006b). Development of hand function and precision grip control in individuals with cerebral palsy: a 13-year follow-up study. *Pediatrics* 118:1723–1725.

Eliasson AC, Forssberg H, Ikuta K, Apel I, Westling G, Johansson R (1995a). Development of human precision grip. V. Anticipatory and triggered grip actions during sudden loading. *Exp Brain Res* 106:425–433.

Eliasson AC, Gordon AM (2000). Impaired force coordination during object release in children with hemiplegic cerebral palsy. *Dev Med Child Neurol* 42:228–234.

Eliasson AC, Gordon AM, Forssberg H (1991). Basic co-ordination of manipulative force of children with cerebral palsy. *Dev Med Child Neurol* 33:661–670.

Eliasson AC, Gordon AM, Forssberg H (1992). Impaired anticipatory control of isometric forces during grasping by children with cerebral palsy. *Dev Med Child Neurol* 34:216–225.

Eliasson AC, Gordon AM, Forssberg H (1995b). Tactile control of isometric fingertip forces during grasping in children with cerebral palsy. *Dev Med Child Neurol* 37:72–84.

Eliasson AC, Krumlinde-Sundholm L, Rosblad B, Beckung E, Arner M, Ohrvall AM, Rosenbaum P (2006a). The Manual Ability Classification System (MACS) for children with cerebral palsy: scale development and evidence of validity and reliability. *Dev Med Child Neurol* 48:549–554.

Eyre J (2007). Corticospinal tract development and its plasticity after perinatal injury. *Neuroscience and Biobehavioral Reviews* 31:1136–1149.

Eyre J, Smith M, Dabydeen L, Clowry G, Petacchi E, Battini R,Guzzetta A, Cioni G (2007). Is hemiplegic cerebral palsy equivalent to amblyopia of the corticospinal system? *Ann Neurol* 62:493–503.

Eyre JA, Taylor JP, Villagra F, Smith M, Miller S (2001). Evidence of activity-dependent withdrawal of corticospinal projections during human development. *Neurology* 57:1543–1554.

Fadiga L, Buccino G, Graighero L, Fogasso L, Gallese V, Pavesi G (1999). Corticospinal excitability is specifically modulated by motor imagery: a magnetic stimulation study. *Neuropsychologia* 37:147–158.

Farmer SF, Harrison LM, Ingram DA, Stephens JA (1991). Plasticity of central motor pathways in children with hemiplegic cerebral palsy. *Neurology* 41:1505–1510.

Fedrizzi E, Oleari G, Inverno M et al. (1994). Motor performance assessment in children with CP. In: Fedrizzi E, Avanzini G, Crenna E (eds), Motor Development in Childhood. London: John Libbey, pp. 51–58.

Fedrizzi E, Pagliano E, Andreucci E, Oleari G (2003). Hand function in children with hemiplegic cerebral palsy: prospective follow-up and functional outcome in adolescence. *Dev Med Child Neurol* 45:85–91.

Feldman AB, Haley SM, Coryell J (1990). Concurrent and construct validity of the Pediatric Evaluation of Disability Inventory. *Phys Ther* 70:602–610.

Ferrari A, Cioni G. (eds). (2010). The Spastic Forms of Cerebral Palsy: A Guide to the Assessment of Adaptive Functions. Springer Verlag Italia.

Ferri R, Elia M, Musumeci SA, Cosentino FII, Roccasalva G, Spada RS, Toscano G (2001). Somatosensory evoked potentials in patients affected by unilateral cerebrovascular lesions with onset during the perinatal period or adulthood. *J Child Neurol* 16:541–547.

Folio M, Fewell R (1983). Peabody Developmental Motor Scales. Chicago: Riverside Publishers.

Fonseca ST, Holt KG, Fetters L, Saltzman E (2004). Dynamic resources used in ambulation by children with spastic hemiplegic cerebral palsy: relationship to kinematics, energetics, and asymmetries. *Phys Ther* 84:344–354.

Forssberg H, Eliasson AC, Kinoshita H, Westling G, Johansson RS (1995). Development of human precision grip. *IV: Tactile adaptation of isometric finger forces to the frictional condition. Exp Brain Res* 104:323–330.

Forssberg H, Eliasson A-C, Redon-Zouitenn C, Mercuri E, Dubowitz L (1999). Impaired grip-lift synergy in children with unilateral brain lesions. *Brain* 122:1157–1168.

Gage JR. (2009). An overview of normal walking. In: Gage J, Schwartz M, Koop S, Novacheck T. (eds), The Identification and Treatment of Gait Problems in Cerebral Palsy (Clinics in Developmental Medicine). London: MacKeith Press.

Gandevia SC, McCloskey DI, Burke D (1992). Kinaesthetic signals and muscle contraction. *Trends Neurosci* 15: 62–65.

Ganesan V, Ng V, Chong WK, Kirkham FJ, Conelly A (1999). Lesion volume, lesion location, and outcome after middle cerebral artery territory stroke. *Arch Dis Child* 81: 295–300.

Gemignani M, DiStefano L, Sebastiani B (2004). Influence of mental motor imagery on the execution of a finger-to-thumb opposition task. *Revues de Biologie* 142:1–9.

Gobel DJ, Brown SH (2009). Dynamic proprioceptive target matching behavior in the upper limb: Effects of speed, task difficulty and arm/hemisphere asymmetries. *Behav Brain Res* 200:7–14.

Goldman PS (1974). An alternative to developmental plasticity: Heterology of CNS structures in infants and adults. In: Stein DG, Rosen JJ, Butters N (eds), Plasticity and Recovery of Function in the Central Nervous System. New York: Academic Press.

Golomb MR, de Veber GA, MacGregor DL, Domi T, Whyte H, Stephens D, Dick PT (2003). Independent walking after neonatal arterial ischemic stroke and sinovenous thrombosis. *J Child Neurol* 18:530–536.

Golomb MR, Garg BP, Saha C, Azzouz F, Williams LS (2008). Cerebral palsy after perinatal arterial ischemic stroke. *J Child Neurol* 23:279–286.

Golomb MR, MacGregor DL, Domi T, Armstrong DC, McCrindle B, Mayank S, deVeber GA (2001). Presumed pre- and perinatal stroke: risk factors and outcomes. *Ann Neurol* 50: 163–168.

Gordon AM, Charles J, Duff SV (1999). Fingertip forces during object manipulation in children with hemiplegic cerebral palsy, II: Bilateral coordination. *Dev Med Child Neurol* 41:176–185.

Gordon AM, Duff SV (1999). Relation between clinical measures and fine manipulative control in children with hemiplegic cerebral palsy. *Dev Med Child Neurol* 41:586–591.

Gordon AM, Forssberg H, Johansson RS, Westling G (1991). Integration of sensory information during the programming of precision grip: comments on the contributions of size cues. *Exp Brain Res* 85:226–229.

Gordon AM, Lewis SR, Eliasson AC, Duff SV (2003). Object release under varying task constraints in children with hemiplegic cerebral palsy. *Dev Med Child Neurol* 45:240–248.

Gordon AM, Steenbergen B (2008). Bimanual coordination in children with cerebral palsy. In: Eliasson AC, Burtner P (eds), Improving Hand Function in Children with Cerebral Palsy: Theory, Evidence and Intervention. Clinics in Developmental Medicine. London: MacKeith Press, pp. 160–175.

Govaert P, Matthys E, Zecic A, Roelens F, Oostra A, Vanzieleghem B (2000). Perinatal cortical infarction within middle cerebral artery trunks. *Arch Dis Child Fetal Neonatal* 82:F59–F63.

Govaert P, Zingman A, Jung YH, Dudink J, Swarte R, Zecic A, Meersschaut V, van Engelen S, Lequin M (2008). Network injury to pulvinar with neonatal arterial ischemic stroke. *NeuroImage* 39:1850–1857.

Greaves S, Imms C, Dodd K, Krumlinde-Sundholm L (2010). Assessing bimanual performance in young children with hemiplegic cerebral palsy: a systematic review. *Dev Med Child Neurol* 52:413–421.

Green JB (1967). An electromyographic study of mirror movements. *Neurology* 7:91–94.

Guzzetta A, Bonanni P, Biagi L, Tosetti M, Montanaro D, Guerrini R, Cioni G (2007). Reorganization of the somatosensory system after early brain damage. *Clin Neurophysiol* 118:1110–1121.

Guzzetta A, Mercuri E, Rapisardi G, Ferrari F, Roversi MF, Cowan F, Rutherford M, Paolicelli PB, Einspieler C, Boldrini A, Dubowitz L, Prechetl HFR, Cioni G (2003). General movements detect early signs of hemiplegia in term infants with neonatal cerebral infarction. *Neuropediatrics* 34:61–66.

Guzzetta A, Pizzardi A, Belmonti V, Boldrini A (2010). Hand movements at 3 months predict later hemiplegia in term infants with neonatal stroke. *Dev Med Child Neurol* 52:767–772.

Hanna S, Law M, Rosenbaum P, King GA, Walter SD, Pollock N, Russell DJ (2003). Development of hand function among children with cerebral palsy: growth curve analysis for ages 16 to 70 months. *Dev Med Child Neurol* 45:448–455.

Hega N, Heijden-Maessen H, van Hoorn J, et al. (2007). Test-retest and inter- and intra-rater reliability of the quality of the upper extremity skills test in preschool-aged children with cerebral palsy. *Arch Phys Med Rehab* 88:1686–1688.

Herrmsdoerfer J, Nowak DA (eds). (2009). Sensorimotor Control of Grasping: Physiology and Pathophysiology. New York: Cambridge University Press.

Himmelmann K, Beckung E, Hagberg G, Uvebrant P (2007). Bilateral spastic cerebral palsy-Prevalence through four decades, motor function and growth. *Eur J Paediatr Neurol* 11: 215–222.

Holmefur M, Krumlinde-Sundholm L, Bergstr J, Eliasson A-C (2010). Longitudinal development of hand function in children with unilateral cerebral palsy. *Dev Med Child Neurol* 52:352–357.

Holmstrom L, Lennartsson F, Eliasson AC, Flodmark O, Clark C, Tedroff K, Forssberg H, Vollmer B (2011). Diffusion MRI in corticofugal fibers correlates with hand function in unilateral cerebral palsy. *Neurology* 77:775–783.

Holmström L, Vollmer B, Tedroff K, Islam M, Persson JK, Kits A, Forssberg H, Eliasson AC (2010). Hand function in relation to brain lesions and corticomotor-projection pattern in children with unilateral cerebral palsy. *Dev Med Child Neurol* 52: 145–152.

Hoon AH, Lawrie WT, Melhem ER, Reinhardt EM, Van Zijl PC, Solaiyappan M, Jiang H, Johnston MV, Mori S (2002). Diffusion tensor imaging of periventricular leukomalacia shows affected sensory cortex white matter pathways. *Neurology* 59:752–756.

Hoon AH, Stashinko EE, Nagae LM, Lin DD, Keller J, Bastian A, Campbell M, Levey E, Mori S, Johnston M (2009). Sensory and motor deficits in children with cerebral palsy born preterm correlate with diffusion tensor imaging abnormalities in thalamocortical pathways. *Dev Med Child Neurol* 51:697–704.

Hubers A, Orekhov Y, Ziemann U (2008). Interhemipshereic motor inhibition. *Eur J Neurosci* 28:363–371.

Humphreys P, Whiting S, Pham B (2000). Hemiparetic cerebral palsy: clinical pattern and imaging in prediction of outcome. *Can J Neurol Sci* 27:210–219.

Hung YC, Charles J, Gordon AM (2004). Bimanual coordination during a goal-directed task in children with hemiplegic cerebral palsy. *Dev Med Child Neurol* 46:746–753.

Hung YC, Charles J, Gordon AM (2010). Influence of accuracy constraints on bimanual coordination during a goal-directed task in children with hemiplegic cerebral palsy. *Exp Brain Res* 201:421–428.

Husson B, Hertz-Pannier L, Renaud C, Allard D, Presles E, Landrieu P, Chabrier S (2010). Motor outcomes after neonatal arterial ischemic stroke related to early MRI data in a prospective study. *Pediatrics* 126:912–918.

Jankowska E, Edgley S (2006). How can corticospinal tracts contribute to ipsilateral movements? *Neuroscientist* 12:67–79.

Janneke LM, Bruggink M, Cioni G, Einspieler C, Maathuis C, Pascale R, Bos A. (2009): Early motor repertoire is related to level of self-mobility in children with cerebral palsy at school age. *Developmental Medicine & Child Neurology* 51: 878–885

Janssen L, Beuting M, Meulenbroek M, Steenbergen B (2009). Combined effects of planning and execution constraints on bimanual task performance. *Exp Brain Res* 192:61–73

Jeannerod M (1984). The timing of natural prehension movements. *J Mot Behav* 16:235–254.

Johansson RS, Westling G (1990). Tactile afferent signals in the control of precision grip. In: Jeannerod M (ed), Attention and Performance. Hillsdale, NJ: Erlbaum, 13:677–713.

Juenger H, Grodd W, Krägeloh-Mann I, Staudt M (2008). (Re-) organization of basal ganglia in congenital hemiparesis with ipsilateral cortico-spinal projections. *Neuropediatrics* 39:252–258.

Juenger H, Linder-Lucht M, Walther M, Berweck S, Mall V, Staudt M (2011). Early determination of somatosensory cortex. *Cerebral Cortex* 21:1827–1831.

Kato T, Okumura A, Hayakawa F, Kuno K, Watanabe K (2004). Electroencephalographic aspects of periventricular hemorrhagic infarction in preterm infants. *Neuropediatrics* 35: 161–166.

Kennard M (1940). Relation of age to motor impairment in man and in subhuman primates. *Arch Neurol Psychiatry* 44:377–397.

Kirton A, de Veber G (2006). Cerebral palsy secondary to perinatal ischemic stroke. *Clin Perinatol* 33:367–386.

Kirton A, de Veber G, Pontigon AM, Macgregor D, Shroff M (2008). Presumed perinatal ischemic stroke: vascular classification predicts outcomes. *Ann Neurol* 63:436–443.

Kirton A, Shroff M, Pontigon AM, deVeber G (2010). Perinatal arterial stroke and perinatal venous infarction. *Arch Neurol* 67:842–848.

Kirton A, Shroff M, Visvanathan T, deVeber G (2007). Quantified corticospinal tract diffusion restriction predicts neonatal stroke outcome. *Stroke* 38:974–980.

Koelfen W, Freund M, Varnholt V (1993). Neonatal stroke involving the middle cerebral artery in term infants: clinical presentation, EEG and imaging studies, and outcome. *Dev Med Child Neurol* 37:204–212.

Kostovic I, Jovanov-Milosevic N (2006). The development of cerebral connections during the first 20–45 weeks' gestation. *Semin Fetal Neonatal Med* 11:415–422.

Kostovic I, Judas M (2010). The development of the subplate and thalamocortical connections in the human foetal brain. *Acta Paediatr* 99:1119–1127.

Krageloh-Mann I, Horber V (2007). The role of magnetic resonance imaging in elucidating the pathogenesis of cerebral palsy: a systematic review. *Dev Med Child Neurol* 49:144–156.

Krakauer J (2005). Arm function after stroke: from physiology to recovery. *Semin Neurol* 25: 384–395.

Krumlinde-Sundholm L, Eliasson A-C (2002). Comparing tests of tactile sensibility: aspects relevant to testing children with spastic hemiplegia. *Dev Med Child Neurol* 44:604–612.

Krumlinde Sundholm L, Eliasson A-C, Forssberg H (1998). Obstetric brachial plexus injuries: assessment protocol and functional outcome at age 5 years. *Dev Med Child Neurol* 40: 4–11.

Krumlinde-Sundholm L, Holmefur M, Kottorp A, Eliasson A-C (2007). The Assisting Hand Assessment: current evidence of validity, reliability and responsiveness to change. *Dev Med Child Neurol* 49:259–264.

Kuhtz-Buschbeck J, Krumlinde-Sundholm L, Eliasson A-C, Forssberg H (2000). Quantitative assessment of mirror movements in children and adolescents with hemiplegic cerebral palsy. *Dev Med Child Neurol* 42:728–736.

Laugesaar R, Kolk A, Tomberg T, Metsvaht T, Lintrop M, Varendi H, Talvik T (2007). Acutely and retrospectively diagnosed perinatal stroke: a population-based study. *Stroke* 38: 2234–2240.

Lee J, Croen LA, Lindan C, Nash KB, Yoshida CK, Ferriero DM, Barkovich AJ, Wu YW (2005). Predictors of outcome in perinatal arterial stroke: a population-based study. *Ann Neurol* 58:303–308.

Lemon R (2008). Descending pathways in motor control. *Annu Rev Neurosci* 31:195–218.

Lesný I, Stehliak A, Cek JT, Tománková A, Havlíĉek.I. (1993) Sensory disorders in cerebral palsy; two-point discrimination. *Developmental Medicine & Child Neurology*. 35; 402–405.

Lesny I, Stehlik A, Tomasek J, Tomankova A, Havlicek I (1993). Sensory disorders in cerebral palsy: Two-point discrimination. *Dev Med Child Neurol* 35:402–405.

Lotze M, Sauseng P, Staudt M (2009). Functional relevance of ipsilateral motor activation in congenital hemiparesis as tested by fMRI-navigated TMS. *Exp Neurol* 217:440–443.

Ludemann NA, Berman JI, Wu YW, Jeremy RJ, Kornak J, Bartha AI, Barkovich AJ, Ferriero DM, Henry RG, Glenn OA (2008). Diffusion tensor imaging of the pyramidal tracts in infants with motor dysfunction. *Neurology* 71:1676–1682.

Macdonell RA, Jackson GD, Curatolo JM, Abbott DF, Berkovic SF, Carey LM, Syngeniotin A, Fibinyi GC, Scheffer IE (1999). Motor cortex localization using functional MRI and transcranial magnetic stimulation. *Neurology* 53:1462–1467.

Mackey AH, Walt SE, Stott NS (2006). Deficits in upper-limb task performance in children with hemiplegic cerebral palsy as defined by 3-dimensional kinematics. *Arch Phys Med Rehab* 87:207–215.

Maegaki Y, Maeoka Y, Ishii S, Shiota M, Takeuchi A, Yoshino K, Takeshita A (1997). Mechanisms of central motor reorganization in pediatric hemiplegic patients. *Neuropediatrics* 28:168–174.

Martin J, Friel KM, Salimi I, Chakrabarty S (2009). Corticospinal development. In: Squire L (ed), Encyclopedia of Neuroscience. Oxford: Academic Press, pp. 203–214.

Martin JH (2005). The corticospinal system: From development to motor control. *Neuroscientist* 11:161–173.

Martin JH, Friel KM, Salimi I, Chakraberty S (2007). Activity- and use-dependent plasticity of the developing corticospinal system. *Neurosci Biobehav Rev* 31:1125–1135.

McCloskey DI, Prochazka A (1993). The role of sensory information in the guidance of movement control: reflections on a symposium held at the 22nd Annual Meeting of the Society of Neuroscience. *Somatosensory Motor Res* 11:69–76.

McLaughlin JF, Felix SD, Nowbar S, Ferrel A, Bjornson K, Hays RM (2005). Lower extremity sensory function in children with cerebral palsy. *Pediatr Rehab* 8:45–52.

Mercuri E, Barnett A, Rutherford M, Guzzetta A, Haataja L, Cioni G, Cowan F, Dubowitz L (2004). Neonatal cerebral infarction and neuromotor outcome at school age. *Pediatrics* 113:95–100.

Mercuri E, Jongmans M, Bouza H, Haataja L, Rutherford M, Henderson S, Dubowitz L (1999). Congenital hemiplegia in children at school age: assessment of hand function in the non-hemiplegic hand and correlation with MRI. *Neuropediatrics* 30:8–13.

Mihran O, Tachdjian MD (1958). Sensory disturbances in the hands of children with cerebral palsy. *J Bone Joint Surg [Am]* 40:85–90.

Moberg E (1962). Criticism and study of methods for examining sensibility in the hand. *Neurology* 12:8–19.

Moberg E. (1990) Two-point discrimination test. A valuable part of hand surgical rehabilitation, e.g. in tetraplegia. *Scandinavian Journal of Rehabilitation Medicine* 22: 127–34.

Moberg E. (1991) The unsolved problem – how to test the functional value of the hand sensibility. *Journal of Hand Therapy* 4: 105–10.

Muller RA, Rothermel RD, Behen ME, Muzik O, Mangner TJ, Chugani HT (1998a). Differential patterns of language and motor reorganization following early left hemisphere lesion: a PET study. *Arch Neurol* 55:1113–1119.

Muller RA, Rothermel RD, Behen ME, Muzik O, Mangner TJ, Chugani HT (1998b). Developmental changes of cortical and cerebellar motor control: a clinical positron emission tomography study with children and adults. *J Child Neurol* 13:550–556.

Murakami, A, Morimoto M, Yamada K, Kizu O, Nishimura A, Nishimura T, Sugimoto T (2008). Fiber-tracking techniques can predict the degree of neurologic impairment for periventricular leukomalacia. *Pediatrics* 122:500.

Mutsaarts M, Steenbergen B, Bekkering H (2005). Anticipatory planning of movement sequences in hemiparetic cerebral palsy. *Motor Control* 9:435–454.

Mutsaarts M, Steenbergen B, Bekkering H (2006). Anticipatory planning deficits and task context effects in hemiparetic cerebral palsy. *Exp Brain Res* 172:151–162.

Mutsaarts M, Steenbergen B, Bekkering H (2007). Impaired motor imagery in right hemiparetic cerebral palsy. *Neuropsychologia* 45:853–859.

Nagae LM, Hoon AH, Stashinko E, Lin D, Zhang W, Levey E, Wakana S, Jiang H, Leite CC, Lucato LT, VanZijl PC, Johnston MV, Mori S (2007). Diffusion tensor imaging in children with PVL: Variability of injuries of white matter tracts. *AJNR Am J Neuroradiol* 28:1213–1222.

Nass R (1985). Mirror movement asymmetries in congenital hemiparesis: the inhibition hypothesis revisited. *Neurology* 35:1059–1062.

Nelson KB, Ellenberg JH (1982). Children who "outgrew" cerebral palsy. *Pediatrics* 69:529–536.

Neville B, Goodman R (eds) (2006). Hand function in CP. In: Congenital Hemiplegia. London: Mac Keith Press, pp. 65–80.

Nezu A, Kimura S, Takeshita S, Tanaka M (1999). Functional recovery in hemiplegic cerebral palsy: ipsilateral electromyographic responses to focal transcranial magnetic stimulation. *Brain Dev* 21:162–165.

Nirkko AC, Rösler KM, Ozdoba C, Heid O, Schroth G, Hess CW (1997). Human cortical plasticity: functional recovery with mirror movements. *Neurology* 48:1090–1093.

Norton JA, Thompson A, Chan KM, Wilman A, Stein R (2008). Persistent mirror movements for over sixty years. *Clin Neurophysiol* 119:80–87.

O'Leary DDM, Kroll TK (2009). Neural patterning: arealization of the cortex. In: Squire LR (ed), Encyclopedia of Neuroscience. Oxford: Academic Press, 2:189–197.

Ounpuu S, DeLuca PA, Davis RB (2001). Gait analysis. In: Nevile B, Goodman R (eds), Congenital Hemiplegia. London: Mac Keith Press, pp. 81–97.

Ounpuu S, Thomason P, Harvey A, Graham H (2009). Classification of cerebral palsy and patterns of gait pathology. In: Gage J, Schwartz M, Koop S, Novacheck T (eds), The Identification and Treatment of Gait Problems in Cerebral Palsy (Clinics in Developmental Medicine). London: MacKeith Press, pp. 147–166.

Pagliano E, Andreucci E, Bono R, Semorile C, Brollo L, Fedrizzi E (2001). Evolution of upper limb function in children with congenital hemiplegia. *Neurol Sci* 22:371–375.

Peacock W (2009). The pathophysiology of spasticity. In: Gage J, Schwartz M, Koop S, Novacheck T (eds), The Identification and Treatment of Gait Problems in Cerebral Palsy (Clinics in Developmental Medicine). London: MacKeith Press, pp. 89–98.

Ponten E, Friden J, Thornell LE, Lieber RL (2005). Spastic wrist flexors are more severely affected than wrist extensors in children with cerebral palsy. *Dev Med Child Neurol* 47: 384–389.

Punt TD, Riddoch MJ, Humphreys GW (2005). Don't think twice it's all right—contralesional dependency for bimanual prehension movements. *Neuropsychologia* 43:1547–1558.

Ragazzoni A, Cincotta M, Borgheresi A, Zaccara G, Ziemann U (2002). Congenital hemiparesis: different functional reorganization of somatosensory and motor pathways. *Clin Neurophysiol* 113:1273–1278.

Riad J, Coleman S, Lundh D, Brostrom E (2011). Arm posture score and arm movement during walking: a comprehensive assessment in spastic hemiplegic cerebral palsy. *Gait & Posture* 33:48–53.

Riquelmea I, Montoya P (2010). Developmental changes in somatosensory processing in cerebral palsy and healthy individuals. *Clin Neurophysiol* 121: 1314–1320.

Rodda J, Graham HK (2001). Classification of gait patterns and spastic hemiplegia and spastic diplegia; a basis for management algorithm. *Eur J Neurol* 8:98–108.

Rosenbaum DA, Meulenbroek RJ, Vaughan J, Jansen C (2001). Posture-based motion planning: applications to grasping. *Psychol Rev* 108:709–734.

Rosenbaum PL, Walter SD, Hanna SE, Palisano RJ, Russell DJ, Raina P, Wood E, Bartlett DJ, Galuppi BE (2002). Prognosis for gross motor function in cerebral palsy: creation of motor development curves. *JAMA* 288:1357–1363.

Sakzewski L, Ziviani J, Boyd R (2010). The relationship between unimanual capacity and bimanual performance in children with congenital hemiplegia. *Dev Med Child Neurol* 58: 811–816.

Scrutton D (2000). Physical assessment and aims of treatment. In: Neville B, Goodman R (eds), Congenital Hemiplegia. London: Mac Keith Press, pp. 65–80.

Sreenan C, Bhargava R, Robertson CM (2000). Cerebral infarction in the term newborn: clinical presentation and long-term outcome. *J Pediatr* 137:351–355.

Staudt M (2007a). (Re-) organization of the developing human brain following periventricular white matter lesions. *Neurosci Biobehav Rev* 31:1150–1156.

Staudt M (2007b). Reorganization of the developing human brain after early lesions. *Dev Med Child Neurol* 49:564.

Staudt M (2010a). Reorganization after pre- and perinatal brain lesions. *J Anat* 217:469–474.

Staudt M (2010b). The role of transcranial magnetic stimulation in the characterization of congenital hemiparesis. *Dev Med Child Neurol* 52:113–114.

Staudt M, Braun C, Gerloff C, Erb M, Grodd W, Krageloh-Mann I (2006a). Developing somatosensory projections bypass periventricular brain lesions. *Neurology* 67:522–525.

Staudt M, Erb M, Braun C, Gerloff C, Grodd W, Krägeloh-Mann I (2006b). Extensive perilesional connectivity in congenital hemiparesis. *Neurology* 66:771–778.

Staudt M, Gerloff C, Grodd W, Holthausen H, Niemann G, Krageloh-Mann I (2004). Reorganization in congenital hemiparesis acquired at different gestational ages. *Ann Neurol* 56:854–863.

Staudt M, Grodd W, Gerloff C, Erb M, Stitz J, Krageloh-Mann I (2002). Two types of ipsilateral reorganization in congenital hemiparesis: A TMS and fMRI study. *Brain* 125:2222–2237.

Staudt M, Krageloh-Mann I, Grodd W (2005). Ipsilateral corticospinal pathways in congenital hemiparesis on routine magnetic resonance imaging. *Pediatr Neurol* 32:37–39.

Staudt M, Niemann G, Grodd W, Krageloh-Mann I (2000). The pyramidal tract in congenital hemiparesis: Relationship between morphology and function in periventricular lesions. *Neuropediatrics* 31:257–264.

Staudt M, Pieper T, Grodd W, Winkler P, Holthausen H, Krageloh-Mann I (2001). Functional MRI in a 6-year-old boy with unilateral cortical malformation: concordant representation of both hands in the unaffected hemisphere. *Neuropediatrics* 32:159–161.

Steenbergen B, Bekkering H (2006). Anticipatory planning deficits and context effects in hemiparetic cerebral palsy. *Exp Brain Res* 172:151–162.

Steenbergen B, Charles J, Gordon AM (2008) Fingertip force control during bimanual object lifting in hemiplegic cerebral palsy. *Exp Brain Res* 186:191–201.

Steenbergen B, Gordon AM (2006). Activity limitation in hemiplegic cerebral palsy: evidence for disorders in motor planning. *Dev Med Child Neurol* 48:780–783.

Steenbergen B, Hulstijn W, Lemmens I.H, Meulenbroek RG (1998). The timing of prehensile movements in subjects with cerebral palsy. *Dev Med Child Neurol* 40:108–114.

Steenbergen B, Meulenbroek RG (2006). Deviations in upper-limb function of the less-affected side in congenital hemiparesis. *Neuropsychologia* 44:2296–2307.

Steenbergen B, Meulenbroek RG, Rosenbaum DA (2004). Constraints on grip selection in hemiparetic CP: effects of lesion side, end point accuracy and context. *Cognitive Brain Res* 19:145–159.

Steenbergen B, Van der Kamp J (2004). Control of prehension in hemiparetic cerebral palsy: Similarities and differences among the ipsi- and contra-lesional side of the body. *Dev Med Child Neurol* 46:325–332.

Steenbergen B, van Nimwegen M, Crajé C (2007). Solving a mental rotation task in congenital hemiparesis: motor imagery versus visual imagery. *Neuropsychologia* 45:3324–3328.

Steenbergen B, Van Thiel E, Hulstijn W, Meulenbroek RGJ (2000). The coordination of reaching and grasping in spastic hemiparesis. *Hum Mov Sci* 19:75–105.

Stinear CM, Fleming MK, Barber PA, Byblow WD (2007). Lateralization of motor imagery following stroke. *Clin Neurophysiol* 118:1794–1801.

Tachdjian MO, Minear WL (1958). Sensory disturbances in the hands of children with cerebral palsy. *J Bone Joint Surg [Am]* 40A:85–90.

Taub E (1976). Movement in nonhunman primates deprived of somatosensory feedback. *Exercise Sports Science Review* 4:335–374.

Taub E, Wolf SL (1997). Constraint-induced (CI) movement techniques to facilitate upper extremity use in stroke patients. *Topics Stroke Rehab* 3:38–61.

Thickbroom GW, Byrnes ML, Archer SA, Nagarajan L, Mastaglia FL (2001). Differences in sensory and motor cortical organization following brain injury early in life. *Ann Neurol* 49:320–327.

Tizard JP, Paine RS, Crothers B (1954). Disturbances of sensation in children with hemiplegia. *JAMA* 155:628–632.

Trauner DA (2003). Hemispatial neglect in young children with early unilateral brain damage. *Dev Med Child Neurol* 45:160–166.

Trauner DA, Chase C, Walker P, Wulfeck B (1993). Neurologic profiles of infants and children after perinatal stroke. *Pediatr Neurol* 9:383–386.

Trauner DA, Mannino FL (1986). Neurodevelopmental outcome after neonatal cerebrovascular accident. *J Pediatr* 108:459–461.

Trombly CA (1993). Observations of improvement of reaching in five subjects with hemiparesis. *J Neurol Neurosurg Psychiatry* 56:40–45.

Tükel Kavak S, Eliasson AC (2011). Development of handwriting skill in children with hemiplegic CP. *Disabil Rehabil.* 33(21–22):2084–91.

Utley A, Steenbergen B (2006). Discrete bimanual co-ordination in children and young adolescents with hemiparetic cerebral palsy: recent findings, implications and future research directions. *Pediatr Res* 9:127–136.

Utley A, Steenbergen B, Sugden DA (2004). The influence of object size on discrete bimanual co-ordination in children with hemiplegic cerebral palsy. *Disabil Rehabil* 26:603–613.

Utley A, Sugden D (1998). Interlimb coupling in children with hemiparetic cerebral palsy during reaching and grasping at speed. *Dev Med Child Neurol* 40:396–404.

Uvebrant P (1988). Hemiplegic cerebral palsy. *Aetiology and outcome. Acta Paediatr Scand Suppl* 345:1–100.

Vandermeeren Y, Olivier E, Sebire G, Cosnard G, Bol A, Sibomama M, Michel C, DeVolder AG (2002). Increased FDG uptake in the ipsilateral sensorimotor cortex in congenital hemiplegia. *Neuroimage* 15:949–960.

Van Elk M, Craje C, Beeren M, Steenbergen B, van Schie HT, Bekkering H (2010). Neural evidence of compromised motor imagery in right hemiparetic CP. *Frontiers Neurol* 30:150.

Van Heest AE, House J, Putnam M (1993). Sensibility deficiencies in the hands of children with spastic hemiplegia. *J Hand Surg* 18:278–281.

Van Roon D, Steenbergen B, Meulenbroek RGJ (2005). Trunk use and co-contraction in cerebral palsy as regulatory mechanisms for accuracy control. *Neuropsychologia* 43:497–508.

Van Thiel E, Meulenbroek RGJ, Smeets JBJ, Hulstijn W (2002). Fast adjustments of ongoing movements in hemiparetic cerebral palsy. *Neuropsychologia* 40:16–27.

Van Thiel E, Steenbergen B (2001). Shoulder and hand displacements during hitting, reaching, and grasping movements in hemiparetic cerebral palsy. *Motor Control* 5:166–182.

Vulliemoz S, Raineteau O, Jabaudon D (2005). Reaching beyond the midline: why are human brains cross wired? *Lancet Neurol* 4:87–99.

Weinstein S. (1993) Fifty years of somatosensory research: from the Semmes-Weinstein monofilaments to the Weinstein Enhanced Sensory Test. *Journal of Hand Therapy* 6: 11–22.

Westmacott R, MacGregor D, Askalan R, DeVeber G (2009). Late emergence of cognitive deficits after unilateral neonatal stroke. *Stroke* 40:2012–2019.

Wilke M, Staudt M, Juenger H, Grodd W, Braun C, Krageloh-Mann I (2009). Somatosensory system in two types of motor reorganization in congenital hemiparesis: topography and function. *Hum Brain Mapp* 30:776–788.

Wilson BC, Wilson JJ (1967a). Sensory and perceptual functions in the cerebral palsied. I. Pressure thresholds and two-point discrimination. *J Nervous Mental Dis* 145:53–60.

Wilson BC, Wilson JJ (1967b). Sensory and perceptual functions in the cerebral palsied. II. Stereognosis. *J Nervous Mental Dis* 145:61–68.

Wingert JR, Burton H, Sinclair RJ, Brunstrom JE, Damiano D (2008). Tactile sensory abilities in cerebral palsy: deficits in roughness and object. *Dev Med Child Neurol* 50:832–838.

Wingert JR, Burton H, Sinclair RJ, Brunstrom JE, Damiano DL (2009). Joint-position sense and kinesthesia in cerebral palsy. *Arch Phys Med Rehabil* 90:447–453.

Woods BT, Teuber HL (1978). Mirror movements after childhood hemiparesis. *Neurology* 28:1152–1158.

Wren TAL, Rethlefsen S, Kay RM (2005). Prevalence of specific gait abnormalities in children with cerebral palsy: influence of cerebral palsy subtype, age, and previous surgery. *J Pediatr Orthop* 25:79–83.

Wu YW, Linda CE, Henning LH, Yoshida CK, Fullerton HJ, Ferriero DM, Barkovich AJ, Croen LA (2006). Neuroimaging abnormalities in infants with congenital hemiparesis. *Pediatr Neurol* 35:191–196.

Wu YW, Lynch JK, Nelson KB (2005). Perinatal arterial stroke: understanding mechanisms and outcomes. *Semin Neurol* 25:424–434

Wu YW, March WM, Croen LA, Grether JK, Escobar GJ, Newman TB (2004). Perinatal stroke in children with motor impairment: a population-based study. *Pediatrics* 114:612–619.

Yakovlev PI, Lecours AR (1967). The myelogenetic cycles of regional maturation of the brain. In: Minkowski A (ed), Regional Development of the Brain in Early Life. Boston: Blackwell Scientific Publications, pp. 3–70.

Yekutiel M, Jariwala M, Stretch P (1994). Sensory deficit in the hands of children with cerebral palsy: a new look at assessment and prevalence. *Dev Med Child Neurol* 36:61–24.

Yokochi K, Hosoe A, Kodama M, Kodama K (1992). Assessment of upper and lower extremity movements in hemiplegic children. *Brain Dev* 14:18–22.

Yokochi K, Yokochi M, Kodama K (1995). Motor function in infants with spastic hemiplegia. *Brain and Development* 17:42–48.

Zancolli EA, Goldner LJ, Swanson AB (1983). Surgery of the spastic hand in cerebral palsy: report of the committee on spastic hand evaluation. *J Hand Surg* 8:766–772.

5

Visuospatial Processes

VISUAL INPUT IS a rich and diverse source of knowledge about the spatial world. It provides information about everything from the structure of objects and scenes to their location or movement in space. Visuospatial processing encompasses a wide variety of neurocognitive abilities ranging from tracking moving objects, to localizing and attending to objects or events in a spatial array, to analyzing how the parts or features of an object combine to form an organized whole. Visuospatial processing also allows us to mentally transform objects and arrays—to visualize what an object will look like when rotated, what a cross-section of an object looks like, or what a scene would look like from another vantage point. Visuospatial processing is supported by a complex neural architecture that involves dozens of interrelated visual areas in the posterior cortices (Van Essen, Anderson, & Felleman, 1992). In the early 1980s, Ungerleider and Mishkin (1982) proposed a model for understanding the organization of this complex set of cortical areas and functions. According to their model, the cortical visual system can be anatomically and functionally subdivided into two principal processing streams (Fig. 5.1), the ventral and dorsal pathways. The ventral stream is primarily involved in processing information about patterns and objects, while the dorsal stream mediates spatial processing associated with attention to movement and location. More recently the characterization of dorsal stream function has been extended to encompass visually guided movement (e.g., Andersen, Snyder, Bradley, & Xing, 1997; Goodale & Milner, 1992; Goodale & Westwood, 2004; Rizzolatti & Matelli, 2003).

This chapter begins with a summary of the neuroarchitecture of the two primary visual streams. The summary focuses on the flow of visual information beginning, for both streams, in primary visual cortex and then extending to the temporal and parietal lobes for the ventral and dorsal streams, respectively. The connections between the two major visual pathways, as well as connections with the frontal lobes, are also considered. The second section discusses the effects of localized injury to the ventral and dorsal systems in adult patients. Patient data have been an important source of information on the functional organization of the two major visual pathways. Many of the original characterizations of the functional organization of the ventral and dorsal streams were derived from studies of adult patients with localized

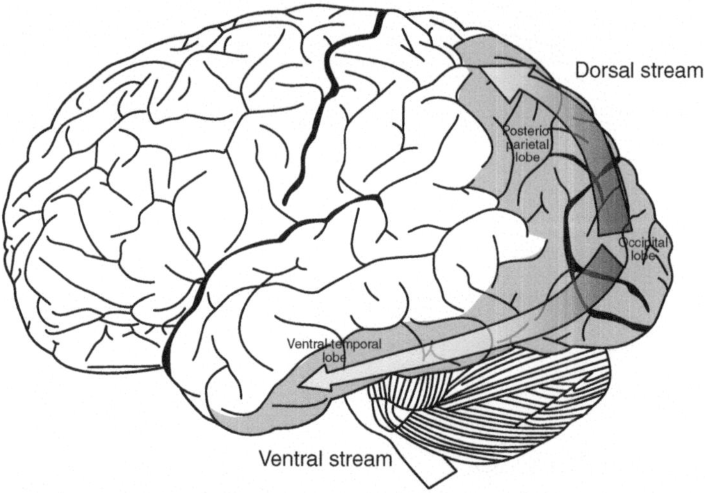

FIGURE 5.1 Dorsal and ventral visual streams. (Image adapted with permission from Wikimedia Commons. en.wikipedia.org/wiki/File:Ventral-dorsal_streams.svg. This file is licensed under the Creative Commons Attribution 2.0 Generic license.)

injury to various neural subsystems within the principal cortical visual pathways. The third section will provide an overview of the available literature on the typical profiles of development for visuospatial functions. It begins with a summary of the developmental trajectories of cognitive functions thought to be subserved by each of the two visual systems separately. It then turns to a discussion of the literature comparing the relative rates of development of the two systems. There is controversy about whether there is developmental priority for ventral versus dorsal stream functions, and whether a relative lag in the development of the dorsal stream may play a role in the enhanced vulnerability of associated dorsal stream functions that has been reported for a range of neurodevelopmental disorders (Atkinson & Braddick, 2011). The outcome of that controversy may have important implications for understanding the effects of early injury on the development of specific visuospatial abilities. The fourth and largest section of this chapter focuses on the effects of early brain injury on the development of visuospatial processing. The body of data concerning the development of ventral stream functions following early brain injury is more extensive than that focused on the dorsal stream. Nonetheless, it is clear that the effects of early injury on visuospatial functions associated with both visual streams are more pronounced than those observed for language, and the relationship between site of injury and type of deficit is more similar to the profiles observed among adult patient populations.

ANATOMICAL ORGANIZATION OF THE PRIMARY CORTICAL VISUAL PATHWAY

The organization of the primary visual pathways has been most fully described for Rhesus Macaque, so the description presented here uses the nomenclature typically used for nonhuman primates. However, the basic pathways in human and monkeys appear to be largely homologous (Brewer, 2002; Orban, 2004). The ventral visual pathway begins at the retina and projects via the lateral geniculate nucleus (LGN) of the thalamus to primary visual cortex, area V1. From there the pathway proceeds to extrastriate visual areas V2 and V4, and then projects ventrally to the posterior (PIT) and anterior (AIT) regions of the inferior temporal lobe. Input to the ventral pathway is derived principally, though not exclusively, from P-type retinal ganglion cells that project to the parvocellular layers of the LGN and then to layer 4C beta of V1. Parvocellular input to V1 organizes into distinct areas called the blob and interblob regions (Kaas & Collins, 2004; Livingstone & Hubel, 1984; Wong-Riley, 1979). Cells in the blob regions are maximally sensitive to form, while cells in the interblob regions respond principally to color. The ventral stream processes information about visual properties of objects and patterns and has been described as the "what" pathway.

The dorsal visual pathway also begins at the retina and projects via the LGN to area V1. From there the pathway proceeds to extrastriate areas V2 and V3, then projects dorsally to the medial (MT/V5) and medial superior (MST) regions of the temporal lobe, and then to the ventral inferior-parietal lobe (IP). Input to the dorsal pathway is derived principally, though not exclusively, from the large M-type retinal ganglion cells that project to the magnocellular layers of LGN and then to layer 4C alpha of V1. Cells in this pathway are maximally sensitive to movement and direction and are less responsive to color or form. The original functions identified for the dorsal stream involved processing of information about spatial location, optic flow, and motion, as well as allocation and maintenance of spatial attention. It was thus described as the "where" pathway. More recently, work examining the dorsal stream's role in visually guided movements suggests that the function of this pathway is more complex than this characterization suggests, as it also involves the integration of visual and motor functions (e.g., Andersen et al., 1997; Goodale & Milner, 1992; Rizzolatti & Matelli, 2003).

Both the dorsal and ventral pathways project rostrally to both common and adjacent areas of the prefrontal cortex. Imaging studies suggest that these networks are involved in a variety of dorsal and ventral stream functions. For example, spatial working memory and attention rely on networks connecting dorsolateral prefrontal cortex and posterior parietal cortex (Awh & Jonides, 2001; Corbetta, Kincade, & Shulman, 2002; Curtis, 2006), while object memory relies on systems connecting prefrontal cortex with inferior temporal areas (Ranganath, 2006; Ranganath, Cohen, Dam, & D'Esposito, 2004; Ranganath & D'Esposito, 2005). In addition, there is substantial evidence that the two pathways are richly interconnected and at least partially overlapping in both the mature (e.g., Dobkins & Albright, 1994, 1995, 1998; Marangolo, Di Pace, Rafal, & Scabini, 1998; Merigan & Maunsell, 1993; Rosa et al., 2009; Sincich & Horton, 2005; Thiele, Dobkins, & Albright, 2001) and the developing visual system (Dobkins & Anderson, 2002; Dobkins & Teller, 1996a, 1996b). Finally, recent work suggests that the dissociation of function across the two pathways may be less complete than originally thought. There is an emerging body of evidence suggesting that subregions within each system may respond to functions typically associated with the other pathway (Husain & Nachev, 2007; Kawasaki, Watanabe, Okuda, Sakagami, & Aihara, 2008; Konen & Kastner, 2008; Lehky & Sereno, 2007).

ADULT PATIENT STUDIES OF VISUOSPATIAL FUNCTIONING

Studies of adults with localized brain injury have been an important source of data on the organization of the human brain. These studies typically use a kind of subtractive approach to investigate brain function. Specifically, they ask what functions are impaired or lost following injury to particular brain regions, and by inference attribute those functions or at least some component of those functions to the injured brain system. The adult studies provide a measure of the endpoint of typical developmental processes. Thus, they provide a means for assessing the effects brain injury in the perinatal lesion (PL) population that can tap both similarities and differences in function when injury occurs early in life.

Ventral Stream Functions

A major function of the ventral visual stream is the analysis of pattern information. Behaviorally, visuospatial analysis is defined as the ability to specify the parts and the overall configuration of a visually presented pattern, and to understand how the parts are related to form an organized whole (e.g., Delis, Kiefner, & Fridlund, 1988; Delis, Robertson, & Efron, 1986; Palmer, 1977, 1980; Palmer & Bucher, 1981; Robertson & Delis, 1986; Smith & Kemler, 1977; Vurpillot, 1976). It thus involves the ability both to segment a pattern into a set of constituent parts (referred to as featural or local-level processing) and to integrate those parts into a coherent whole (configural or global-level processing). Studies of visuospatial processing within the ventral stream have shown systematic differences in the distribution of global- and local-level processing across the cerebral hemispheres. Specifically, right posterior temporal regions dominate for global processing, while left posterior temporal regions dominate for local processing.

Global–Local Processing

Differential laterality for global and local processing is well documented in adults and shows right hemisphere (RH) dominance for global processing and left hemisphere (LH) dominance for local processing (e.g., Han et al., 2002; Martin, 1979; Martinez et al., 1997; Sergent, 1982; Volberg & Hubner, 2004; Yovel, Levy, & Yovel, 2001). Sergent (1982) suggested that these differences stem from differential processing of lower spatial frequencies in the RH and higher spatial frequencies in the LH. In accordance with this view, a number of experiments have presented sinusoidal gratings containing a single spatial frequency to the right visual field (RVF) or the left visual field (LVF). Low spatial frequencies elicit faster responses when presented to the LVF-RH than the RVF-LH, while high spatial frequencies elicit the opposite pattern (Kitterle, Christman, & Hellige, 1990; Kitterle, Hellige, & Christman, 1992; Kitterle & Selig, 1991). Event-related potential (ERP) and functional imaging studies have supported these basic patterns of lateralization (e.g., Fink et al., 1997; Heinze, Hinrichs, Scholz, Burchert, & Mangun, 1998; Martinez et al., 1997).

Consistent with findings of lateralized visual field studies with typical adults, studies of adult patients have shown that left posterior versus right posterior focal brain injury results in dissociable disorders of spatial analytic functioning (e.g., Arena & Gainotti, 1978; Delis et al., 1986, 1988; Gainotti & Tiacci, 1970; Ivry & Robertson, 1998; Lamb, Robertson, & Knight, 1989, 1990; McFie & Zangwill, 1960; Robertson & Delis, 1986; Robertson, Lamb, & Knight, 1988; Swindell, Holland, Fromm, & Greenhouse, 1988). Left posterior injury disrupts local-level processing and results in disorders involving difficulty processing the parts of a spatial array. For example, in drawing, patients with left posterior lesions tend to oversimplify spatial patterns and omit details, while on perceptual judgment tasks they rely upon overall configural cues and ignore specific elements. By contrast, patients with right posterior lesions have difficulty with global-level processing that disrupts the configural aspects of spatial analysis. For example, in drawing, they include details but fail to maintain a coherent organization among the elements, while on perceptual judgment tasks, they focus on the parts of the pattern and ignore the overall form.

Face Processing

The ventral stream also plays a critical role in processing a particularly important class of socially relevant stimuli, faces. Effective social communication and organization depends on the ability to recognize other members of one's social group. Humans recognize members of our species primarily by visual cues. A large body of neuroimaging work has focused on the role of a specific cortical region in face processing. This region is located in the lateral fusiform gyrus of the ventral occipital temporal lobe and has been dubbed the fusiform face area (FFA) (Gauthier, Behrmann, & Tarr, 1999; Gauthier et al., 2000; Kanwisher, McDermott, & Chun, 1997; Kanwisher & Yovel, 2006; Tarr & Gauthier, 2000; Yovel & Kanwisher, 2004). Prosopagnosia is the clinical term that describes a specific disruption of face recognition. It can occur as an isolated disturbance or in combination with other visual processing dysfunctions, though in such cases the impact on face processing is more severe (Barton, 2003). Prosopagnosia is caused by lesions of the fusiform and lingual gyri (Damasio, Damasio, & Van Hoesen, 1982). Lateralized differences in responsivity to face stimuli have also been reported, suggesting that face discrimination may rely more on the holistic and configural processing capacity of the RH than on the featural processing system of the LH (Hillger & Koenig, 1991; Rhodes, 1993; Rossion et al., 2000). Consistent with these findings, more reliable activation of right than left FFA is often reported in neuroimaging studies of face processing (Kanwisher et al., 1997; McCarthy, Puce, Gore, & Allison, 1997). In addition, while prosopagnosic patients often have bilateral lesions, cases of prosopagnosia associated with isolated RH lesions have been reported (Barton, 2008; Wilkinson et al., 2009). Consistent with evidence suggesting a greater role for the RH injury in cases of prosopagnosia, impairment of face processing has been associated with more pronounced disruption of configural processing than featural processing (Barton, 2009; Barton, Press, Keenan, & O'Connor, 2002; Rivest, Moscovitch, & Black, 2009; Wilkinson et al., 2009).

Dorsal Stream Functions

A variety of spatial functions have been associated with the dorsal stream; however, data on the effects of PL on dorsal stream functioning have focused primarily on spatial localization and spatial attention. Data from adult patients with localized brain injury have contributed to our understanding of the neural systems that mediate these two functions. In this chapter, only the first of these important dorsal stream function will be considered. The review of spatial attention will be incorporated into the more general discussion of memory and attentional functions in Chapter 6.

Spatial Localization

Spatial localization is a complex, multimodal process that engages a wide array of both cortical and subcortical brain systems. Evidence from both human and animal studies has shown that the dorsal stream plays a critical role in perceptual localization (Belger et al., 1998; Chiba, Kesner, & Jackson, 2002). Positron emission tomography (PET) and functional magnetic resonance imaging (fMRI) studies with adult humans have also implicated the parietal region in episodic memory for spatial location (Belger et al., 1998; Wagner, Shannon, Kahn, & Buckner, 2005). Haxby examined profiles of posterior brain activation that required participants to compare the location of objects in two visually presented arrays (Haxby et al., 1991, 1994). The basic activation findings of Haxby's experiments are consistent with animal studies (Colby & Duhamel, 1996; Colby & Goldberg, 1999; Rizzolatti & Matelli, 2003) and have been largely replicated in subsequent fMRI, PET, and transcranial magnetic stimulation (TMS) studies using a variety of perceptual and working memory tasks (Belger et al., 1998; Casey et al., 1998; Ellison & Cowey, 2006; Jonides et al., 1993; Nelson et al., 2000; Oliveri et al., 2001; Smith, Jonides, & Koeppe, 1996; Smith et al., 1995). Haxby's studies showed that in the most posterior brain regions, areas of extrastriate cortex are activated bilaterally; these include the dorsolateral occipital (area 19), the calcarine, and medial and lateral areas of the occipital lobe. Within the parietal lobe, activation was observed bilaterally in posterior superior parietal areas, extending rostrally to the intraparietal sulcus (Brodmann's area 7). In addition, subsequent studies also identified the inferior parietal lobe as important in perceptual processing of location (Colby & Duhamel, 1996; Courtney, Ungerleider, Keil, & Haxby, 1996). Finally, a large number of functional neuroimaging studies have demonstrated the importance of frontal regions in spatial working memory for locations. Two regions that appear to be particularly important for spatial working memory in humans are superior frontal cortex (SFC; Courtney, Petit, Maisog, Ungerleider, & Haxby, 1998; Curtis, 2006; Haxby, Petit, Ungerleider, & Courtney, 2000; Sala, Rama, & Courtney, 2003) and dorsolateral prefrontal cortex (DLPFC, Curtis, 2006; Postle, Berger, Taich, & D'Esposito, 2000).

Categorical vs. Coordinate Processing

Spatial localization is essential for processing the relationships among elements in a visual scene. Location processing relies on the computation of two distinct types of relation, categorical and coordinate (Kosslyn 1987, 2006; Kosslyn, Chabris, Marsolek, & Koenig, 1992; Kosslyn et al., 1989). Categorical relations provide generalized abstract positional information about the relative location of two elements such as above/below or right/left that are often captured with single lexical terms in language. In contrast, coordinate relations provide precise metric information about spatial relations, including the exact spacing between objects and relative position in coordinate space (e.g., a mapmaker might say that city A is 2.75 miles north-northeast of city B). Neuroimaging studies have implicated posterior parietal regions for both categorical and coordinate relational processing (Kosslyn, et al., 1998; Trojano et al., 2002), but the laterality of the two processes appears to differ. Specifically, categorical processing is left dominant, while coordinate processing is right dominant (Kosslyn, 2006; Kosslyn et al., 1989; Kosslyn, Maljkovic, Hamilton, Horwitz, & Thompson, 1995). A recent imaging study more specifically linked activation of the left intraparietal lobule (IPL) to categorical processing (Amorapanth et al., 2010).

Studies of adult patients with lesions encompassing either the right or left parietal lobe provide support for the idea that categorical and coordinate relations exhibit significant laterality. In an early study, Laeng (1994) showed that patients with left parietal injury were impaired in categorical judgments and patients with right parietal injury were impaired in coordinate judgments. Subsequent studies have generally supported that model, with some caveats. Van Asselen et al. (van Asselen, Kessels, Kappelle, & Postma, 2008) reported findings very similar to Laeng's when the task required location memory only, but when memory for object *and* memory for location were required, there were no laterality differences. Subsequent analysis suggested that injury to both right parietal and right hippocampal areas results in a selective deficit of coordinate processing; and injury to left parietal and left or right hippocampal areas selectively affects categorical processing (Postma, Kessels, & van Asselen, 2008). Palmero et al. (Palermo, Bureca, Matano, & Guariglia, 2008) have reported a somewhat different pattern in which left parietal injury impairs categorical but not coordinate processing, but right parietal injury affects performance on both tasks. Finally, Amorapanth (Amorapanth, et al, 2010) reported a somewhat more complex pattern of results based on voxel-based lesion-symptom mapping (VLSM). They reported that injury to a wide variety of both RH and LH brain areas can affect performance on both categorical and coordinate processing tasks. However, the magnitude of deficit when controlling for overall performance on both tasks follows the generally reported pattern. Specifically, while patients may show some degree of deficit on both tasks, patients with LH lesions were more impaired on the categorical tasks, and those with RH lesions were more impaired on the coordinate tasks. Further, when the sample was divided into patients whose lesions either did or did not involve the IPL, only those with significant compromise of the IPL showed the patterns of task-specific, lateralized deficits. Together these findings provide general support for the lateralized model of spatial location processing, but suggest that regions beyond the parietal lobe may contribute to location coding and thus to the particular patterns of deficit.

THE DEVELOPMENT OF VISUOSPATIAL FUNCTIONS IN TYPICAL CHILDREN

The next section will examine the developmental trajectories for both dorsal and ventral stream functions, incorporating available data from neuroimaging studies that can provide insight into the associated changes in the neural substrate that occur across development. While there is strong evidence for very early emerging visuospatial processing abilities, it is also clear that mature levels of processing develop slowly through the school-age period and into adolescence. Overall, this protracted pattern of developmental change is evident for both dorsal and ventral stream functions. Data on the relative rates of change across the two visual streams are mixed and present a somewhat contradictory picture of the relation between the two streams across development.

The Development of Ventral Stream Processes

The ability to analyze spatial patterns begins to emerge in the first year of life. Newborns exhibit both configural preferences and rudimentary part-whole processing (Cassia, Simion, Milani, & Umilta, 2002; Farroni, Valenza, Simion, & Umilta 2000; Quinn, Burke, & Rush, 1993; Slater, Mattock, Brown, & Bremner, 1991). Across the first year of life there are dramatic changes in the complexity of visual pattern processing that reflect systematic improvement of the infant's ability to process global- and local-level pattern information (Cohen & Younger, 1984). Further, these patterns of change appear to reflect early hemispheric differences in processing. Infants as young as 4 months exhibit lateralized processing differences on global and local processing tasks that are similar to those observed in adult neuroimaging studies (Deruelle & de Schonen, 1991, 1998).

Change in the complexity and sophistication of spatial analytic processing continues through the preschool and school-age periods. Data from a large series of studies using different measures and testing children ranging in age from 3 to 12 years show that initially children segment out well-formed, independent parts and use simple combinatorial rules to integrate the parts into the overall configuration (Akshoomoff & Stiles, 1995a, 1995b; Feeney & Stiles, 1996; Stiles & Stern, 2001; Tada & Stiles, 1996). However, across this period, change is observed in both the nature of the parts and the relations children use to organize the parts.

Developmental Studies of Global- vs. Local-Level Processing

Studies using standard hierarchical form stimuli (Fig. 5.2; Navon, 1977) have consistently documented a protracted period of developmental change in global–local processing that extends well into adolescence (Dukette & Stiles, 1996, 2001; Harrison & Stiles, 2009; Mondloch, Geldart, Maurer, & de Schonen, 2003; Moses et al., 2002; Porporino, Shore, Iarocci, & Burack, 2004). An important characteristic of adult performance on hierarchical form tasks is the "global precedence effect," which is observed in the common finding that inconsistent or competing information at the global level interferes with local processing, but inconsistent local information does not affect global processing (Navon, 1977). These data suggest that for adults, global-level information takes precedence over local-level information. However, the evidence for a robust global precedence effect among children is mixed. While some studies have reported a global processing bias for children (Cassia et al., 2002; Mondloch

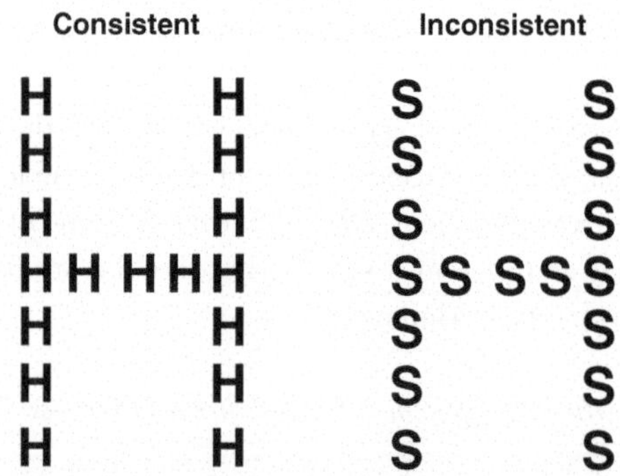

FIGURE 5.2 Hierarchical form stimuli consist of a large, global-level letter or form composed of appropriately arranged small, local-level forms. For the consistent hierarchical form stimulus (left) the letter or form at the global level is the same as those that make up the local level. For the inconsistent stimulus (right), the global and local levels differ.

et al., 2003; Moses et al., 2002; Porporino et al., 2004), others report more modest effects. For example, both increases in task demands (Harrison & Stiles, 2009) and selective degradation of the global-level information induce a shift in processing bias from the global to the local level that is much more pronounced in children than in adults (Dukette & Stiles, 1996).

Functional imaging data suggest similar patterns of developmental change in the neural systems that support global–local processing. Neuroimaging studies of children in the school-age and early adolescent period (e.g., 8 to 14 years) report bilateral activation that tends to be greater on the right than the left during both global and local processing, rather than the pattern of differential lateralization observed for adults (Moses et al., 2002). In addition, overall activation is greater for children, and they show considerably more bilateral activation, particularly on the local processing tasks, than adults. These findings suggest an early, immature pattern of neural engagement that is relatively undifferentiated by the nature of the spatial processing task. Increasing neural lateralization is observed with development, mirroring adult-like behavioral and neural patterns by adolescence.

The combined behavioral and neuroimaging data from the studies of hierarchical form processing show that children are clearly able to engage in both global- and local-level processing from a very early age. However, stable and mature levels of visuospatial processing emerge very slowly, and for a protracted period of development, variations in stimulus and task demands play an important role in modulating the dominant level of processing. Specialization within the neural systems that support global and local processing also develops gradually. Initially children engage the full bilateral posterior network for either global or local processing. As behavioral proficiency emerges, it is accompanied by increasing lateralization of the neural systems that support global and local processing. These findings are consistent with reports from other domains of a developmental shift from diffuse to focal patterns of neural activation (Durston et al., 2006).

Development of Face Processing

Faces are an important class of social stimuli. Preference for face stimuli has been documented from the first hours of life (Johnson, Dziurawiec, Ellis, & Morton, 1991). Infants as young as 2 to 3 months show selective cortical responses to faces (Halit, Csibra, Volein, & Johnson, 2004; Tzourio-Mazoyer et al., 2002). Some studies suggest that infants show a RH bias for faces (de Schonen & Deruelle, 1991; de Schonen, Deruelle, Mancini, & Pascalis, 1996; de Schonen & Mathivet, 1990). However, despite these early competencies there is overwhelming evidence for developmental change in face processing that extends at least through the school-age period (Chung & Thomson, 1995; Taylor, Edmonds, McCarthy, & Allison, 2001). Early studies suggested that changes in face processing might reflect a shift from a more feature-based to a more configural strategy (Carey & Diamond, 1977; Diamond & Carey, 1986; Tanaka & Farah, 1993). Research suggests that this shift is associated with the emergence of a RH advantage in processing unfamiliar faces at ages 9 to 10, coupled with an earlier RH advantage (by age 7) for the processing of familiar faces (Levine, 1985).

Recent work supports a pattern of gradual, quantitative age-related change (Itier & Taylor, 2004; Taylor, McCarthy, Saliba, & Degiovanni, 1999) and more effective use of the same types of cues used by adults (Baenninger, 1994; Freire & Lee, 2001; Pedelty, Levine, & Shevell, 1985) This kind of change may be associated with the acquisition of greater expertise in processing faces and other visual objects (Carey, 1996; Diamond & Carey, 1986; Gauthier & Nelson, 2001). Some researchers suggest that the changes in the neural system underlying age-related performance improvements involve increases in cortical specialization, with increasing specificity of systems for face processing (Johnson, 2002). Recent developmental fMRI studies of face processing support this proposition (Aylward et al., 2005; Gathers, Bhatt, Corbly, Farley, & Joseph, 2004; Golarai et al., 2007; Grill-Spector, Golarai, & Gabrieli, 2008; Passarotti et al., 2003). Most studies have focused on a region of fusiform gyrus in the ventral occipital temporal region referred to as the fusiform face area (FFA). These studies generally report increases in the size of the FFA with age (Golarai et al., 2007; Golarai, Liberman, Yoon, & Grill-Spector, 2010; Peelen, Glaser, Vuilleumier, & Eliez, 2009) and in the intensity of activation within this region from the early school-age period through adulthood (Cohen Kadosh, Cohen Kadosh, Dick, & Johnson, 2010; Golarai et al., 2007, 2010; Joseph, Gathers, & Bhatt, 2010). Further, the reported increases in size and intensity of activation correlate with improvement in recognition memory for faces (Golarai et al., 2007, 2010). Other studies have reported change in the larger face network organization involving change in the neural components of the face network (Joseph et al., 2010) as well as in the strength of connectivity among face network components (Cohen Kadosh et al., 2010).

The Development of Dorsal Stream Processes

The ability to process the location of objects and events is an essential spatial function. There is evidence that even very young children can solve simple object localization problems, but facility with these complex processes continues to develop well into adolescence. As discussed earlier, a frontoparietal circuit has been implicated in location processing. Data from a number of different domains suggest that this circuit undergoes substantial development and refinement over the period of infancy through adolescence.

Location Processing in Infancy

One of the largest bodies of data on early visuospatial processing comes from a simple, spatial hiding task introduced by Piaget (1952). In this task, infants watch as a toy is hidden under one of two screens (A and B), and then they are encouraged to retrieve it. In a typical test sequence, the object is first hidden at A for two or three trials, but on the next trial the hiding location is changed to B, again as the infant watches. Eight-month-olds easily retrieve the object hidden under A (but also see Lew, Hopkins, Owen, & Green, 2007; Smith, Thelen, Titzer, & McLin, 1999), but when the object is then hidden under B, they continue to search at A. This error has been termed the A not B error (AB error). The AB error is observed on the standard task between 8 and 12 months. However, children's experience outside the task setting can influence the likelihood of making the error (see Hauser, 1999). The experience of self-locomotion, either naturally occurring or through the use of an infant walker, significantly reduces the likelihood of the AB error (Bertenthal & Campos, 1990; Horobin & Acredolo, 1986; Kermoian & Campos, 1988).

Although still limited, the body of neuropsychological data on the AB task has begun to define the neural changes that contribute to the changes in task performance. Together they suggest that a complex network of neural systems emerges across the first year to support performance on this seemingly simple task (Baird et al., 2002). The data point to changes in both frontal and parietal regions within the dorsal stream (Diamond, 1991; Diamond, Werker, & Lalonde, 1994; Lew et al., 2007). As Johnson has noted, the changes within these different neural regions are unlikely to be unitary events. Rather, neural development is likely to reflect a more gradual "coming online" of the different components of the complex neural system that progressively comes to support the range of behaviors involved in this visual search task (Johnson, Mareschal, & Csibra, 2001).

Location Processing in Toddlers

Huttenlocher et al. (Huttenlocher & Lourenco, 2007b; Huttenlocher, Newcombe, & Sandberg, 1994) examined location coding in typically developing toddlers using a task in which children watched as a toy was buried in a long narrow sandbox and were then asked to indicate where the toy was hidden. Based on a theory of location coding developed by Huttenlocher, Hedges, and Duncan (Huttenlocher, Hedges, & Duncan, 1991), they hypothesized that young children would show evidence of hierarchical encoding of spatial location information, combining their fine-grained, inexact memory for the precise location of the toy with categorical information about the region in which the toy was located. Indeed, they found that the responses of 16- to 24-month-olds, the youngest children tested, were biased toward the center of the space in which the toy was buried, indicating that they treated the space as a single category with a prototypical location at the center (Fig. 5.3A). Somewhat older typically developing children, 3- to 5-year-olds, also showed evidence of hierarchical encoding, but unlike the younger children, they subdivided the space into two categories (left half, right half), each with a prototypical location at its center (i.e., a quarter of the way across the whole space, and three-quarters of the way across the whole space). Thus, children in this age group bias their responses for locations in the left half of the space toward the center of that category and their responses for locations in the right half of the space toward the center of that category (Fig. 5.3B). Huttenlocher et al. (1991) argue that categorical combination serves to increase the accuracy of response when the fine-grained location information is imprecise. Building on this work, others (Recker, Plumert, Hund, & Reimer, 2007; Spencer & Hund, 2003) have provided evidence that the degree to which object location memory depends on fine-grained location information versus categorical information depends on the ease of encoding these different kinds of information. Ease of coding, in turn, depends on subjects' cognitive abilities (e.g., variations in the ability to remember individual locations and to form spatial categories) as well as differences in the structure of the memory task (e.g., variations in the degree to which the location of individual objects vs. categories of objects are highlighted in particular tasks). Ultimately, accuracy of location memory is determined by the relative weighting that is given to memory for individual locations and category structure (for reviews see Huttenlocher & Lourenco, 2007a; Plumert, Hund, & Recker, 2007).

Location Processing in Older Children

Neural specialization of categorical and coordinate location coding in adults was originally tested using visual hemifield tasks (Kosslyn, Thompson, Kim, & Alpert, 1995) in which participants made decisions about the location of a target probe presented on either a blank grid (categorical task) or a bracketed square (coordinate task; Fig. 5.4A). Specifically, prior to

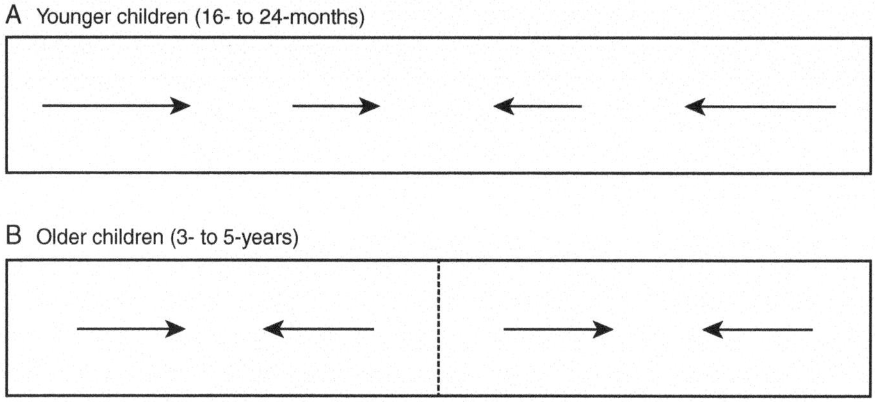

FIGURE 5.3 Location coding strategies observed among older and younger typically developing children. During the task a toy was hidden, in full view of the child, at a target location in the rectangular sandbox. After a brief delay, the child was encouraged to retrieve the toy. Throughout the preschool period (16 months to 5 years) children show evidence of categorical encoding of spatial locations, which involves combining their fine-grained, imprecise memory for the location of the hidden toy with their categorical information about the spatial region in which the toy was hidden. (A) Between 16 and 24 months typically developing children were biased toward the center of space, indicating that they treat space as a single category with a prototypical location at the center. (B) By 3 to 5 years children's coding of space is more complex. They subdivide space into two categories, left and right, with a prototypical center in the center of each space.

testing, participants studied a series of stimuli depicting a capital, block letter positioned on a grid. During test participants decided whether a probe mark (X), presented on a blank grid (categorical task) or bracketed square (coordinate task), would have appeared on the previously studied block letter (Fig. 5.4B). Target grids or brackets were presented to either the right (RVF) or left visual hemifield (LVF). The task was designed to elicit mental image generation of the block letter. To assess whether participants mentally generated the target letter, the probe location was varied. "Early" probes appeared on letter segments that are first produced when the letter is copied, while "late" probes appeared on later-produced segments (see Fig. 5.4B caption for details). For adults, the grid task elicits a LH "categorical" advantage, while the bracket task elicits a RH "coordinate" advantage.

Among typically developing control children, laterality effects in the categorical/coordinate processing task were affected by both age and probe location. For the 10-year-olds, early probe locations elicited a strong RH advantage for both tasks, whereas late probe locations produced a significant hemispheric dissociation consistent with those reported for adults. For the 8-year-olds, the early probes also elicited a strong RH advantage for both categorical and coordinate tasks, but performance on the late probes was poor (mean error rates near 30% compared to 10% for early probe trials presented to the LVF/RH), and there was no evidence of a task-related hemispheric dissociation on late probe trials (Reese & Stiles, 2005). The early probe location task may have facilitated performance by allowing subjects to use a strategy focused on global boundary information. Because the early "Yes" probe locations appeared on the edges of the stimuli, participants could use this boundary information,

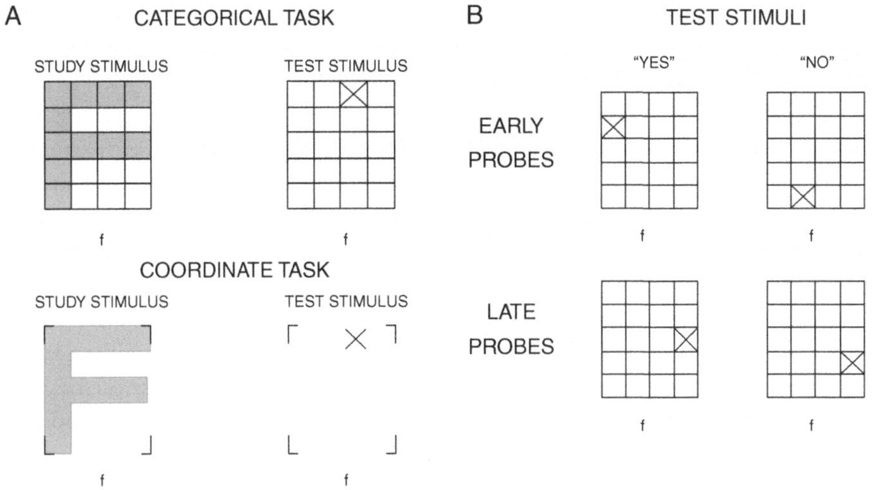

FIGURE 5.4 (A) Examples of the categorical (grids) and coordinate (brackets) stimuli (adapted from Kosslyn, Maljkovic, Hamilton, Horwitz, Thompson, 1995). Before the test, participants studied examples of the test stimuli presented on paper. When they indicated that they had familiarized themselves with the stimuli, they were asked to draw the letter on a separate sheet within a grid or bracket frame. This was repeated three times. The procedure they used to draw the letter was recorded to ensure that all participants produced the components in the canonical order so that their production of the component letters would conform to the definition of early and late probes. The two task conditions (grids and brackets) were presented in blocks and the order was counterbalanced across participants. (B) Stimuli were presented equally to the two visual half-fields. The subject's task was to read the small letter and determine whether the corresponding block letter would have covered the target probes (x). The two examples of stimuli presented in the categorical condition illustrate the "early" versus "late" positioning of the target probes. The typical procedure for drawing a block letter "F" is to begin in the upper left corner and draw the vertical line, then the top horizontal from left to right, and finally the lower horizontal from left to right. Thus the upper panels illustrate an "early" probe position for the yes and no responses and the lower panels the "late" probe position. (Adapted with permission from Reese & Stiles, 2005, Figs. 1 and 2.)

responding "Yes" if the probe fell on the outer edge of the figure and "No" if it did not. The finding of a developmentally early LVF/RH advantage for both categorical and coordinate processing is consistent with the finding discussed earlier of a RH fMRI activation bias for both global- and local-level processing (Moses & Stiles, 2002). It appears that both local-level pattern processing and categorical spatial processing are later-emerging aspects of neurobehavioral specialization. It is not until early adolescence that strongly lateralized patterns of neural mediation emerge in each of these task domains. The principal shift in neural mediation is the emergence of specialized LH systems for local and categorical processing.

Trajectories of Dorsal and Ventral Stream Development

Although many studies have examined the development of ventral or dorsal stream functions separately, work comparing the developmental trajectories of these two systems is more limited. Further, the available data present contradictory views of the relative rates of maturation of the two visual systems. One body of data that draws largely from studies of infants younger than a year suggests that dorsal stream functions involved in motion and location processing emerge earlier than ventral stream functions involved in feature processing. In contrast to this view, studies of older children tend to support the view that the ventral stream matures earlier than the dorsal stream.

Much of the evidence for the early maturation of the dorsal stream comes from infant studies of object individuation in which spatiotemporal cues involving motion and location processing are pitted against featural cues (Mash, Novak, Berthier, & Keen, 2006; Xu & Carey, 1996). The common finding from these experiments is that infants under about 12 months of age (Krojgaard, 2007; Wilcox & Baillargeon, 1998) recognize spatiotemporal violations but fail to notice featural changes (Bonatti, Frot, Zangl, & Mehler, 2002; Van de Walle, Carey, & Prevor, 2000; Xu & Carey, 1996; Xu, Carey, & Quint, 2004). These results have led to the suggestion that the dorsal system, which is responsible for processing spatiotemporal information, develops ahead of the ventral stream. Other evidence indicates that it is only toward the end of the first year of life that ventral stream information, such as color, is incorporated into object processing (Kaldy & Leslie, 2003; Leslie, Xu, Tremoulet, & Scholl, 1998).

In contrast to the infant work, studies of older preschool and school-aged children generally report that the development of the dorsal stream lags behind the ventral stream. In a series of ERP studies, Neville and colleagues (Armstrong, Neville, Hillyard, & Mitchell, 2002; Coch, Skendzel, Grossi, & Neville, 2005; Mitchell & Neville, 2004) reported significant developmental changes in response latency for motion but not color stimuli that extended from childhood through adulthood. However, visual evoked potential (VEP) studies that contrasted stimuli that varied in spatial frequency (Gordon & McCulloch, 1999) and chromaticity (Madrid & Crognale, 2000) provide evidence of a developmental lag in ventral stream functioning, in line with infant studies reported above. Still other studies have tested thresholds for motion and form coherence and report that ventral stream-mediated form coherence matures significantly ahead of dorsal stream-mediated motion coherence (Atkinson et al., 2005; Braddick, Atkinson, & Wattam-Bell, 2003; Gunn et al., 2002). Behavioral studies of children using the dual-stream framework comparing "what" versus "how" (Milner & Goodale, 1995) are rare. Atkinson (1998) reported data from a small sample of 4- to 7-year-old children using Milner and Goodale's (1995) "postbox" task, which requires manual posting of a letter into a slot at a particular angle (dorsal) or visual matching of the perceived angle of the slot (ventral). They report significantly better performance with the perceptual matching task. A second study using the same task but focused on 3- to 4-year-old children reported a very similar pattern of results (Dilks, Hoffman, & Landau, 2008), suggesting a ventral stream advantage.

The mixed and often contradictory results from studies comparing the relative rates of development of dorsal and ventral streams have led a number of investigators to suggest that it may be misleading to treat the development of either visual system as a unitary event. Quinn (Quinn & Bhatt, 2006) has suggested that the global dichotomy likely overlooks more subtle changes that occur within each stream across development. In addition, Johnson, Mareschal, and colleagues (Johnson et al., 2001; Kaufman, Csibra, & Johnson, 2003; Mareschal & Johnson, 2003) suggest that the inconsistency between the infant studies and the studies involving school-age children may arise from another factor related to the immaturity of the visual system. In particular, while there is good evidence that both streams are functional from very early in development, there are few data suggesting that information from the two streams becomes integrated until late in the first year. This lack of integration may account for some of the findings of the early dominance of spatiotemporal information in the infant literature.

THE DEVELOPMENT OF VISUOSPATIAL PROCESSES IN CHILDREN WITH PERINATAL LESIONS

The overview of the basic anatomical and functional organization of the mature dorsal and ventral pathways presented at the beginning of this chapter provides a template for evaluating the effects of perinatal brain injury on the development of these important systems. The data on the typical development of major processes associated with two visual streams suggests that the mature organization of the visual system emerges slowly, over much of the childhood and early adolescent periods. The developmental trajectories for the two pathways appear to emerge roughly in parallel, though there is evidence of both very early and later developmental offset in at least some tasks involving dorsal and ventral stream processing. Very little is known about the interaction of the two systems during development, although there is evidence that as early as 16 months of age, children combine categorical and metric (coordinate) information in location coding. The developmental data provide important benchmarks for evaluating the effects of early injury on the development of visuospatial processing. Our discussion of the development of visuospatial processing following early perinatal brain injury will be guided by the following questions:

1. Is there evidence of systematic early-emerging deficits in visuospatial processing in children with PL?
2. If so, how do they compare with those of adults with homologous lesions? Is the pattern of site of lesion to type of spatial deficit similar in adults and children?
3. Do the data from the PL population provide insight into the relationship between the developmental trajectories of the dorsal and ventral visual streams?
4. Do the deficits change over time either qualitatively or by degree?

The Development of Ventral Stream Processes in Children with Perinatal Lesions

The ventral visual stream is a system for processing a wide array of visual patterns from objects, to scenes, to faces. Analysis of any visual pattern requires specification of both the parts and the overall configuration. As discussed earlier, studies with adults have shown that different patterns of spatial deficit are associated with LH damage and RH damage (e.g., Arena & Gainotti, 1978; Delis et al., 1986, 1988; Gainotti & Tiacci, 1970; McFie & Zangwill, 1960; Piercy, Hecaen, & De Ajuriaguerra, 1960; Ratcliff, 1982; Swindell et al., 1988; Warrington, James, & Kinsbourne, 1966), with the LH dominant for featural processing and the RH for configural processing. Data from children with PL suggest that the basic organization of the ventral stream occipitotemporal system is established early but is capable of at least limited adaptive organization. Studies of children with PL report patterns of deficit that are consistent with those observed among adults, though the severity of deficit is less pronounced. There is also clear evidence for improvements in performance from the preschool to late adolescent period, suggesting that children may be better able to compensate for their spatial processing deficits than adults with comparable injury.

Ventral Stream Processing in the Preschool Period

The first study to explicitly establish a specific disorder of spatial integrative ability in children with right PL examined spatial classification in very young preschoolers (Stiles-Davis, Sugarman, & Nass, 1985). In this task, 2- to 3-year-old children were presented with stimulus sets containing two classes of objects (e.g., blocks and small plates) and were simply encouraged to play. This procedure elicits systematic class grouping activity in both typically developing children and children with PL, but among children with right PL the organization and complexity of the spatial groupings were limited. Specifically, while children with right PL would stack objects or place one object in another in a manner that demonstrated their sensitivity to *object* categories, their use of spatial relations such as adjacency was lacking. While typically developing children and children with left PL regularly place objects next to each other in orderly rows as early as 24 months, children with right PL failed to do so even at 36 to 42 months.

The findings from this very basic spatial classification task were examined in greater depth in a longitudinal study of 3- to 5-year-old children within the context of a block construction task (Stiles, Stern, Trauner, & Nass, 1996; Vicari, Stiles, Stern, & Resca, 1998). In the task the children were given unlimited time to copy models of simple block constructions (e.g., lines, stacks, arches). The study assessed both the accuracy of constructions the children generated (the products) as well as how they went about producing them (the processes). Among typically developing 2- to 4-year-old children there is systematic change in the procedures children use in block construction. Up to about 18 months, children produce only single relations within a construction (stacking or aligning). Between 24 and 36 months children combine several types of relations, but they do so sequentially, completing one component (e.g., stack or line) before beginning another. By 36 to 42 months, their spatial grouping procedures become flexible and they shift between both relation types and parts of the emerging construction. This task provided evidence of spatial impairment in both left PL and right PL groups. Children with left PL were initially delayed in their construction, producing only very simple constructions using simple procedures. By age 4, they showed an interesting dissociation in performance. Most of the children were able to produce accurate copies of the target constructions, but the procedures they used in copying the forms were greatly simplified. This dissociation between product and process persisted at least through age 6. Children with right PL were also initially delayed. By age 4, they produced disordered, poorly configured constructions, but at this age the procedures they used to generate their ill-formed constructions were comparable to age-matched controls. However, at age 6 there was a striking change in their construction activities, marked by both improved construction accuracy and compensation for their deficit. Specifically, the children with right PL were able to accurately copy the target constructions, but now, like their left PL peers and unlike their own earlier performance, they used simple procedures to generate these constructions. This study suggests that early injury to either the RH or LH results in impaired spatial processing, but there is also some capacity for compensation with development.

Studies of drawing also provide an index of spatial impairment, particularly among children with right PL. In a simple free drawing task, children were asked to draw a house (Stiles-Davis, 1988). Typically developing 3.5- to 4-year-olds produced well-organized houses, with an outer form representing the building and appropriately positioned inner features representing doors and windows. Children with left PL produced drawings that were indistinguishable from those of controls by age 5 (Fig. 5.5A). By contrast, throughout the preschool period, drawings of children with right PL were disordered and lacked integration (Fig. 5.5B). Their drawings were much like those of adults with RH injury that have been described as "scattered, fragmented, and disorganized . . . subjects often overscored lines and added extraneous scribblings" (Swindell et al., 1988, p. 19). However, longitudinal evaluation of children with right PL reveals improvement in their drawings that is not observed among adult patients, but the improvement appeared to reflect the use of a particular compensatory strategy, graphic formulas.

Graphic formulas are common in the normal development course of drawing, beginning in the earliest drawings and persisting through adulthood (Stiles, 1995), but in typical

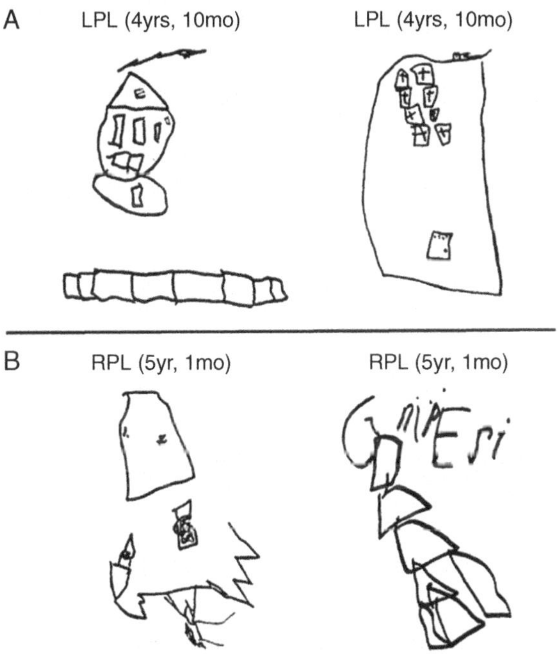

FIGURE 5.5 Free drawings of houses by four 5-year-old children with PL. (A) The free drawings of houses by two children with left PL (LPL) look very much like those of typically developing children. They have an outer frame and appropriately arranged inner features. (B) The free drawings by two children with right PL (RPL) lack organization and integration. In the drawing on the left, the door is below the house and the chimney below that. The figure to the right of the chimney is a "person in the house" according to the child. In the drawing on the right, the rooms are arranged linearly. As he drew each, he labeled them "my mother's room, my brother's room, my brother's room, my sister's room, my sister's room, my brother's room, my room" (from the top, counterclockwise). (Adapted with permission from Stiles-Davis et al., 1988.)

children development formulas are one tool among many used for drawing. For children with right PL, the mastery of graphic formulas appears to provide a useful compensatory strategy that allows them to represent common objects while minimizing the spatial processing demands. If the children's improvement on the drawing task is achieved through the compensatory strategy of graphic formula production, then they should be more dependent on formulaic representation than normally developing children. Reliance on graphic formulas was tested using a task developed by Karmiloff-Smith (Karmiloff-Smith, 1990) in which children are asked to first draw a house, and then an impossible house (Stiles, Trauner, Engel, & Nass, 1997). The most common solution to this task among typically developing children and children with left PL is to distort the spatial configuration of the house (Fig. 5.6A), a strategy rarely used by the children with right PL. Instead, the children with right PL derived a number of equally implausible but non-configurational solutions for solving the problem, including inversion, impossible placement, verbal descriptions, formula substitution, size reduction, and invisibility (Fig. 5.6B). Once again, these findings indicate that while these children are developing and their performance on specific spatial tasks improves, the processes

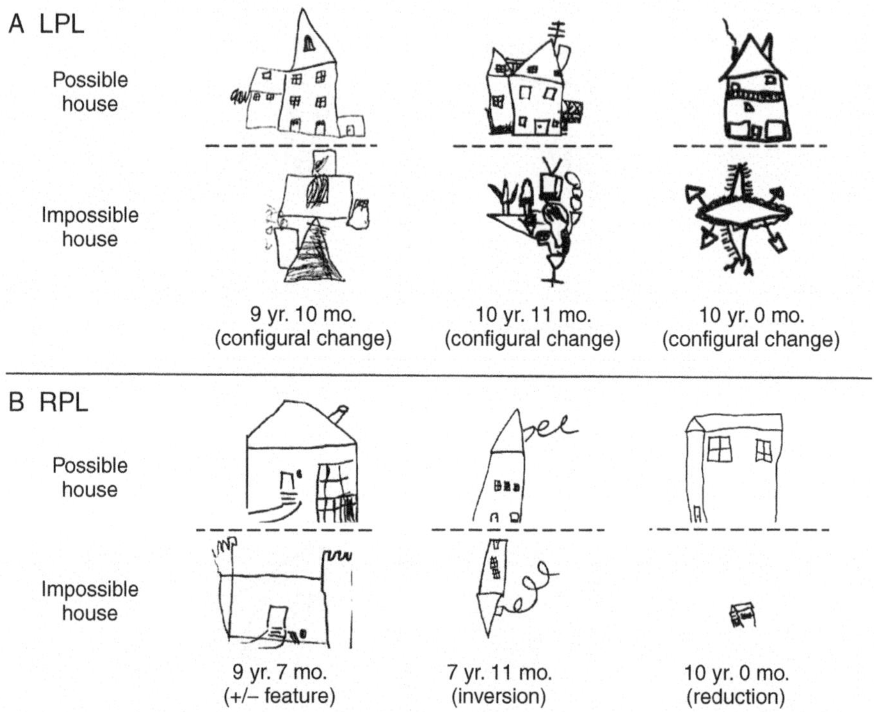

FIGURE 5.6 The test of graphic formula production asked children to first draw a house, and then to draw an "impossible house, a house that could not be." (A) Three examples of possible and impossible house drawing from children with left PL represent the responses of the majority of children in this population and the population of typically developing children, which is to alter the overall configuration of the house. (B) Children with right PL rarely altered the configuration of the house. The drawings of the three children shown here represent the more common responses of children with right PL. The children produced the basic house form but altered its features, inverted it, or made it very small. (Adapted with permission from Stiles et al., 1997.)

by which they master these tasks differ from those of typically developing children. This suggests a pattern of specific, subtle, and persistent deficit in spatial processing as well as compensation.

Ventral Stream Processing in School-age Children and Adolescents

Through the school-age and adolescent period evidence of persistent subtle spatial processing deficits are observed against a continuing background of developmental improvement. Children appear to find means for mastering tasks that are challenging for a particular developmental period but show evidence of continuing impairment when more difficult tasks are introduced. Such a pattern is evident for children with both left and right PL on tasks that tap global–local-level processing.

Visual patterns can be conceived of as a structured hierarchy consisting of local-level elements and more global-level assemblies. A common stimulus in many experimental tests of global–local processing are large letters composed of appropriately arranged smaller letters, such as a large H made up of small Ss (see Fig. 5.2). These "hierarchical stimuli" have been used in studies of normal adults (e.g., Kinchla & Wolfe, 1979; Martin, 1979; Navon, 1977; Palmer, 1980; Palmer & Bucher, 1981) and children (Dukette & Stiles, 1996, 2001; Harrison & Stiles, 2009; Stiles, Delis, & Tada, 1991). They also have been used to identify differential patterns of spatial deficit in adults with focal left and right posterior brain injury (Delis, et al., 1986, 1988; Lamb & Robertson, 1988, 1989; Robertson & Delis, 1986). As reviewed earlier in this chapter, adult patients with RH damage have difficulty processing the global level of the form, while patients with LH damage have difficulty processing the local level.

Data from a large study of hierarchical form processing in children with left or right PL are consistent with data from adult patients (Stiles et al., 2008). In this task children were asked to study and remember a hierarchical pattern. After a brief distracter task they were asked to reproduce the form from memory. Typically developing children are equally accurate in producing the global and local levels of the patterns (Fig. 5.7A,B). Two age groups of children with PL were tested, 5- to 7-year-olds, and 9- to 11-year-olds. The younger children with left PL had difficulty producing both the global and the local level of pattern structure, while the younger children with right PL were able to accurately produce the local-level elements but had difficulty with the global-level ones (Fig. 5.8). Older children with left PL were impaired only with production of local-level elements, and older children with right PL continued to show impairment with the global level. For each group, the level of impairment was more pronounced for the younger than the older children. For the young children with left PL, the severe impairment in ability to produce local elements also affects their ability to generate a well-configured global form. The reverse profile was not observed for the young children with right PL: it was possible for them to accurately generate local-level elements, even though they were unable to configure them appropriately.

The Rey-Osterrieth Complex Figure (ROCF; Osterrieth, 1944) task requires participants to first copy a model of the figure, and after a delay reproduce it from memory (Fig. 5.9). The task is challenging for children with PL (Akshoomoff, Feroleto, Doyle, & Stiles, 2002; Akshoomoff & Stiles, 2003), as illustrated in a longitudinal study of 6- to 13-year-olds. On the copying task, both children with right PL and with left PL performed worse than controls. Deficits were particularly evident among the youngest children (age 6), but did not

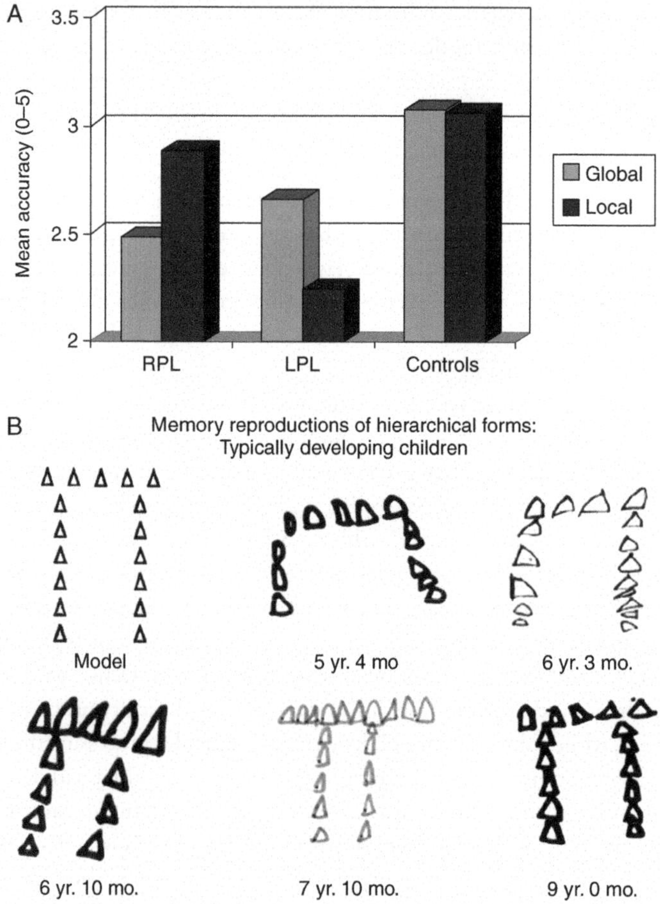

FIGURE 5.7 In the memory task, children were shown four hierarchical form stimuli one at a time and after a brief delay they were asked to reproduce them from memory. (A) The reproduction accuracy of the hierarchical forms was assessed with two, matched 5-point (0–5) scales, one for local processing and one for global (see Dukette & Stiles, 2001, for details). While the 5- to 12-year-old controls were comparably accurate at the global and local levels, the PL children showed systematic differences that reflect a local processing deficit for the left PL group and a global processing deficit for the right PL group. (Reprinted with permission from Stiles et al., 2008.) (B) Examples of the reproduction from five typically developing children ranging in age from 5 to 9 years. Note the improvement in accuracy at both levels with age.

differ by side of lesion (Fig. 5.9). Performance improved such that by 10 years the children's copies were accurate, but they were produced using the most immature and piecemeal strategy (see Fig. 5.9 figure caption for description of strategies). The failure to find differences between the right and left PL groups likely reflects underlying task demands that place equal emphasis on segmentation and integration. Thus, a deficit in either process would disrupt performance on the task. However, in contrast to the findings from the copy task, the memory task did distinguish between the lesion groups. When the copy and memory data from the oldest children in the sample were compared, few differences were observed for the

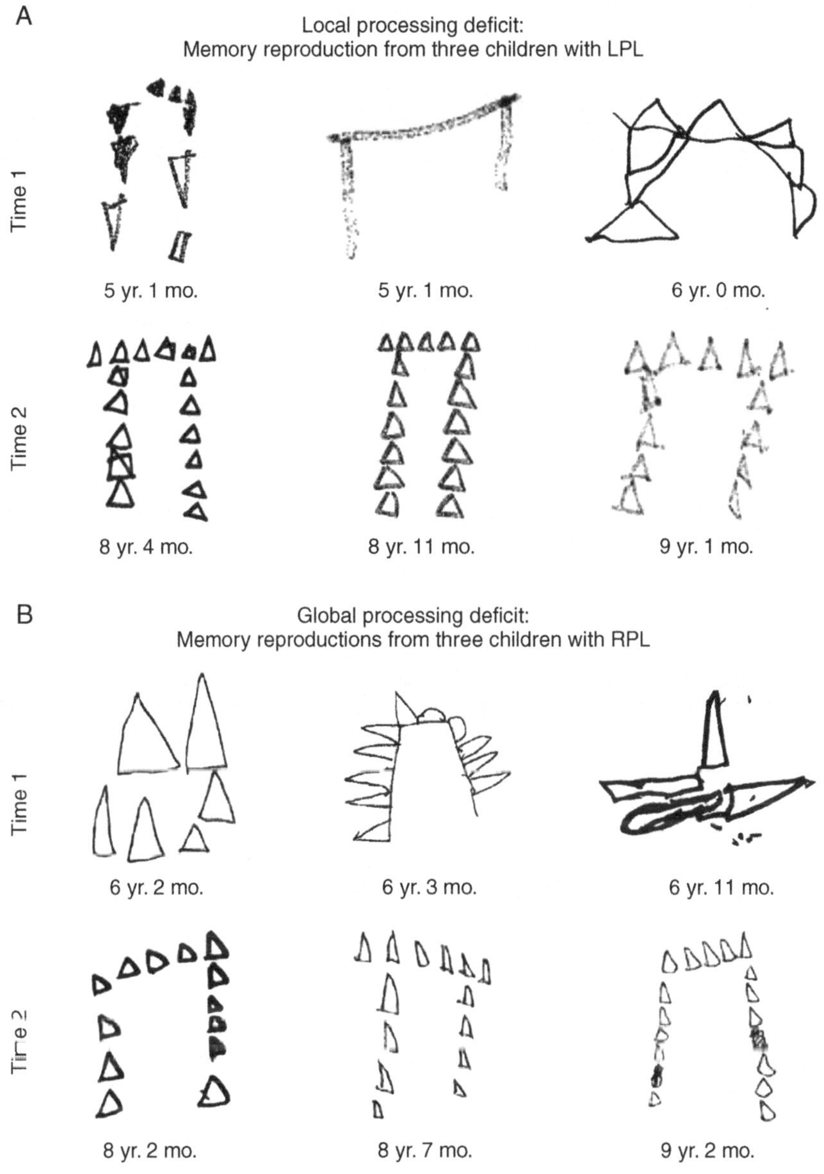

FIGURE 5.8 Longitudinal data from six children with PL on the hierarchical forms memory reproduction task. (A) Young children (top row) with left PL show marked deficits in local-level processing. By later childhood (bottom row) improvement is noted, but local accuracy continues to lag behind global accuracy. (B) Young children (top row) with right PL show marked deficits in global-level processing. By later childhood (bottom row) improvement is noted, but global accuracy continues to lag behind local.

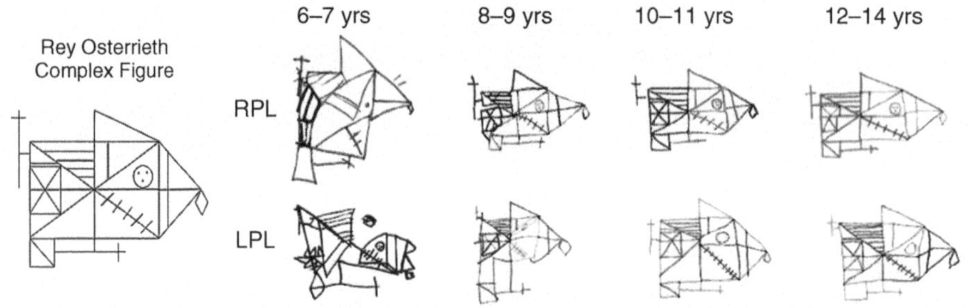

FIGURE 5.9 The longitudinal data from the copy version of the Rey-Osterrieth Complex Figure task are presented for two representative children, one with left PL (LPL) and one with right PL (RPL). Note the very disordered drawings for both children at 6 and 7 years of age. Improvement is observed over the subsequent years in the overall organization of the copies. However, the children continue to use the most immature "piecemeal strategy" even as young adolescents. Typically developing children organize their drawings around larger and larger subcomponents of the form with age. At age 5 and 6 they use a piecemeal strategy, by age 9 and 10 organization reflects the right and left sides of the figure, and finally by early adolescence they organize their drawings around the core rectangle, thus adopting the adult strategy (see Akshoomoff, et al 1995a, for details). It is notable that neither the right PL nor the left PL child changed his drawing strategy over a period of 6 years. (Adapted with permission from Akshoomoff et al., 2002.) (See color insert.)

children with right PL (Fig. 5.10). Under both task conditions they produced accurate reproductions using a piecemeal reproduction strategy. However, a dramatic shift in the reproduction strategies of the children with LH injury was observed in the memory task (Fig. 5.10). Unlike the copy task, children organized their memory reproductions around the core rectangle and produced relatively few additional details. The demands of the memory

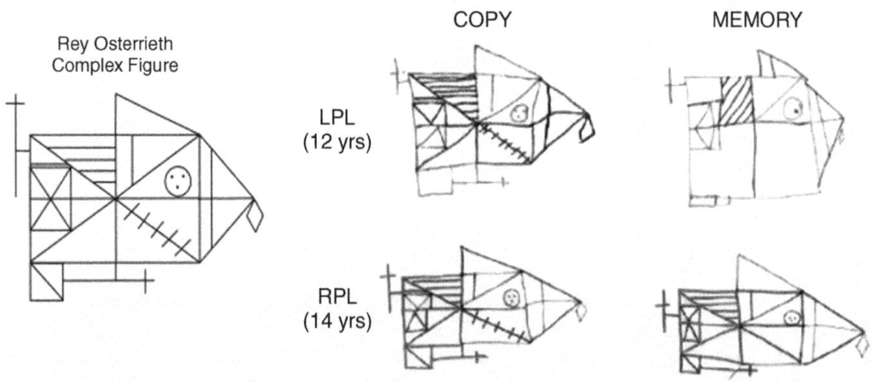

FIGURE 5.10 The data from the Rey-Osterrieth copy and memory tasks are shown for the same two children whose longitudinal copy data were shown in Figure 5.9. In contrast to the copy data, where the performance of the two children did not differ, clear contrasts are seen in the memory task data. The memory reproduction for the child with left PL (LPL) is strikingly different from his copy. While he used a piecemeal strategy when copying a model, his memory reproduction is sparse and includes the core rectangle and only a few other details. The memory reproduction for the child with right PL (RPL) is strikingly similar to his copy, and he uses a very similar piecemeal strategy. (Adapted with permission from Akshoomoff et al., 2002.) (See color insert.)

task thus revealed the characteristic left PL featural processing deficit, while the copying task captured the children's strategies for compensating for that deficit.

Face Processing

A growing body of evidence suggests that face processing is affected by early brain injury. However, the evidence suggests that impairment is not confined to children with right PL and can extend to children with left PL as well. De Schonen and colleagues (de Schonen, Mancini, Camps, Maes, & Laurent, 2005; Mancini, de Schonen, Deruelle, & Massoulier, 1994) reported a series of studies examining different aspects of face processing in school-age children with PL. Deficits in face processing were common in their population of children and as common among the children with left PL as right PL. A similar pattern of performance on the Benton Face task, which requires participants to match a black-and-white photograph of a target to one of six black-and-white photos in a test array, was also reported by Ballantyne (Ballantyne & Trauner, 1999). The severity of the face processing deficits reported in these studies suggests that face processing may be established very early and may be less plastic than other aspects of visuospatial processing. Data from a study of somewhat older children and adolescents with PL are consistent with these findings. Paul (Paul et al., in preparation; Stiles, Paul, & Hesselink, 2006) examined reaction time and accuracy in a face identity-matching task. Children and adolescents with right PL were significantly slower and less accurate in identifying faces than typical controls. Performance of the left PL group was marginally worse than controls but did not differ significantly from the right PL group, suggesting that early lesions to either hemisphere affect face processing but perhaps less markedly in the case of left PL lesions. Together the data suggest that face processing is vulnerable to the effects of early injury, manifesting significant impairments that extend well into adolescence.

The Development of Dorsal Stream Processes in Children with Perinatal Lesions

Spatial localization is an important dorsal stream function. Consistent with data from ventral stream functioning, studies of children with PL report patterns of deficit for dorsal stream function that are consistent with those observed among adult patients with unilateral lesions, though the severity of deficit is less pronounced. And again, there is also clear evidence for performance improvements from the preschool to late adolescent period, suggesting that children may be better able to compensate for their spatial processing deficits than adults with comparable injury.

Dorsal Stream Processing in the Preschool Period

The data on dorsal stream processing in children with PL is more limited than data on ventral stream processing, particularly in the preschool period. Lourenco & Levine (Lourenco & Levine, 2009, in preparation) have adapted a task developed by Huttenlocher et al. (Huttenlocher et al., 1994) to examine location coding in children with PL. Recall that Huttenlocher et al.'s findings show that by 16 months of age, typically developing children combine metric (distance from the edge or center of the space) and categorical information (right, left) in coding location in their search for toys hidden in a sandbox. In the adapted task, toys were placed on a 60-inch-long rug for a brief period and then removed; the children then indicated the location on the rug where the toy had been placed. Findings show that both children with left PL and right PL perform this task differently than typically developing children, and differently from each other, in ways that are broadly consistent with findings on the lateralization of metric and categorical coding in adult patients. In particular, throughout the 3- to 5-year age range, children with right PL show evidence of categorical combination in their location coding, whereas this is not the case for children with left PL. However, even at 5 years of age, children with right PL use a simpler category structure than typically developing children, treating the rug as a single category. That is, they bias their responses toward the center of the rug, as was the case for typically developing 16- to 24-month-olds in Huttelocher et al.'s (Huttenlocher et al., 1994) sandbox study (Fig. 5.11 A). Using this immature category structure, children with right PL are quite accurate by age 5, although still somewhat less accurate than typically developing 5-year-olds.

In contrast, children with left PL do not show any evidence of using categorical information in their location coding at ages 3 to 4 years. That is, their location errors are not biased toward the center of the whole space like younger typically developing children or children with right PL, nor toward the center of the left half or right half of the space like older typically developing children. At 5 years of age, children with left PL show some evidence of hierarchical coding of location but use an atypical category structure. In particular, their coding of locations near the endpoints of the rug (the 10-inch and 50-inch locations) are biased toward the respective ends of the rug (i.e., away from the center of the rug), their

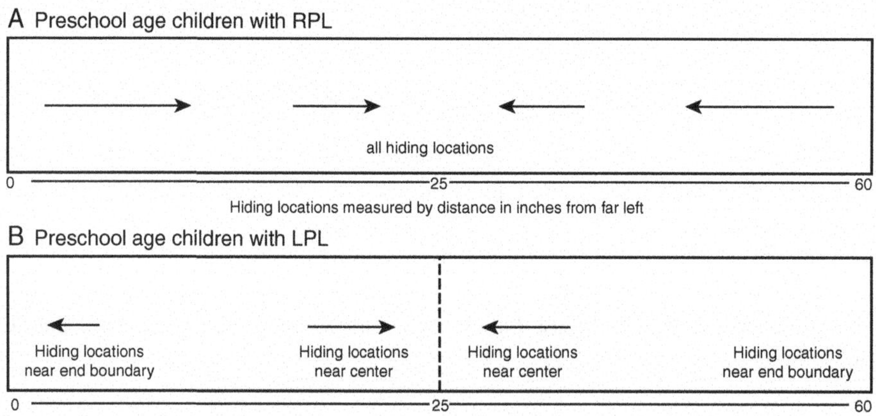

FIGURE 5.11 Schematic drawings of location coding observed for preschool-age children with PL on a modified version of the sandbox task. Here toys were placed on a rectangular rug (60 inches in length), and after a brief delay they were removed. The child's task was to indicate where the toy had been. Hiding locations were centered vertically, and at positions 10, 20, 30, 40, and 50 inches from the left border along the horizontal axis. (A) Children with right PL (RPL) adopt the location coding strategy of typically developing young children. They are biased toward the center of space, indicating that they treat space as a single category with a prototypical location at the center. (B) Children with left PL (LPL) adopt very different coding strategies. When objects are hidden near the outer boundary, their search shifts toward that boundary, and when objects are hidden near the center of the box, their search shifts toward the center.

responses to the 20-inch and 40-inch locations are biased toward the center of the rug, and their responses to the central 30-inch location are extremely accurate (Fig. 5.11B). Thus, by age 5, children with left PL appear to combine their approximate memories for the location of objects with three categories, the two endpoints and the center of the space. Of note, by 5 years of age, the responses of children with left PL, like those of children with right PL, are very accurate, but somewhat less accurate than typically developing 5-year-olds. The performance levels of children with left PL and right PL do not significantly differ at any of the time points examined, even though they apply different strategies to location coding. Although both groups perform somewhat less accurately than typically developing children, they continue to show improvements in accuracy throughout the 3- to 5-year period.

These findings on location coding, a prototypical dorsal stream task, are reminiscent of findings on the ventral stream tasks described above, which show that the product achieved by children with early brain injury can reach or approach the level of typically developing children using different processes (Stiles, Stern, Trauner, & Nass, 1996; Vicari et al, 1998). Thus, we see that children with right PL achieve near-normal performance on the location coding task by age 5 using an immature category structure, and children with left PL achieve near-normal performance by age 5 using an atypical category structure.

Dorsal Stream Processing in School-age Children and Adolescents

As was the case with ventral stream processes, evidence of persistent subtle dorsal stream spatial processing deficits is observed against a background of developmental improvement. Although preschool-age children initially show deficits on spatial location tasks, by age 5 their performance is close to the level of their typically developing peers in terms of accuracy. However, when more challenging tasks are introduced with older children, evidence of hemisphere-specific deficits for different aspects of spatial location processing emerges in the school-age and early adolescent period.

Categorical and coordinate coding has been examined in adolescents with PL (Reese & Stiles, submitted) using the child adaptation (Reese & Stiles, 2005) of Kosslyn's visual hemifield mental image generation task. Among typical adults, categorical probes are processed more efficiently when presented to the RVF/LH and coordinate probes are processed more efficiently when presented to the LVF/RH (Kosslyn et al., 1989). Among typically developing children, early probe locations elicited a strong LVF/RH advantage for both tasks, whereas late probe locations produced the mature pattern of hemispheric dissociation among 10-year-olds, but not 8-year-olds.

The left PL and right PL groups showed different patterns of performance. The left PL group showed an overall LVF/RH advantage, regardless of task or probe location; indeed, performance on all probes presented to the RVF/LH was poor. The RH advantage for both categorical and coordinate processing among the left PL group is similar to that of young typical children for the early probe trials but distinctly different from any age group for the late probe trials. By contrast, overall accuracy for the right PL group was only slightly poorer than the controls, but they showed no evidence of hemispheric specialization for either task or probe location. Rather, accuracy and response times were comparable across stimulus types and side of presentation. Thus, largely spared level of performance but lack of typical task-related laterality characterized the performance of children with right PL.

This combination of findings may reflect the effects of several developmental events working in concert. First, as discussed earlier, the data from typically developing children appear to reflect the comparatively late emergence of LH specialization for categorical processing. Thus, consistent with findings from other domains, the brain systems for location processing appear to be relatively inefficient and distributed early in development, and become more focused and specialized with age. Further, several studies of adults with focal brain damage suggest that while LH injury impairs categorical but not coordinate processing, RH injury affects both processes (Amorapanth et al., 2010; Palermo, Bureca, Matano, & Guariglia, 2008). Thus, the mature RH appears to be a neural substrate that can support both categorical and coordinate processing, at least to some degree. The combination of developmental flexibility coupled with the apparent multifunctionality of the RH affords the possibility of establishing both categorical and coordinate spatial processing within a single intact RH, and that is consistent with the findings from the left PL group. The reason for the more general sparing of both categorical and coordinate processing in the absence of clear evidence for lateralization in the right PL group is less clear. However, it may be related to the later course of specialization for the LH that is reported for both global–local and categorical–coordinate processing in typically developing children. This prolonged period of development could provide a window of plasticity that allows for alternative patterns of organization to arise. Because the LH is less well suited to coordinate processing, the alternative organization may also take advantage of any remaining RH resources and utilize them in a distributed fashion, giving rise to the relatively spared performance and lack of laterality in the right PL group. This kind of profile is similar to the pattern of reorganization observed for language functioning following early brain injury (see Chapter 8). These findings suggest that the visual spatial processing system maintains at least some degree of neural plasticity during development.

SUMMARY OF VISUOSPATIAL PROCESSING IN CHILDREN WITH PERINATAL LESIONS

This section began with a series of questions about the effects of perinatal brain injury on the development of visuospatial functions. The first two questions asked whether there was evidence of early deficit and whether the patterns of deficits relative to site of lesion were similar to those observed among adults with similar patterns of brain injury. The short answer to both of those questions is yes: there is evidence of specific spatial deficit from very early in development, and the associations between site of injury and specific type of deficit are broadly similar for adults and children whose lesions were acquired late and early in life, respectively. Given the differences in the nature of the lesions in the different age groups, the characterization of "similarity" is very general and refers largely to patterns of deficit associated with laterality of injury in both adults and children. Consistent with the data from typically developing children, these findings suggest that the basic organization of the visuospatial system emerges very early in development, and that early lateralized lesions systematically affect the development of specific functions in ways that generally mirror the organization of the mature system.

One notable difference between the effects of perinatal and adult-onset lesions concerns the extent and specificity of the lesion within a cerebral hemisphere. Among children with brain injury the lateralized differences on tasks involving functions such as global–local or categorical–coordinate processing are associated with lesions to widely distributed cortical regions. In part this is due to the fact that many of the child lesions involve much of the MCA distribution and are thus quite large. But even in cases of smaller cortical lesions, including those that do not directly involve the primary dorsal and ventral stream pathways, evidence of specific visuospatial deficits is apparent and conforms to the general, lateralized pattern of deficit. The exception to this finding involves children with smaller lesions confined to mainly subcortical regions, who often present with much milder profiles of visuospatial deficit overall. These generalized effects of cortical injury may reflect the interruption of neural development within a hemisphere that results from the early injury. Consistent with this finding is a study that examined the distribution of white matter abnormalities in a small number of cases of children with isolated anterior lesions. That study reported reduced levels of white matter in the posterior portions of the major association pathways (Stiles, Moses, & Paul, 2006; Stiles, Nass, Levine, Moses, & Reilly, 2009). Such white matter abnormalities could account for findings of specific posterior temporal or parietal processing deficits in the absence of frank lesions to those regions.

The third question raised at the beginning of this section concerned possible insights into the relative trajectories of development for the dorsal and ventral streams emerging from the PL data. Evidence of systematic, lateralized deficits is observed for both dorsal and ventral stream functions, and for both systems the patterns of deficit broadly mirror those seen in adults with localized brain injury. While it is difficult to draw strong conclusions in the absence of well-matched dorsal and ventral streams tasks administered at the same developmental points, the available data from children with PL injury do not thus far support the relative sparing of one system over the other. Major functions associated with both systems are affected by early injury, suggesting at least rudimentary establishment of both visual processing streams very early in development.

The final question raised in the beginning paragraph broached the issue of developmental plasticity. It asked whether there is evidence of qualitative or quantitative change in the patterns of deficit over developmental time. There is little evidence to suggest qualitative change in the patterns of deficit across development. While there are many instances of developmental improvement on a particular spatial task, there is little evidence to suggest significant change in the nature of the underlying deficit. Rather, the most striking differences between adult and child lesion patients' visuospatial processing abilities are the magnitude of their deficits. While the lesion-specific profiles of deficit for adults and children are qualitatively similar, the severity of deficit among children with PL is notably reduced relative to adults, and performance generally improves over developmental time. For both dorsal and ventral stream processing, the characteristic pattern of developmental change involves gradual mastery of tasks that are intentionally designed to challenge typical children of a particular age. Thus, during the targeted age window, the spatial tasks are challenging for both typical children and children with PL, but the patterns of error differ, revealing specific deficits among the PL group. For example, the memory for hierarchical forms task is challenging for typically developing 4- to 5-year-olds, but their errors are equally distributed across the global and local levels of the forms, and their reproductions of both levels improve with development. By contrast, the distribution of errors in the PL groups reveals their underlying deficits. Children with RH lesions make many more errors at the global level and children with

LH lesion err more at the local level. As children with PL develop and gradually master the specific task, evidence of their deficit declines, but the subtle differences in errors persist through at least early adolescence.

The data suggest that the path to mastery on a particular visuospatial task may diverge from normal. While the children may eventually succeed in producing the "right answer," their success may involve the use of alternative strategies such as the use of graphic formulas in drawing; or it may involve the effective marshalling of simpler but still effective strategies typical of younger children, such as those observed in the block construction and Rey-Osterrieth Complex Figure tasks; or it may involve the use of simpler or atypical category structures on location coding tasks. The persistence of deficit is captured developmentally when similar but more difficult versions of tasks are introduced. Thus, preschool children show initial specific deficits or the use of simpler or atypical category structures in simple spatial location tasks, but they master them by the early school-age period. However, when older children are confronted with a much more difficult location processing task such as Kosslyn's categorical–coordinate processing task, the original profile of deficit is again evident. Thus, the behavioral profiles that have emerged from the studies of children with PL are best characterized by subtle but persistent lesion-specific deficits that can be tracked against a backdrop of development, adaptation, and compensation. Children appear to compensate for subtle persistent spatial cognitive processing deficits by using simplified, less complicated cognitive procedures and strategies. And they do so successfully, as measured by their mastery of specific tasks. The critical questions raised by these data are: why are these simplified procedures necessary, and what are the neural mechanisms that mediate them? While these questions derive from and are articulated by the behavioral evidence, they cannot be addressed by behavioral tests alone. Rather, they require an understanding of both the status of the neural substrate and the functional neural organization that emerges in the wake of early injury.

As discussed in Chapter 8, these crucial neural processing data for language processing have begun to emerge from the fMRI studies. While somewhat variable, those studies point to the emergence of alternative patterns of brain organization to support the critical functions of language. In the case of LH injury, optimal outcomes appear to involve activation of remaining, uninjured language regions within the LH, in coordination with recruitment of generally homologous regions of the RH. Interestingly, the data from younger typically developing children also suggest early bilateral mediation of language processing. Thus, the pattern of neural recruitment for language observed in the PL group may reflect an alternative developmental pathway in which earlier, perhaps less efficient but nonetheless effective, neural systems are recruited and retained to support functional language in the wake of early stroke.

While the data on the neural substrates of visuospatial processing in children with PL are extremely limited, the small bit of case study data is consistent with the findings from the language studies described above. In the typical course of development, children engage bilateral posterior brain regions for both global- and local-level processing in hierarchical forms tasks. With development the lateralized profiles of greater right activation for global and greater left activation for local processing begin to emerge, suggesting greater neural efficiency as the task is mastered. Data from two case studies of adolescents with PL, one with LH and one with RH injury, show that both global processing and local processing activate the intact hemisphere. But in these two cases the activation is in opposite hemispheres, depending on side of injury. One interpretation of these data that would accord with the interpretation of the language studies is that the PL children in the visuospatial task, like their typically developing peers, initially recruit all available neural resources when given the task of processing a form at the global or local level. However, for the PL children, "all available resources" are contained within the intact hemisphere, creating a situation in which the non-injured hemisphere would assume the role of mediating both global and local processing. The effects of the early injury would, however, diminish the capacity for specialization observed in typically developing children and immature processing strategies would thus persist, creating the stabilization of a functional neural system in which the processing of both global and local information would continue to be carried out largely within a single hemisphere. Thus, as in the case for language, alternative neural networks would arise via alterations in developmental trajectories that are conditioned by the early neural pathology as well as by typical developmental constraints.

REFERENCES

Akshoomoff NA, Feroleto CC, Doyle RE, Stiles J. (2002). The impact of early unilateral brain injury on perceptual organization and visual memory. *Neuropsychologia* 40(5):539–561.

Akshoomoff NA, Stiles J. (1995a). Developmental trends in visuospatial analysis and planning: I. *Copying a complex figure. Neuropsychology* 9(3):364–377.

Akshoomoff NA, Stiles J. (1995b). Developmental trends in visuospatial analysis and planning: II. *Memory for a complex figure. Neuropsychology* 9(3):378–389.

Akshoomoff NA, Stiles J. (2003). Children's performance on the ROCF and the development of spatial analysis. In Knight JA, Kaplan, E (eds), The Handbook of Rey-Osterrieth Complex Figure Usage: Clinical and Research Applications (pp. 393–409). Lutz, FL: Psychological Assessment Resources, Inc.

Amorapanth PX, Widick P, Chatterjee A. (2010). The neural basis for spatial relations. *J Cogn Neurosci* 22(8):1739–1753.

Andersen RA, Snyder LH, Bradley DC, Xing J. (1997). Multimodal representation of space in the posterior parietal cortex and its use in planning movements. *Annu Rev Neurosci* 20:303–330.

Arena R, Gainotti G. (1978). Constructional apraxia and visuoperceptive disabilities in relation to laterality of cerebral lesions. *Cortex* 14(4):463–473.

Armstrong BA, Neville HJ, Hillyard SA, Mitchell TV. (2002). Auditory deprivation affects processing of motion, but not color. *Brain Res Cogn Brain Res* 14(3):422–434.

Atkinson J. (1998). The "where and what" or "who and how" of visual development. In Simion F, Butterworth G (Eds), The Development of Sensory, Motor and Cognitive Capacities in Early Infancy: From Perception to Cognition (pp. 3–24). Hove, England: Psychology Press/Erlbaum (UK) Taylor & Francis.

Atkinson JH, Braddick O. (2011). From genes to brain development to phenotypic behavior: "dorsal-stream vulnerability" in relation to spatial cognition, attention, and planning of actions in Williams syndrome (WS) and other developmental disorders. *Progress Brain Res* 189: 261–283.

Atkinson J, Nardini M, Anker S, Braddick O, Hughes C, Rae S. (2005). Refractive errors in infancy predict reduced performance on the movement assessment battery for children at 3 1/2 and 5 1/2 years. *Dev Med Child Neurol* 47(4):243–251.

Awh E, Jonides J. (2001). Overlapping mechanisms of attention and spatial working memory. *Trends Cogn Sci* 5(3):119–126.

Aylward EH, Park JE, Field KM, Parsons AC, Richards TL, Cramer SC, et al. (2005). Brain activation during face perception: evidence of a developmental change. *J Cogn Neurosci* 17(2): 308–319.

Baenninger M. (1994). The development of face recognition: Featural or configurational processing? *J Exp Child Psychol* 57(3):377–396.

Baird AA, Kagan J, Gaudette T, Walz KA, Hershlag N, Boas DA. (2002). Frontal lobe activation during object permanence: data from near-infrared spectroscopy. *NeuroImage* 16(4): 1120–1125.

Ballantyne AO, Trauner DA. (1999). Facial recognition in children after perinatal stroke. *Neuropsychiatry Neuropsychol Behav Neurol* 12(2):82–87.

Barton JJ. (2003). Disorders of face perception and recognition. *Neurol Clin* 21(2):521–548.

Barton JJ. (2008). Structure and function in acquired prosopagnosia: lessons from a series of 10 patients with brain damage. *J Neuropsychol* 2(Pt 1):197–225.

Barton JJ. (2009). What is meant by impaired configural processing in acquired prosopagnosia? *Perception* 38(2):242–260.

Barton JJ, Press DZ, Keenan JP, O'Connor M. (2002). Lesions of the fusiform face area impair perception of facial configuration in prosopagnosia. *Neurology* 58(1):71–78.

Belger A, Puce A, Krystal JH, Gore JC, Goldman-Rakic P, McCarthy G. (1998). Dissociation of mnemonic and perceptual processes during spatial and nonspatial working memory using fMRI. *Hum Brain Mapp* 6(1):14–32.

Bertenthal BI, Campos JJ. (1990). A systems approach to the organizing effects of self-produced locomotion during infancy. *Advances Infancy Res* 6, 1–60.

Bonatti L, Frot E, Zangl R, Mehler J. (2002). The human first hypothesis: identification of conspecifics and individuation of objects in the young infant. *Cogn Psychol* 44(4):388–426.

Braddick O, Atkinson J, Wattam-Bell J. (2003). Normal and anomalous development of visual motion processing: motion coherence and "dorsal-stream vulnerability". *Neuropsychologia* 41(13):1769–1784.

Brewer, A.A., Press, W.A., Logothetis, N.K., & Wandell, B.A. (2002). Visual Areas in Macaque Cortex Measured Using Functional Magnetic Resonance Imaging. *Journal of Neuroscience*, 22(23), 10416–10426.

Carey S. (1996). Perceptual classification and expertise. In Gelman R, Kit-Fong T (Eds), Perceptual and Cognitive Development (pp. 49–69). San Diego, CA: Academic Press, Inc.

Carey S, Diamond R. (1977). From piecemeal to configurational representation of faces. *Science* 195(4275):312–314.

Casey BJ, Cohen JD, O'Craven K, Davidson RJ, Irwin W, Nelson CA, et al. (1998). Reproducibility of fMRI results across four institutions using a spatial working memory task. *NeuroImage* 8(3):249–261.

Cassia VM, Simion F, Milani I, Umilta C. (2002). Dominance of global visual properties at birth. *J Exp Psychol Gen* 131(3):398–411.

Chiba AA, Kesner RP, Jackson PA. (2002). Two forms of spatial memory: a double dissociation between the parietal cortex and the hippocampus in the rat. *Behav Neurosci* 116(5):874–883.

Chung M-S, Thomson DM. (1995). Development of face recognition. *Br J Psychol* 86(1):55–87.

Coch D, Skendzel W, Grossi G, Neville H. (2005). Motion and color processing in school-age children and adults: an ERP study. *Dev Sci* 8(4):372–386.

Cohen LB, Younger BA. (1984). Infant perception of angular relations. *Infant Behav Dev* 7(1):37–47.

Cohen Kadosh K, Cohen Kadosh R, Dick F, Johnson MH. (2010). Developmental changes in effective connectivity in the emerging core face network. *Cerebral Cortex [e-pub Nov. 2].*

Colby CL, Duhamel JR. (1996). Spatial representations for action in parietal cortex. *Brain Res Cogn Brain Res* 5(1–2):105–115.

Colby CL, Goldberg ME. (1999). Space and attention in parietal cortex. *Annu Rev Neurosci* 22:319–349.

Corbetta M, Kincade JM, Shulman GL. (2002). Neural systems for visual orienting and their relationships to spatial working memory. *J Cogn Neurosci* 14(3):508–523.

Courtney SM, Petit L, Maisog JM, Ungerleider LG, Haxby JV. (1998). An area specialized for spatial working memory in human frontal cortex. *Science* 279(5355):1347–1351.

Courtney SM, Ungerleider LG, Keil K, Haxby JV. (1996). Object and spatial visual working memory activate separate neural systems in human cortex. *Cerebral Cortex* 6(1):39–49.

Curtis CE. (2006). Prefrontal and parietal contributions to spatial working memory. *Neuroscience* 139(1):173–180.

Damasio AR, Damasio H, Van Hoesen GW. (1982). Prosopagnosia: anatomic basis and behavioral mechanisms. *Neurology* 32(4):331–341.

de Schonen S, Deruelle C. (1991). Hemispheric specialization and recognition of shapes and faces by the baby. *Annee Psychologique* 91(1):15–46.

de Schonen S, Deruelle C, Mancini J, Pascalis O. (1996). Pattern processing in infancy: Hemispheric differences and brain maturation. In Vital-Durand F, Atkinson J, et al. (Eds), Infant Vision (pp. 327–344). Oxford, UK: Oxford University Press.

de Schonen S, Mancini J, Camps R, Maes E, Laurent A. (2005). Early brain lesions and face-processing development. *Dev Psychobiol* 46(3):184–208.

de Schonen S, Mathivet E. (1990). Hemispheric asymmetry in a face discrimination task in infants. *Child Dev* 61(4):1192–1205.

Delis DC, Kiefner MG, Fridlund AJ. (1988). Visuospatial dysfunction following unilateral brain damage: Dissociations in hierarchical hemispatial analysis. *J Clin Exp Neuropsychol* 10(4): 421–431.

Delis DC, Robertson LC, Efron R. (1986). Hemispheric specialization of memory for visual hierarchical stimuli. *Neuropsychologia* 24(2):205–214.

Deruelle C, de Schonen S. (1991). Hemispheric asymmetries in visual pattern processing in infancy. *Brain Cogn* 16(2):151–179.

Deruelle C, de Schonen S. (1998). Do the right and left hemispheres attend to the same visuospatial information within a face in infancy? *Dev Neuropsychol* 14(4):535–554.

Diamond A. (1991). Frontal lobe involvement in cognitive changes during the first year of life. In Gibson KR, Petersen AC, et al. (Eds), Brain Maturation and Cognitive Development: Comparative and Cross-Cultural Perspectives (pp. 127–180). New York: Aldine De Gruyter.

Diamond A, Werker JF, Lalonde C. (1994). Toward understanding commonalities in the development of object search, detour navigation, categorization, and speech perception. In Dawson G, Fischer KW, et al. (Eds), Human Behavior and the Developing Brain (pp. 380–426). New York: The Guilford Press.

Diamond R, Carey S. (1986). Why faces are and are not special: an effect of expertise. *J Exp Psychol Gen* 115(2):107–117.

Dilks DD, Hoffman JE, Landau B. (2008). Vision for perception and vision for action: normal and unusual development. *Dev Sci* 11(4):474–486.

Dobkins KR, Albright TD. (1994). What happens if it changes color when it moves? The nature of chromatic input to macaque visual area MT. *J Neurosci* 14(8):4854–4870.

Dobkins KR, Albright TD. (1995). Behavioral and neural effects of chromatic isoluminance in the primate visual motion system. *Vis Neurosci* 12(2):321–332.

Dobkins KR, Albright TD. (1998). The influence of chromatic information on visual motion processing in the primate visual system. In Watanabe T, et al. (Eds), High-Level Motion Processing: Computational, Neurobiological, and Psychophysical Perspectives (pp. 53–94). Cambridge, MA: The MIT Press.

Dobkins KR, Anderson CM. (2002). Color-based motion processing is stronger in infants than in adults. *Psychol Sci* 13(1):76–80.

Dobkins KR, Teller DY. (1996a). Infant contrast detectors are selective for direction of motion. *Vis Res* 36(2):281–294.

Dobkins KR, Teller DY. (1996b). Infant motion: Detection (M:D) ratios for chromatically defined and luminance-defined moving stimuli. *Vis Res* 36(20):3293–3310.

Dukette D, Stiles J. (1996). Children's analysis of hierarchical patterns: Evidence from a similarity judgment task. *J Exp Child Psychol* 63(1):103–140.

Dukette D, Stiles J. (2001). The effects of stimulus density on children's analysis of hierarchical patterns. *Dev Sci* 4(2):233–251.

Durston S, Davidson MC, Tottenham N, Galvan A, Spicer J, Fossella JA, et al. (2006). A shift from diffuse to focal cortical activity with development. *Dev Sci* 9(1):1–20.

Ellison A, Cowey A. (2006). TMS can reveal contrasting functions of the dorsal and ventral visual processing streams. *Exp Brain Res* [e-pub July 4].

Farroni T, Valenza E, Simion F, Umilta C. (2000). Configural processing at birth: Evidence for perceptual organisation. *Perception* 29(3):355–372.

Feeney SM, Stiles J. (1996). Spatial analysis: An examination of preschoolers' perception and construction of geometric patterns. *Dev Psychol* 32(5):933–941.

Fink GR, Halligan PW, Marshall JC, Frith CD, Frackowiak RSJ, Dolan RJ. (1997). Neural mechanisms involved in the processing of global and local aspects of hierarchically organized visual stimuli. *Brain* 120(10):1779–1791.

Freire A, Lee K. (2001). Face recognition in 4- to 7-year-olds: processing of configural, featural, and paraphernalia information. *J Exp Child Psychol* 80(4):347–371.

Gainotti G, Tiacci C. (1970). Patterns of drawing disability in right and left hemispheric patients. *Neuropsychologia* 8(3):379–384.

Gathers A. D Bhatt, R Corbly C. R Farley A. B., Joseph, J. E. (2004). Developmental shifts in cortical loci for face and object recognition. *Neuroreport* 15(10):1549–1553.

Gauthier I, Behrmann M, Tarr MJ. (1999). Can face recognition really be dissociated from object recognition? *J Cogn Neurosci* 11(4):349–370.

Gauthier I, Nelson CA. (2001). The development of face expertise. *Curr Opinion Neurobiol* 11(2):219–224.

Gauthier I, Tarr MJ, Moylan J, Anderson AW, Skudlarski P, Gore JC. (2000). Does visual subordinate-level categorisation engage the functionally defined fusiform face area? Cognitive Neuropsychology. *Special Issue: The Cognitive Neuroscience of Face Processing* 17(1–3):143–163.

Golarai G, Ghahremani DG, Whitfield-Gabrieli S, Reiss A, Eberhardt JL, Gabrieli JD, et al. (2007). Differential development of high-level visual cortex correlates with category-specific recognition memory. *Nat Neurosci* 10(4):512–522.

Golarai G, Liberman A, Yoon JM, Grill-Spector K. (2010). Differential development of the ventral visual cortex extends through adolescence. *Frontiers Hum Neurosci* 3:80.

Goodale MA, Milner AD. (1992). Separate visual pathways for perception and action. *Trends Neurosci* 15(1, 163):20–25.

Goodale MA, Westwood DA. (2004). An evolving view of duplex vision: separate but interacting cortical pathways for perception and action. *Curr Opin Neurobiol* 14(2):203–211.

Gordon GE, McCulloch DL. (1999). A VEP investigation of parallel visual pathway development in primary school age children. *Doc Ophthalmol* 99(1):1–10.

Grill-Spector K, Golarai G, Gabrieli J. (2008). Developmental neuroimaging of the human ventral visual cortex. *Trends Cogn Sci* 12(4):152–162.

Gunn A, Cory E, Atkinson J, Braddick O, Wattam-Bell J, Guzzetta A, et al. (2002). Dorsal and ventral stream sensitivity in normal development and hemiplegia. *Neuroreport* 13(6): 843–847.

Halit H, Csibra G, Volein A, Johnson MH. (2004). Face-sensitive cortical processing in early infancy. *J Child Psychol Psychiatry* 45(7):1228–1234.

Han S, Weaver JA, Murray SO, Kang X, Yund EW, Woods DL. (2002). Hemispheric asymmetry in global/local processing: effects of stimulus position and spatial frequency. *NeuroImage* 17(3):1290–1299.

Harrison TB, Stiles J. (2009). Hierarchical forms processing in adults and children. *J Exp Child Psychol* 103(2):222–240.

Hauser MD. (1999). Perseveration, inhibition and the prefrontal cortex: a new look. *Curr Opinion Neurobiol* 9(2):214–222.

Haxby JV, Grady CL, Horwitz B, Ungerleider LG, Mishkin M, Carson RE, et al. (1991). Dissociation of object and spatial visual processing pathways in human extrastriate cortex. *Proc Natl Acad Sci U S A* 88(5):1621–1625.

Haxby JV, Horwitz B, Ungerleider LG, Maisog JM, Pietrini P, Grady CL. (1994). The functional organization of human extrastriate cortex: a PET-rCBF study of selective attention to faces and locations. *J Neurosci* 14(11 Pt 1):6336–6353.

Haxby JV, Petit L, Ungerleider LG, Courtney SM. (2000). Distinguishing the functional roles of multiple regions in distributed neural systems for visual working memory. *NeuroImage* 11(2):145–156.

Heinze HJ, Hinrichs H, Scholz M, Burchert W, Mangun GR. (1998). Neural mechanisms of global and local processing. *A combined PET and ERP study. J Cogn Neurosci* 10(4):485–498.

Hillger LA, Koenig O. (1991). Separable mechanisms in face processing: Evidence from hemispheric specialization. *J Cogn Neurosci. Special Issue: Face Perception* 3(1):42–58.

Horobin K, Acredolo L. (1986). The role of attentiveness, mobility history, and separation of hiding sites on Stage IV search behavior. *J Exp Child Psychol* 41(1):114–127.

Husain M, Nachev P. (2007). Space and the parietal cortex. *Trends Cogn Sci* 11(1):30–36.

Huttenlocher J, Hedges LV, Duncan S. (1991). Categories and particulars: prototype effects in estimating spatial location. *Psychol Rev* 191(3):352–376.

Huttenlocher J, Lourenco SF. (2007a). Coding location in enclosed spaces: is geometry the principle? *Dev Sci* 10(6):741–746.

Huttenlocher J, Lourenco SF. (2007b). Using spatial categories to reason about location. In Plumert J, Spencer J (Eds),The Emerging Spatial Mind (pp. 3–24). New York: Oxford University Press.

Huttenlocher J, Newcombe N, Sandberg EH. (1994). The coding of spatial location in young children. *Cogn Psychol* 27(2):115–148.

Itier RJ, Taylor MJ. (2004). Face recognition memory and configural processing: a developmental ERP study using upright, inverted, and contrast-reversed faces. *J Cogn Neurosci* 16(3): 487–502.

Ivry RB, Robertson LC. (1998). The Two Sides of Perception. Cambridge, MA: The MIT Press.

Johnson MH. (2002). The development of visual attention: A cognitive neuroscience perspective. In Johnson MH, Munakata Y, Gilmore RO (Eds), Brain Development and Cognition: A Reader (pp. 134–150). Malden, MA: Blackwell Publishers.

Johnson MH, Dziurawiec S, Ellis H, Morton J. (1991). Newborns' preferential tracking of face-like stimuli and its subsequent decline. *Cognition* 40(1–2):1–19.

Johnson MH, Mareschal D, Csibra G. (2001). The functional development and integration of the dorsal and ventral visual pathways: a neurocomputational approach. In Nelson CA, Luciana M (Eds), Handbook of Developmental Cognitive Neuroscience (pp. 339–351). Cambridge, MA: The MIT Press.

Jonides J, Smith EE, Koeppe RA, Awh E, Minoshima S, Mintun MA. (1993). Spatial working memory in humans as revealed by PET. *Nature* 363(6430):623–625.

Joseph JE, Gathers AD, Bhatt RS. (2010). Progressive and regressive developmental changes in neural substrates for face processing: testing specific predictions of the Interactive Specialization account. *Dev Sci* 14(2):227–241.

Kaas JH, Collins CE. (Eds.). (2004). The Primate Visual System. Boca Raton FL: CRC Press.

Kaldy Z, Leslie AM. (2003). Identification of objects in 9-month-old infants: Integrating "what" and "where" information. *Dev Sci* 6(3):360–373.

Kanwisher N, McDermott J, Chun MM. (1997). The fusiform face area: a module in human extrastriate cortex specialized for face perception. *J Neurosci* 17(11):4302–4311.

Kanwisher N, Yovel G. (2006). The fusiform face area: a cortical region specialized for the perception of faces. *Philos Trans R Soc Lond B Biol Sci* 361(1476):2109–2128.

Karmiloff-Smith A. (1990). Constraints on representational change: Evidence from children's drawing. *Cognition* 34(1):57–83.

Kaufman J, Csibra G, Johnson MH. (2003). Representing occluded objects in the human infant brain. *Proc Biol Sci* 270 Suppl 2, S140–143.

Kawasaki M, Watanabe M, Okuda J, Sakagami M, Aihara K. (2008). Human posterior parietal cortex maintains color, shape and motion in visual short-term memory. *Brain Res* 1213:91–97.

Kermoian R, Campos JJ. (1988). Locomotor experience: A facilitator of spatial cognitive development. *Child Dev* 59(4):908–917.

Kinchla RA, Wolfe JM. (1979). The order of visual processing: "Top-down," "bottom-up," or "middle-out." *Perception Psychophysics* 25(3):225–231.

Kitterle FL, Christman S, Hellige JB. (1990). Hemispheric differences are found in the identification, but not the detection, of low versus high spatial frequencies. *Perception Psychophysics* 48(4):297–306.

Kitterle FL, Hellige JB, Christman S. (1992). Visual hemispheric asymmetries depend on which spatial frequencies are task relevant. *Brain Cognition* 20(2):308–314.

Kitterle FL, Selig LM. (1991). Visual field effects in the discrimination of sine-wave gratings. *Perception Psychophysics* 50(1):15–18.

Konen CS, Kastner S. (2008). Two hierarchically organized neural systems for object information in human visual cortex. *Nat Neurosci* 11(2):224–231.

Kosslyn SM. (1987). Seeing and imagining in the cerebral hemispheres: a computational approach. *Psychol Rev* 94(2):148–175.

Kosslyn, S. M., Koenig, O., Barrett, A., Cave, C. B., Tang, J., & Gabrieli, J. D. (1989). Evidence for two types of spatial representations: hemispheric specialization for categorical and coordinate relations. *J Exp Psychol Hum Percept Perform*, 15(4), 723–735.

Kosslyn, S. M., Thompson, W. L., Gitelman, D. R., & Alpert, N. M. (1998). Neural systems that encode categorical vs. coordinate spatial relations: PET investigations. *Psychobiology*, 26, 333–347.

Kosslyn SM. (2006). You can play 20 questions with nature and win: categorical versus coordinate spatial relations as a case study. *Neuropsychologia* 44(9):1519–1523.

Kosslyn SM, Chabris CF, Marsolek CJ, Koenig O. (1992). Categorical versus coordinate spatial relations: computational analyses and computer simulations. *J Exp Psychol Hum Percept Perform* 18(2):562–577.

Kosslyn SM, Koenig O, Barrett A, Cave CB, Tang J, Gabrieli JD. (1989). Evidence for two types of spatial representations: hemispheric specialization for categorical and coordinate relations. *J Exp Psychol Hum Percept Perform* 15(4):723–735.

Kosslyn SM, Maljkovic V, Hamilton SE, Horwitz G, Thompson WL. (1995). Two types of image generation: evidence for left and right hemisphere processes. *Neuropsychologia* 33(11):1485–1510.

Kosslyn SM, Thompson WL, Kim IJ, Alpert NM. (1995). Topographical representations of mental images in primary visual cortex. *Nature* 378(6556):496–498.

Krojgaard P. (2007). Comparing infants' use of featural and spatiotemporal information in an object individuation task using a new event-monitoring design. *Dev Sci* 10(6):892–909.

Laeng, B. (1994). Lateralization of Categorical and Coordinate Spatial Functions: A Study of Unilateral Stroke Patients. *Journal of Cognitive Neuroscience*, 6(3), 189–203.

Lamb MR, Robertson LC. (1988). The processing of hierarchical stimuli: Effects of retinal locus, locational uncertainty, and stimulus identity. *Perception Psychophysics* 44(2):172–181.

Lamb MR, Robertson LC. (1989). Do response time advantage and interference reflect the order of processing of global- and local-level information? *Perception Psychophysics* 46(3): 254–258.

Lamb MR, Robertson LC, Knight RT. (1989). Attention and interference in the processing of global and local information: Effects of unilateral temporal-parietal junction lesions. *Neuropsychologia* 27(4):471–483.

Lamb MR, Robertson LC, Knight RT. (1990). Component mechanisms underlying the processing of hierarchically organized patterns: Inferences from patients with unilateral cortical lesions. *J Exp Psychol: Learning, Memory, Cognition* 16(3):471–483.

Lehky SR, Sereno AB. (2007). Comparison of shape encoding in primate dorsal and ventral visual pathways. *J Neurophysiol* 97(1):307–319.

Leslie AM, Xu F, Tremoulet PD, Scholl BJ. (1998). Indexing and the object concept: Developing "what" and "where" systems. *Trends Cogn Sci* 2(1):10–18.

Levine SC. (1985). Developmental change in right hemisphere involvement in face recognition. In Best C (Ed), Developmental Neuropsychology and Education: Hemispheric Function and Collaboration (pp. 157–191). New York: Academic Press.

Lew AR, Hopkins B, Owen LH, Green M. (2007). Postural change effects on infants' AB task performance: visual, postural, or spatial? *J Exp Child Psychol* 97(1):1–13.

Livingstone MS, Hubel DH. (1984). Anatomy and physiology of a color system in the primate visual cortex. *J Neurosci* 4(1):309–356.

Lourenco SF, Levine SC. (2009). Location representation following early unilateral brain injury: evidence of distinct deficits and degrees of plasticity. Paper presented at the Society for Research in Child Development.

Lourenco SF, Levine SC. (in preparation). Location representation following early unilateral brain injury: evidence of distinct deficits and degrees of plasticity.

Madrid M, Crognale MA. (2000). Long-term maturation of visual pathways. *Vis Neurosci* 17(6):831–837.

Mancini J, de Schonen S, Deruelle C, Massoulier A. (1994). Face recognition in children with early right or left brain damage. *Dev Med Child Neurol* 36(2):156–166.

Marangolo P, Di Pace E, Rafal R, Scabini D. (1998). Effects of parietal lesions in humans on color and location priming. *J Cogn Neurosci* 10(6):704–716.

Mareschal D, Johnson MH. (2003). The "what" and "where" of object representations in infancy. *Cognition* 88(3):259–276.

Martin M. (1979). Hemispheric specialization for local and global processing. *Neuropsychologia* 17(1):33–40.

Martinez A, Moses P, Frank L, Buxton R, Wong E, Stiles J. (1997). Hemispheric asymmetries in global and local processing: evidence from fMRI. *Neuroreport* 8(7):1685–1689.

Mash C, Novak E, Berthier NE, Keen R. (2006). What do two-year-olds understand about hidden-object events? *Dev Psychol* 42(2):263–271.

McCarthy G, Puce A, Gore JC, Allison T. (1997). Face-specific processing in the human fusiform gyrus. *J Cogn Neurosci* 9(5):605–610.

McFie J, Zangwill OL. (1960). Visual-constructive disabilities associated with lesions of the left cerebral hemisphere. *Brain* 83:243–259.

Merigan WH, Maunsell JH. (1993). How parallel are the primate visual pathways? *Annu Rev Neurosci* 16:369–402.

Milner AD, Goodale MA. (1995). The Visual Brain in Action. New York: Oxford University Press.

Mitchell TV, Neville HJ. (2004). Asynchronies in the development of electrophysiological responses to motion and color. *J Cogn Neurosci* 16(8):1363–1374.

Mondloch CJ, Geldart S, Maurer D, de Schonen S. (2003). Developmental changes in the processing of hierarchical shapes continue into adolescence. *J Exp Child Psychol* 84(1):20–40.

Moses P, Roe K, Buxton RB, Wong EC, Frank LR, Stiles J. (2002). Functional MRI of global and local processing in children. *NeuroImage* 16(2):415–424.

Moses P, Stiles J. (2002). The lesion methodology: contrasting views from adult and child studies. *Dev Psychobiol* 40(3):266–277.

Navon D. (1977). Forest before trees: The precedence of global features in visual perception. *Cogn Psychol* 9(3):353–383.

Nelson CA, Monk CS, Lin J, Carver LJ, Thomas KM, Truwit CL. (2000). Functional neuroanatomy of spatial working memory in children. *Dev Psychol* 36(1):109–116.

Oliveri M, Turriziani P, Carlesimo GA, Koch G, Tomaiuolo F, Panella M, et al. (2001). Parieto-frontal interactions in visual-object and visual-spatial working memory: evidence from transcranial magnetic stimulation. *Cereb Cortex* 11(7):606–618.

Orban, G. A., Van Essen, D., & Vanduffel, W. (2004). Comparative mapping of higher visual areas in monkeys and humans. *Trends in cognitive sciences*, 8(7), 315–324.

Osterrieth PA. (1944). Le test de copie d'une figure complexe. Contribution a 1'*etude de la perception et de la memoire. Archive de Psychologie* 30:206–353.

Palermo L, Bureca I, Matano A, Guariglia C. (2008). Hemispheric contribution to categorical and coordinate representational processes: a study on brain-damaged patients. *Neuropsychologia* 46(11):2802–2807.

Palmer SE. (1977). Hierarchical structure in perceptual representation. *Cogn Psychol* 9(4): 441–474.

Palmer SE. (1980). What makes triangles point: Local and global effects in configurations of ambiguous triangles. *Cogn Psychol* 12(3):285–305.

Palmer SE, Bucher NM. (1981). Configural effects in perceived pointing of ambiguous triangles. *J Exp Psychol: Human Perception Performance* 7(1):88–114.

Passarotti AM, Paul BM, Bussiere JR, Buxton RB, Wong EC, Stiles J. (2003). The development of face and location processing: An fMRI study. *Dev Sci* 6(1):100–117.

Paul B, Appelbaum, M, Carapetian S, Hesselink J, Nass R, Trauner D, Stiles J. (in preparation). Face and location processing in children with early unilateral brain injury.

Pedelty L, Levine SC, Shevell S. (1985). Developmental changes in face processing: Results from multidimensional scaling. *J Exp Child Psychol* 39:421–436.

Peelen MV, Glaser B, Vuilleumier P, Eliez S. (2009). Differential development of selectivity for faces and bodies in the fusiform gyrus. *Dev Sci* 12(6):F16–25.

Piaget J. (1952). The Origins of Intelligence in Children. New York: International Universities Press.

Piercy M, Hecaen H, De Ajuriaguerra J. (1960). Constructional apraxia associated with unilateral cerebral lesions: left- and right-sided cases compared. *Brain* 83:225–242.

Plumert, J, Hund A. M., Recker, K. M. (2007). Organism-environment interaction in spatial development: Explaining categorical bias in memory for location. In Plumert J, Spencer J (Eds), The Emerging Spatial Mind (pp. 25–52). New York: Oxford University Press.

Porporino M, Shore DI, Iarocci G, Burack JA. (2004). A developmental change in selective attention and global form perception. *Intl J Behav Dev* 28(4):358–364.

Postle BR, Berger JS, Taich AM, D'Esposito M. (2000). Activity in human frontal cortex associated with spatial working memory and saccadic behavior. *J Cogn Neurosci* 12(Suppl 2):2–14.

Postma A, Kessels RP, van Asselen M. (2008). How the brain remembers and forgets where things are: the neurocognition of object-location memory. *Neurosci Biobehav Rev* 32(8):1339–1345.

Quinn PC, Bhatt RS. (2006). Are some gestalt principles deployed more readily than others during early development? The case of lightness versus form similarity. *J Exp Psychol Hum Percept Perform* 32(5):1221–1230.

Quinn PC, Burke S, Rush A. (1993). Part-whole perception in early infancy: Evidence for perceptual grouping produced by lightness similarity. *Infant Behav Dev* 16(1):19–42.

Ranganath C. (2006). Working memory for visual objects: complementary roles of inferior temporal, medial temporal, and prefrontal cortex. *Neuroscience* 139(1):277–289.

Ranganath C, Cohen MX, Dam C, D'Esposito M. (2004). Inferior temporal, prefrontal, and hippocampal contributions to visual working memory maintenance and associative memory retrieval. *J Neurosci* 24(16):3917–3925.

Ranganath C, D'Esposito M. (2005). Directing the mind's eye: prefrontal, inferior and medial temporal mechanisms for visual working memory. *Curr Opin Neurobiol* 15(2):175–182.

Ratcliff G. (1982). Disturbances of spatial orientation associated with cerebral lesions. In Potegal M (Ed), Spatial Abilities: Development and Physiological Foundations. (pp. 301–331). New York: Academic Press.

Recker KM, Plumert JM, Hund AM, Reimer R. (2007). How do biases in spatial memory change as children and adults are learning locations? *J Exp Child Psychol* 98(4):217–232.

Reese CJ, Stiles J. (2005). Hemispheric specialization for categorical and coordinate spatial relations during an image generation task: Evidence from children and adults. *Neuropsychologia* 43(4):517–529. Reese, CJ, Stiles, J. (submitted). The effects of perinatal brain injury on processing of categorical and coordinate spatial relations.

Rhodes G. (1993). Configural coding, expertise, and the right hemisphere advantage for face recognition. *Brain Cognition* 22(1):19–41.

Rivest J, Moscovitch M, Black S. (2009). A comparative case study of face recognition: The contribution of configural and part-based recognition systems, and their interaction. *Neuropsychologia* [e-pub June 12*]*.

Rizzolatti G, Matelli M. (2003). Two different streams form the dorsal visual system: anatomy and functions. *Exp Brain Res* 153(2):146–157.

Robertson LC, Delis DC. (1986). "Part-whole" processing in unilateral brain-damaged patients: Dysfunction of hierarchical organization. *Neuropsychologia* 24(3):363–370.

Robertson LC, Lamb MR, Knight RT. (1988). Effects of lesions of temporal-parietal junction on perceptual and attentional processing in humans. *J Neurosci* 8(10):3757–3769.

Rosa MG, Palmer SM, Gamberini Mm Burman KJ, Yu HH, Reser DH, et al. (2009). Connections of the dorsomedial visual area: pathways for early integration of dorsal and ventral streams in extrastriate cortex. *J Neurosci* 29(14):4548–4563.

Rossion B, Dricot L, Devolder A, Bodart JM, Crommelinck M, De Gelder B, et al. (2000). Hemispheric asymmetries for whole-based and part-based face processing in the human fusiform gyrus. *J Cogn Neurosci* 12(5):793–802.

Sala JB, Rama P, Courtney SM. (2003). Functional topography of a distributed neural system for spatial and nonspatial information maintenance in working memory. *Neuropsychologia. Special Issue: Functional Neuroimaging of Memory* 41(3):341–356.

Sergent J. (1982). The cerebral balance of power: Confrontation or cooperation? *J Exp Psychol: Human Perception Performance* 8(2):253–272.

Sincich LC, Horton JC. (2005). The circuitry of V1 and V2: integration of color, form, and motion. *Annu Rev Neurosci* 28 303–326.

Slater A, Mattock A, Brown E, Bremner JG. (1991). Form perception at birth: Cohen and Younger (1984) revisited. *J Exp Child Psychol* 51(3):395–406.

Smith EE, Jonides J, Koeppe RA. (1996). Dissociating verbal and spatial working memory using PET. *Cerebral Cortex* 6(1):11–20.

Smith EE, Jonides J, Koeppe RA, Awh E, Schumacher EH., Minoshima S. (1995). Spatial versus object working memory: PET investigations. *J Cogn Neurosci* 7(3):337–356.

Smith LB, Kemler DG. (1977). Developmental trends in free classification: Evidence for a new conceptualization of perceptual development. *J Exp Child Psychol* 24(2):279–298.

Smith LB, Thelen E, Titzer R, McLin D. (1999). Knowing in the context of acting: the task dynamics of the A-not-B error. *Psychol Rev* 106(2):235–260.

Spencer JP, Hund AM. (2003). Developmental continuity in the processes that underlie spatial recall. *Cogn Psychol* 47(4):432–480.

Stiles J. (1995). Plasticity and development: Evidence from children with early occurring focal brain injury. In Julesz B, Kovács I (Eds), Maturational Windows and Adult Cortical Plasticity (pp. 217–237). Reading, MA: Addison-Wesley.

Stiles J, Delis DC, Tada WL. (1991). Global-local processing in preschool children. *Child Dev* 62(6):1258–1275.

Stiles J, Moses P, Paul BM. (2006). The longitudinal study of spatial cognitive development in children with pre- or perinatal focal brain injury: evidence for cognitive compensation and for the emergence of alternative profiles of brain organization. In Lomber SG, Eggermont J (Eds), Reprogramming the Cerebral Cortex (pp. 415–428). New York: Oxford University Press.

Stiles J, Nass RD, Levine SC, Moses P, Reilly JS. (2009). Perinatal stroke: Effects and outcomes. In Yeates KO, Ris MD, Taylor HG, Pennington B (Eds), Pediatric Neuropsychology: Research, Theory, and Practice (2nd ed, pp. 181–210). New York: The Guilford Press.

Stiles J, Paul B, Hesselink J. (2006). Spatial cognitive development following early focal brain injury: evidence for adaptive change in brain and cognition. In Munakata Y, Johnson MH (Eds), Process of Change in Brain and Cognitive Development. Attention and Performance XXI (pp. 535–561). Oxford: Oxford University Press.

Stiles J, Stern C. (2001). Developmental change in spatial cognitive processing: Complexity effects and block construction performance in preschool children. *J Cogn Dev* 2(2):157–187.

Stiles J, Stern C, Appelbaum M, Nass RD, Trauner DA, Hesselink J. (2008). Effects of early focal brain injury on memory for visuospatial patterns: Selective deficits of global-local processing. *Neuropsychology* 22(1):61–73.

Stiles J, Stern C, Trauner D, Nass R. (1996). Developmental change in spatial grouping activity among children with early focal brain injury: Evidence from a modeling task. *Brain Cognition* 31(1):46–62.

Stiles J, Trauner D, Engel M, Nass R. (1997). The development of drawing in children with congenital focal brain injury: Evidence for limited functional recovery. *Neuropsychologia* 35(3):299–312.

Stiles-Davis J. (1988). Spatial dysfunctions in young children with right cerebral hemisphere injury. In Stiles-Davis J, Kritchevsky M, et al. (Eds), Spatial Cognition: Brain Bases and Development (pp. 251–272): Hillsdale, NJ.

Stiles-Davis J, Sugarman S, Nass R. (1985). The development of spatial and class relations in four young children with right-cerebral-hemisphere damage: Evidence for an early spatial constructive deficit. *Brain Cognition* 4(4):388–412.

Stiles-Davis, Joan, Janowsky, Jeri, Engel, Murray, & Nass, Ruth D. (1988). Drawing ability in four young children with congenital unilateral brain lesions. *Neuropsychologia*, 26(3), 359–371.

Swindell CS, Holland AL, Fromm D, Greenhouse JB. (1988). Characteristics of recovery of drawing ability in left and right brain-damaged patients. *Brain Cognition* 7(1):16–30.

Tada WL, Stiles J. (1996). Developmental change in children's analysis of spatial patterns. *Dev Psychol* 32(5):951–970.

Tanaka JW, Farah MJ. (1993). Parts and wholes in face recognition. *Q J Exp Psychol: Hum Exp Psychol* 46A(2):225–245.

Tarr MJ, Gauthier I. (2000). FFA: a flexible fusiform area for subordinate-level visual processing automatized by expertise. *Nat Neurosci* 3(8):764–769.

Taylor MJ, Edmonds GE, McCarthy G, Allison T. (2001). Eyes first! Eye processing develops before face processing in children. *Neuroreport* 12(8):1671–1676.

Taylor MJ, McCarthy G, Saliba E, Degiovanni E. (1999). ERP evidence of developmental changes in processing of faces. *Clin Neurophysiol* 110(5):910–915.

Thiele A, Dobkins KR, Albright TD. (2001). Neural correlates of chromatic motion perception. *Neuron* 32(2):351–358.

Trojano L, Grossi D, Linden DE, Formisano E, Goebel R, Cirillo S, et al. (2002). Coordinate and categorical judgements in spatial imagery. *An fMRI study. Neuropsychologia* 40(10): 1666–1674.

Tzourio-Mazoyer N, De Schonen S, Crivello F, Reutter B, Aujard Y, Mazoyer B. (2002). Neural correlates of woman face processing by 2-month-old infants. *NeuroImage* 15(2):454–461.

Ungerleider LG, Mishkin M. (1982). Two cortical visual systems. In Ingle DJ, Goodale MA, Mansfield RJW (Eds), Analysis of Visual Behavior (pp. 549–586). Cambridge, MA: The MIT Press.

van Asselen M, Kessels RP, Kappelle LJ, Postma A. (2008). Categorical and coordinate spatial representations within object-location memory. *Cortex* 44(3):249–256.

Van de Walle GA, Carey S, Prevor M. (2000). Bases for object individuation in infancy: Evidence from manual search. *J Cogn Dev* 1(3):249–280.

Van Essen DC, Anderson CH, Felleman DJ. (1992). Information processing in the primate visual system: An integrated systems perspective. *Science* 255(5043):419–423.

Vicari S, Stiles J, Stern C, Resca A. (1998). Spatial grouping activity in children with early cortical and subcortical lesions. *Dev Med Child Neurol* 40(2):90–99.

Volberg G, Hubner R. (2004). On the role of response conflicts and stimulus position for hemispheric differences in global/local processing: an ERP study. *Neuropsychologia* 42(13): 1805–1813.

Vurpillot E. (1976). The Visual World of the Child. New York: International Universities Press.

Wagner AD, Shannon BJ, Kahn I, Buckner RL. (2005). Parietal lobe contributions to episodic memory retrieval. *Trends Cogn Sci* 9(9):445–453.

Warrington EK, James M, Kinsbourne M. (1966). Drawing disability in relation to laterality of cerebral lesion. *Brain* 89(1):53–82.

Wilcox T, Baillargeon R. (1998). Object individuation in infancy: The use of featural information in reasoning about occlusion events. *Cogn Psychol* 37(2):97–155.

Wilkinson D, Ko P, Wiriadjaja A, Kilduff P, McGlinchey R, Milberg W. (2009). Unilateral damage to the right cerebral hemisphere disrupts the apprehension of whole faces and their component parts. *Neuropsychologia* 47(7):1701–1711.

Wong-Riley M. (1979). Changes in the visual system of monocularly sutured or enucleated cats demonstrable with cytochrome oxidase histochemistry. *Brain Res* 171(1):11–28.

Xu F, Carey S. (1996). Infants' metaphysics: the case of numerical identity. *Cogn Psychol* 30(2): 111–153.

Xu F, Carey S, Quint N. (2004). The emergence of kind-based object individuation in infancy. *Cogn Psychol* 49(2):155–190.

Yovel G, Kanwisher N. (2004). Face perception: domain specific, not process specific. *Neuron* 44(5):889–898.

Yovel G, Levy J, Yovel I. (2001). Hemispheric asymmetries for global and local visual perception: effects of stimulus and task factors. *J Exp Psychol Hum Percept Perform* 27(6):1369–1385.

6

Spatial Attention, Working Memory, and Executive Function

SPATIAL ATTENTION, WORKING memory, and executive function are each cognitive functions that are crucial for communicating, learning, and functioning in society. Spatial attention and spatial working memory are closely related cognitive processes that are hypothesized to share some neural substrates. Executive functioning is a complex set of constructs that overlap with aspects of spatial attention and working memory to allow an individual to carry out goal-directed behaviors. They fit within the larger constellation of processes collectively referred to as cognitive control processes (Luna, 2009). As such they are part of a neurobehavioral network that allows information processing and behavior to vary adaptively and adjust to changing contingencies and goals.

Spatial attention is a basic cognitive function that is important for higher-level processes such as navigating in space, attending to relevant stimuli in the environment, and ignoring irrelevant stimuli. Spatial attention consists of three primary components: alerting, orienting, and executive control. Alerting involves a heightened awareness of incoming stimuli and can be facilitated by directing the person's attention to the location of the stimulus (Posner et al., 1980). Orienting involves selecting the relevant stimulus from multiple simultaneous incoming bits of information. Executive control refers to the process of making decisions about the relevant stimulus (what action should be taken based on the stimulus, such as reaching for a cup of coffee) and also error-monitoring (e.g., Was the stimulus relevant after all? Did I react appropriately to it?)

Working memory refers to a basic cognitive process that allows for temporary storage and manipulation of information necessary for numerous complex cognitive tasks such as language, spatial analysis, and decision-making. Spatial attention serves as a selective filter that can control access to working memory that may have limited capacity. Spatial attention may also facilitate rehearsal of information held in spatial working memory through repeated shifts of attention to pertinent locations (e.g., Allen et al., 1997). Working memory is a skill that everyone uses in daily life. For the purposes of this discussion, it is important to keep in mind that children rely on working memory to a vast extent in school, having to retain information that the teacher is presenting and to manipulate it in memory in order to draw conclusions, interpret literary writings, and do math problems, just as a few examples. Thus, impairments in working memory may have a strong negative influence on a child's ability to perform academically and socially.

Executive functioning is a multidimensional construct that includes higher-order cognitive processes such as initiation, planning, problem-solving, cognitive flexibility, behavioral regulation, metacognition, and feedback utilization (Delis, Kaplan, & Kramer, 2001; Powell & Voeller, 2004; Strauss, Sherman, & Spreen, 2006). Executive functions draw upon the individual's more basic cognitive skills, such as perception, attention, and working memory (Delis, Kaplan, & Kramer, 2001), The abilities to select relevant information, retain it, manipulate it, and make judgments about its relative importance are fundamental prerequisites for higher cognitive processes, including social and linguistic function. Spatial attention and working memory are critical links between the sensory and perceptual processes involved in taking in information and using that information in higher cognitive function.

To give an example of how these three cognitive processes interact in the daily life of an individual, imagine going to a social event at which you know very few people. The friend who invited you introduces you to the hosts. The conversation turns to a controversial topic. You listen to people's viewpoints but decide not to make yours known because they differ dramatically from those of the hosts, and you do not want to offend them or get into a heated debate. Spatial attention allowed you to attend to the different points of the conversation; working memory allowed you to recall who was espousing which ideas and viewpoints; and executive functioning guided your decision about whether or not to escalate the debate by voicing your own views.

These cognitive skills play an important role during development as well. They allow children to make new friends, enter into social relationships, and learn to get along in society. Significant deficits in any or all of these areas can impede social and academic development.

There has been considerable work on typical development in each of these domains. One important area of investigation has been the attempt to understand the origins of these essential and complex processes during infancy and the preschool period (see Garon et al., 2008; Korkmaz, 2011; Oakes et al., 2010, for summaries). Studies of developmental change in the neural systems that support these functions have focused primarily on the evidence for shifts in the organization of neural networks, with particular focus on the changing role of frontal cortex across development. Much of this work has focused on later-occurring changes in school-age children and adolescents. Despite this growing body of evidence concerning the typical development of these critical functions, very little is known about how early brain injury affects each of these functions.

SPATIAL ATTENTION

Adult Models

There is a large amount of information describing the neural bases of spatial attention networks in adults. Most studies have focused on aspects of visual spatial attention, with less emphasis on spatial attention in other modalities, such as auditory and tactile. Landmark behavioral studies done by Posner demonstrated that directing a person's attention to a specific location in space facilitated the processing of information at that location (Posner,

Snyder, & Davidson, 1980; Posner, Walker, Friedrich, & Rafal, 1984, 1987). Posner developed a task in which subjects viewed stimuli in one segment of their visual field, either in an area to which they were previously told to attend, or in an area to which they were not directed to attend. He found that responses were much faster to stimuli in the attended location than in the unattended location. Posner's early studies with stroke patients provided a strong link between parietal cortex and spatial attention function, particularly the disengagement of attention from an attended location. Electrophysiological studies done by Hillyard et al. (1998) helped to explain the neurophysiological bases for Posner's findings. Hillyard recorded brain wave electrical activity time-linked to a task the subject was asked to do, and then analyzed the waveform patterns for the groups of stimuli (event-related brain potentials). Using a spatial attention task, he demonstrated that shifting attention to a location in space enhanced sensory responses to information at that location (Hillyard, Vogel, & Luck, 1998; Mangun & Hillyard, 1991, Martínez, Teder-Salejarvi & Hillyard, 2007). These studies provided evidence that visual spatial attention is distributed in a gradient, with the greatest attention-related enhancement at the attended focus and decreasing sensory enhancement with increasing distance from that focus. Consistent with this work are single-cell recordings in macaques demonstrating that spatial attention increases firing of neurons that are processing an attended location and decreases firing of neurons that are processing an unattended location (Luck, Chelazzi, Hillyard, & Desimone, 1997; Martinez-Trujillo & Treue, 2002). Womelsdorf et al. have found wide-ranging modulation of cortical receptive fields associated with shifts of spatial attention affecting the entire visual field (Womelsdorf, Anton-Erxleben, Pieper, & Treue, 2006). They suggest this represents an attention-driven dynamic reallocation of processing resources that enhances processing at attended relative to unattended locations. Recent fMRI studies also show attention-enhanced processing in primary and secondary visual cortex (Jack, Shulman, Snyder, McAvoy, & Corbetta, 2006; Martinez et al., 1999, 2001).

Seminal PET and fMRI studies done by Corbetta, Mesulam, Nobre and others (Corbetta, Miezin, Shulman, & Petersen, 1993; Corbetta, Shulman, Miezin, & Petersen, 1995; Coull & Frith, 1998; Coull & Nobre, 1998; Mesulam, 1981; Nobre et al., 1997) have identified key neural structures involved in spatial attention, including posterior parietal cortex (intraparietal sulcus, right hemisphere and bilateral), frontal eye fields in bilateral premotor cortex, anterior cingulate, temporal-parietal junction, and subcortical circuits (such as the fronto-striato-thalamo-cortical network identified by Goldman-Rakic, 1987). More recent event-related fMRI studies have identified an anterior circuit that involves the anterior cingulate and is specific to spatial attention orienting, a dorsal network that includes the intraparietal sulcus and frontal eye fields and supports the allocation and maintenance of attention at a location (spatial attention and working memory), and a right-sided network that is specific to re-orienting (disengaging) attention and involves the intraparietal sulcus, inferior frontal gyrus, and the temporal-parietal junction (Corbetta, Kincade, & Shulman, 2002; Jack et al., 2006; Thiel, Zilles, & Fink, 2004).

While much less is known about spatial attention in the auditory modality, there are a number of studies showing that spatial cuing also enhances processing of auditory information (e.g., Mondor & Zatorre, 1995; Rhodes, 1987; Schmitt, Postma, & De Haan, 2000; Spence & Driver, 1994). At least one study provides evidence that auditory spatial attention, like visual spatial attention, is distributed in a gradient around the attended location (Mondor & Zatorre, 1995).The neural bases for both auditory and visual spatial attention may involve the same critical networks. There is some evidence that spatial attention systems are not modality-specific, but rather are "supramodal" and maintain representations of space that are independent of sensory modality and motor response (Downar, Crawley, Mikulis, & Davis, 2000; Driver & Spence, 1998; Farah, Wong, Monheit, & Morrow, 1989; Macaluso, Driver, & Frith, 2003; Macaluso, Frith, & Driver, 2002; Mayer, Harrington, Adair, & Lee, 2006; Shomstein & Yantis, 2004).

Studies of adults with unilateral strokes have been crucial in furthering understanding of the neural bases of spatial attention. Adults with parietal or frontal lesions exhibit spatial attention deficits in alerting and orienting. However, only frontal lesions produce deficits in executive control of spatial attention. Numerous studies of adults with focal brain damage, as well as of normal adults, suggest that spatial attention is predominantly mediated through the right parietal cortex (Farah, Wong, Monheit & Morrow, 1989; Petersen, Corbetta, Miezin, & Shulman, 1994; Petersen, Robinson, & Currie, 1989). Some of this knowledge has been gained by studying adults with neglect syndrome. This is a condition in which patients with focal brain damage, typically to the right parietal or frontal cortex, are unable to adequately attend to spatial stimuli, particularly in contra-lesional space. Manifestations of spatial neglect include inattention to visual stimuli and inability to read an entire page in a book (ignoring the words on the contra-lesional side of the page); inability to draw a complete clock (drawing only the ipsi-lesional side of the figure); and inability to localize a sound or a tactile stimulus on the side contralateral to the lesion. These neglect syndromes tend to occur more with right than left hemisphere damage in adults, and may gradually improve over time after the stroke (Heilman & Van Den Abell, 1980; Mesulam, 1981).

Development of Attention

Both function and structure of spatial attention are well specified in adults, but is the adult model of attentional networks valid during brain development? Fairly large changes in brain structure take place from birth through adolescence. Synapses proliferate early in the first 2 to 4 years of life and then gradually reduce in number (Huttenlocher, 1979; Huttenlocher, de Courten, Garey, & Van der Loos, 1982). Cerebral blood flow is higher in 1- to 4-year-olds and then gradually reduces to adult levels in a pattern that approximates that of neuronal proliferation and pruning (Chugani, 1998; Chugani, Phelps, & Mazziotta, 1987). Changes in gray and white matter volumes of the brain are seen throughout childhood, with reduction in gray matter volume in particular during adolescence (Sowell, Trauner, Gamst, & Jernigan, 2002; Toga, Thompson, & Sowell, 2006). Longitudinal studies using structural MRI methodology demonstrate that structural changes parallel cognitive milestones. For example, brain regions subserving primary motor and sensory systems mature earliest; temporal and parietal association areas next; and prefrontal and lateral temporal cortical areas last. These changes are hypothesized to reflect "pruning" or sculpting of the brain, during which synapses and cells "drop out" as cognitive networks become more specified (Chugani, 1998; Chugani, Phelps, & Mazziotta, 1987; Huttenlocher, 1979; Huttenlocher, de Courten, Garey, & Van der Loos, 1982; Sowell, Trauner, Gamst, & Jernigan, 2002; Toga, Thompson, & Sowell, 2006). Given these major structural changes that occur throughout childhood and well into adolescence, the adult model of attentional networks may not be the same as that utilized by the developing brain.

A number of studies have investigated spatial attention in infants and children. Infants as young as 4 months of age can shift visual-spatial attention (Johnson, 1996; Posner et al., 1988; Posner, Rothbart, Thomas-Thrapp, & Gerardi, 1998). A very interesting study by Reid et al. (2004) demonstrated that 4-month-old infants were influenced by direction of eye gaze of another person. In this study, infants were shown images of an adult face with the eyes gazing either towards or away from an object. Brain electrical activity was recorded during the study and responses were time-locked to the stimuli. The children were then shown pictures of the objects separately. Their brain wave activity showed that those pictures that had previously been shown with the adult eyes looking away from them were perceived by the infant as less familiar than those objects that had previously been shown with the eyes looking towards them. The authors conclude that the direction of eye gaze can influence attention in infants, as well as enhance processing of the information. However, the speed and efficiency of attention manipulation increases significantly throughout childhood and adolescence. There is evidence for improvement of attention shifting speed, the ability to disengage attention and control of the attentional field throughout childhood (Enns & Brodeur, 1989; Ridderinkhof & van der Stelt, 2000; Schul, Townsend, & Stiles, 2003). Tasks similar to Posner's original paradigm have been designed for use with children. Schul et al. (2003) used an "E" task in which the letter E was used as the target stimulus, and the child was told to move a joystick in the direction that the E was pointing (up, down, left, or right). The child was told to fixate on a central point, and the target was presented to the left or right side of the fixation point. Prior to the target being presented, a small square was illuminated to one side of the fixation point. The target was then shown either where the square had been presented or on the opposite side. Children had a faster response when the target was presented in the same spot as the square, and both speed and accuracy of attention processing improved with age. This type of paradigm has been used successfully in many studies of children and adults (Fig. 6.1) and nicely demonstrates the development of attentional processes over time. According to the "zoom lens hypothesis" (Eriksen & Yeh, 1985), the field of spatial attention contracts and expands according to task demands, and the efficiency of processing varies inversely with the size of the attentional field. Several authors have suggested that the ability to contract and expand the attentional field improves throughout the school-age years (Enns & Girgus, 1985; Pasto & Burack, 1997). Many researchers have suggested that these age-related improvements in selective attention function are linked to development of the relevant brain systems (Johnson, 2001, 2003).

There are also age-related differences in brain activation during spatial attention and working memory tasks. A recent fMRI study found that when children aged 8 to 12 re-oriented spatial attention, their patterns of activation did not reflect the activation commonly seen in adults, but rather showed decreased activation in the temporal-parietal junction and increased activation in ventro-lateral systems, including the right striatal-insula circuits and the left superior frontal gyrus (Konrad et al., 2005). In this study, children aged 8 to 12 years and adult volunteers were given the same behavioral task, and MRI scans were acquired with image acquisition trials time-locked to the presentation of the stimuli. Stimuli consisted of a vertical array of five arrows, with the middle arrow being the target. The other arrows were pointed in either the same or opposite directions as the middle arrow, and the visual stimuli were presented at different spatial locations with either cued or non-cued trials. MRI brain

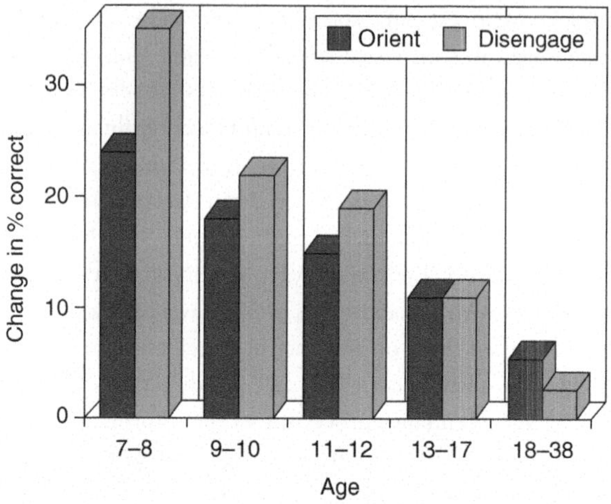

FIGURE 6.1 Development of ability to shift spatial attention from childhood to adults. Younger typically developing children are significantly slower to orient and disengage spatial attention and do not reach adult levels of efficiency until age 18. (Adapted from Schul et al., 2003.)

activation patterns were determined by subtracting baseline conditions from target-response conditions. Children and adults had similar levels of accuracy on this task. The results indicated, however, that children used different brain regions for attention than adults. Specifically, while adults showed activation in the right inferior frontal gyrus, right temporal-parietal junction, and bilateral superior parietal lobes, the activation patterns of the children were much more diffuse and included left superior frontal gyrus, right occipital-temporal gyrus, and left occipital gyrus. They also conducted volumetric analyses of structural MRI scans and found that the children had larger volumes of cortical gray matter in frontal, temporal, and parietal regions than did adults. The authors suggest that the differential pattern of activation reflects an immature process, and that as the brain becomes more mature and unnecessary or inefficient dendritic connections are pruned, more focal and efficient neural networks are established to mediate specific functions such as attention.

As discussed below, results from working memory studies have shown similar patterns of activation in children and adults during spatial working memory operations but different regional levels and distribution of activity; that is, location is similar but differing degrees of activity are found (Casey et al., 1995; Thomas et al., 1999). Both children and adults showed reliable activation of the middle and inferior frontal gyri and regions of inferior and superior parietal cortex, but in children there was greater volume and percent change of prefrontal activity, while in adults levels of parietal activation were greater. In this study, worse performance was associated with greater prefrontal activation. This may reflect less efficient processes in the immature brain; that is, greater activation is required when networks are less well specified. fMRI studies of spatial attention from Townsend et al. (Townsend, Haist,

Adamo, & Stiles, 2003) found that in adults there was bilateral parietal activation during covert attention in the region of the intraparietal sulcus that was greater on the right side and in the inferior temporal gyrus. In children, activation was more widespread and greater in prefrontal and inferior temporal cortices while parietal activation was relatively lower. Johnson has suggested that the cortical substrate for attention is different in infants than in adults and, in the case of spatial attention, relies more heavily on anterior than posterior cortical regions (Johnson, Tucker, Stiles, & Trauner, 1998). According to Johnson, this may reflect a more general principle in which frontal systems are active during learning, and this enhanced frontal activity decreases as proficiency increases. One possibility then is that increased reliance on prefrontal systems in children reflects less efficient attention networks.

There is a great deal of information about changes in brain white matter during normal development. Many recent studies have used diffusion tensor imaging (DTI) to study white matter changes. DTI is a quantitative technique that measures the diffusion of water in white matter fibers. White matter is composed of axonal projections from nerve cell bodies. These fibers become myelinated early in life. Myelin forms a protective sheath around the nerve fiber and restricts diffusion of water from the fiber. Thus, if the fiber is intact and myelin has formed effectively, the amount of diffusion will be low. The measure of movement of water along an axis is called fractional anisotropy (FA). The higher the FA, the more intact the nerve fiber is thought to be. FA increases with age in children and adolescents, both in the pyramidal tracts and in association areas (Schmithorst, Wilke, Dardzinski, & Holland, 2002). In agreement with these findings, mean diffusivity decreases with age in white matter throughout the brain. Other studies have documented evidence of increasing myelination and increasing white matter volume with age throughout childhood (e.g., Bava, Thayer, Jacobus, Ward, Jernigan, & Tapert, 2010; Paus et al., 2001). Much less is known about the relationship of white matter development to cognitive function. A recent study by Schmithorst et al. (Schmithorst, Wilke, Dardzinski, & Holland, 2005) demonstrated positive correlations between IQ scores and FA in white matter association areas bilaterally, in frontal, parietal, and occipital cortex. The authors conclude that these results suggest that increased white matter fiber organization and/or density correlates with cognitive function. Another recent study (Bava, Theilman, Sach, May, Frank, Hesselink, Vu, & Trauner, 2010) found that visual spatial ability correlated positively with increased FA in the right inferior parietal lobule in children with a genetic disorder. Tuch et al. (2005) found that reaction time on a visual attention task correlated positively with FA values in association pathways thought to be involved with visual spatial attention, including right occipital and parietal white matter pathways. Thus, converging evidence from a number of approaches suggests that spatial attention may be mediated more broadly by both anterior and posterior cortical regions during development, whereas adults rely on parietal regions for spatial attention except when executive control of spatial attention is required, necessitating more frontal involvement.

Attention in Children with Early Focal Brain Damage

Numerous studies of children with early unilateral brain damage from ischemic infarcts or bleeds have demonstrated that the location of the lesion does not predict the same cognitive consequences as do similar lesions in adults (e.g., Ballantyne, Spilkin, Hesselink & Trauner, 2008; Bates et al., 2001). There is a paucity of information on spatial attention in children with early focal damage, and those studies that have been done often have too few subjects to draw meaningful conclusions about structure–function relationships. For example, a study of five twin pairs discordant for perinatal stroke (Talib et al., 2008) showed some impairments in visual attention in the stroke group compared to their non-stroke twins, but the number was too small to draw conclusions about the location of the lesion and visual attention deficits. Temporal lobe epilepsy patients scheduled for surgery due to focal lesions demonstrated deficits in visual spatial attention prior to the surgery, whereas another group of children with frontal lobe epilepsy showed no impairments in visual spatial attention (Daniela et al., 2010).

Deficits in spatial attention, including spatial neglect, have been documented in children with early focal brain damage (Laurent-Vannier et al., 2003; Trauner, 2003), but focal brain damage early in development may not mimic the sequelae of damage in adults. While studies of adults with strokes consistently demonstrate the presence of neglect after right but not left hemisphere lesions, a very different pattern has been found in children after perinatal stroke. Trauner (2003) used a novel task in which toddlers were required to remove small toys from a corkboard. The order in which toys were removed and the time taken to remove the objects were recorded. Both typically developing children and children with perinatal stroke were included in the study. They found that typically developing children tended to remove toys from the center of the board first, and then moved outward with no strong right- or left-sided preference. However, children with right hemisphere lesions had a strong preference for removing objects from the right side of the board first, whereas children with left hemisphere lesions had the opposite preference of removing toys from the left side first. Thus, both right- *and* left-hemisphere lesions resulted in similar evidence of contralateral spatial neglect. These findings suggest that neural substrates of spatial attention and neglect are not the same in children as in adults, and that the developing brain may mediate attention in different ways from that of the mature brain. In an ongoing study by Townsend and Trauner (unpublished data), the E task described above is being used to study spatial attention in children with perinatal stroke compared with age-matched controls. Data from this study (Fig. 6.2) suggests that children with parietal lobe damage have difficulty disengaging attention from the side ipsilateral to the lesion to attend to the contralateral side, while patients with frontal lobe lesions have difficulty both orienting to a stimulus in space and disengaging. Although this study is ongoing, results to date do suggest that subtle evidence of spatial inattention to contralateral space is present after perinatal stroke, and that this reduces the ability of the child to orient attention in the case of frontal lesions, and to disengage and shift attention in the case of parietal lesions.

Interestingly, studies of attention and behavior in children with early unilateral brain damage using parent questionnaires show no consistent attention problems, and no correlation between attention problems and the site or side of the lesion (Trauner, Nass, & Ballantyne, 2001). Again, these studies suggest that the brain regions necessary for development of specific cognitive functions may not be the same as those required for maintenance of that function once the brain has developed.

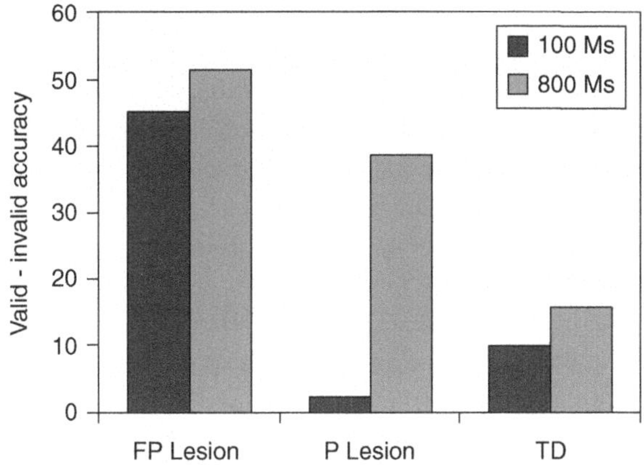

FIGURE 6.2 Spatial attention task in children with perinatal stroke and typically developing controls. Children with parietal lobe lesions (P Les) oriented attention to the cued side as quickly as typically developing controls (TD) but had great difficulty disengaging attention from the visual field ipsilateral to their lesion to respond in the contra-lesional field. Children with lesions that affected both frontal and parietal lobes (FP Les) were slow to orient attention following a cue, and after orienting attention (at 800 ms following the attention-directing cue) were slow to disengage attention from the ipsi-lesional visual field. Dark bars represent attention disengagement (percent correct at validly cued location minus percent correct at the uncued location) with 100 ms to orient attention. Light bars are attention disengagement with 800 ms to orient attention. These data are for responses to contralesional visual field for lesion children and the average across location for TD. (Unpublished data from Townsend J and Trauner DA.)

WORKING MEMORY

Adult Models

Baddeley (Baddeley, 1992) defined working memory as "a brain system that provides temporary storage and manipulation of the information necessary for such complex cognitive tasks as language comprehension, learning, and reasoning," a definition that captures the key elements present in most models of this important cognitive ability. According to Baddeley "working memory stands at the crossroads between memory, attention, and perception." The ability to store and manipulate information "on-line" efficiently is critical to a wide variety of more complex cognitive tasks, from following and discerning the meaning of a paragraph being read to making sure that one's actions are consistent with situational social requirements and longer-term goals. In fact, working memory has been proposed as a key underlying mechanism to executive functions in general (Pennington, Bennetto, McAleer, & Roberts, 1996; Roberts & Pennington, 1996), which include planning, problem-solving, initiation of behavior, self-monitoring, concept shifting, flexibility, inhibitory control, and in general matching one's behavior to environmental contingencies and requirements. Working memory is, in turn, dependent on the integrity of basic perceptual and attentional mechanisms such as maintaining alertness, directing attention in space, and screening out irrelevant stimuli (Postle et al., 2004).

In general, studies from multiple areas (animal and human, behavioral, functional imaging, and event-related brain potentials) all indicate that working memory utilizes a distributed network of posterior parietal and prefrontal cortical areas. Most studies use similar methods for testing working memory, with the subject being required to hold some pieces of information in memory for a short period of time, and sometimes to manipulate that information by reorganizing it or making judgments about it.

Several models of working memory have been proposed that differ from one another in the relationship of working memory to attention, the location of capacity limitations in working memory, whether limitations are modality-specific, and other key issues. Baddeley's seminal model consists of four components: a central executive, which directs attention and is resource-limited; two modality-specific slave systems (phonological loop and visuospatial sketchpad) that store and rehearse information, integrate their contents with information from long-term memory and manipulate representations; and the episodic buffer, a storage component that is not modality-specific. In contrast to Baddeley's model, Just and Carpenter (1992) proposed a model of working memory that combines processing and storage functions and assumes a trade-off in resources allocated to these two functions. Thus, a limited amount of activation is available (the amount varying between individuals) for both maintenance and manipulation of information, and trade-offs occur when demands exceed the available activation. Some authors discuss the primacy and recency effects; that is, when presented with a long list of information items, the individual generally can recall the first item mentioned and then the last several, but has more difficulty recalling the ones in the middle. Buchsbaum, Ye, and D'Esposito (2011) used an fMRI paradigm to study the neural basis of the recency effect. In this study, subjects were presented either with visual word lists presented one at a time, or auditory word lists also presented one at a time. They were to push a button if the word had been presented before. Lateral inferior parietal cortex activity was modulated in response to the recency effect, and the response was dissociable from other parts of the parietal lobe that are thought to be involved in different aspects of memory function. Superior parietal-temporal cortex was activated for verbal working memory maintenance. In their review, Engle et al. (Engle, Tuholski, Laughling, & Conway, 1999) emphasized the "executive attention" nature of working memory and its role in maintaining information (including goal states and task demands) in the face of interference. They, and other authors, also discuss the significant contribution of working memory to individual differences in fluid intelligence and in performing complex cognitive tasks (Fry & Hale, 1996; Jonides & Nee, 2006; Just & Carpenter, 1999).

D'Esposito et al. have used paradigms that separate components of working memory in fMRI studies of normal adults. These paradigms are somewhat complicated. Briefly, they involve maintenance of a series of random letters in working memory for several seconds, during which an MRI is performed. The subject is either told to remember the letters, or in a separate condition, is told to manipulate the letters held in memory by putting them in alphabetical order. Dorsolateral and ventrolateral prefrontal cortex (PFC) were activated while subjects were retaining the letters in memory. However, only dorsolateral PFC was activated during the manipulation of letters into alphabetical order, indicating a specialization of different parts of PFC for different segments of working memory. In another part of the study, subjects are given anywhere from two to six letters to retain in memory so that the effects of memory load could be isolated as well. Right dorsolateral PFC was activated during the memory load trials. Another series of studies was performed using objects rather than letters to be held in working memory, and utilized the same fMRI procedures. Based on these series of studies, D'Esposito et al. have proposed a neurally based, process-specific model of working memory that involves a network of parietal and both ventral and dorsal lateral prefrontal cortex (D'Esposito et al., 1998; D'Esposito, Postle, Ballard, & Lease, 1999). In this model, the organization and maintenance of information that has been received from posterior association areas is performed in both ventral and dorsal lateral PFC. Activity related to maintenance of information tends to be lateralized by information type, with greater right hemisphere ventrolateral PFC activation by spatial tasks, and greater left hemisphere activation by nonspatial tasks. Tasks that require monitoring or manipulation of information in working memory produce additional activation of dorsal, but not ventral, lateral PFC, and this activation tends to be bilateral or lateralized to the right. Thus, a hierarchical organization exists wherein information is passed from ventral to dorsolateral PFC depending on processing requirements. Other investigators have delineated the functions of prefrontal areas by domain rather than process (see Mohr, Goebel, & Linden, 2006).

In an attempt to synthesize the functional neuroimaging literature on working memory, Owen et al. (Owen, McMillan, Laird, & Bullmore, 2005) conducted a meta-analysis of fMRI studies of the *n*-back paradigm, a commonly used working memory task that is appropriate for use in both children and adults. This task requires the subject to monitor a series of stimuli, compare them with previously presented stimuli, and respond when the current stimulus matches one presented *n* trials previously. The number of trials separating the two stimuli to be compared can be manipulated, thus varying the processing and memory load. This complex task involves several components of the working memory network, as well as attentional and motor processes. In their meta-analysis, Owen et al. divided studies into those involving verbal versus nonverbal stimuli, and those requiring comparisons of stimulus identity versus stimulus location. They found consistency across studies in the recruitment of parietal and prefrontal areas (including dorso- and ventrolateral and frontal poles), as well as cingulate/medial premotor cortex and medial cerebellum, but differential activation based on task demands. They suggest that premotor cortex is active during maintenance of visuospatial attention during working memory tasks, while parietal cortex is important for attentional processes. This illustrates the interconnected network that is involved in the performance of attentional and working memory tasks. There is overlap in the networks that subserve spatial attention and spatial working memory (Awh, Vogel, & Oh, 2006; Corbetta, Kincaid, & Shulman, 2002). The synchronization of activity of the areas involved in both verbal and spatial working memory has also begun to receive greater attention (see, for example, Diwadkar, Carpenter, & Just, 2000; Newman, Just, & Carpenter, 2002).

In adults, working memory deficits have been linked to PFC damage (review by Engle et al., 1999). However, there appears to be some specialization of brain regions for specific aspects of working memory. Dorsal frontal areas have been found to be involved in manipulation of information within working memory (D'Esposito, Postle, & Rypma, 2000). A recent study (Baier et al., 2010) demonstrated that basal ganglia damage in adult stroke patients produced working memory deficits by allowing irrelevant stimuli to interfere with working memory function. Right PFC lesions in adults limited the amount of information patients could hold in working memory. These findings as well as earlier work (McNab & Klingberg, 2008) suggest a basal ganglia-PFC circuit for working memory in which the basal ganglia prevent irrelevant information from getting into working memory, and PFC maintains relevant information to be used during working memory tasks.

Working Memory in Typical Development

Studies of infants report rapid development of visual short-term memory in the second half of the first year of life. Before 6 months of age visual short-term memory is quite limited. By 4 months, infants can store features of a single item or a single location (Oakes, Hurley, Ross-Sheehy, & Luck, 2010; Oakes, Messenger, Ross-Sheehy, & Luck, 2009; Ross-Sheehy, Oakes, & Luck, 2003). After 6 months infants are able to store information about multiple objects and track their position at multiple locations.

In typical development, working memory performance improves throughout childhood, with speed and efficiency continuing to develop after accuracy has been attained (Brocki & Bohlin, 2004; Pennington, Bennetto, McAleer, & Roberts, 1996). The underlying mechanism of changes in working memory with age has been under debate. Competing theories have suggested change in capacity, speed of processing, or trade-offs between processing and storage as the key variable, or complex combinations thereof (e.g., Barrouillet, Bernardin, & Camos, 2004; Barrouillet & Camos, 2001; Bayliss, Jarrold, Baddeley, Gunn, & Leigh, 2005; Conlin, Gathercole, & Adams, 2005; Gavens & Barrouillet, 2004; Towse & Hitch, 1995). fMRI studies in children by Casey and others have found both similarities and differences in the patterns of activation in children and adults, with the degree of activation in different parts of the network also differing between children and adults (Casey et al., 1995; Crone, Wendelken, Donohue, van Leijenhorst, & Bunge, 2006; Klingberg, Forssberg, & Westerberg, 2002; Kwon, Reiss, & Menon, 2002; Olesen, Macoveanu, Tegner, & Klingberg, 2007; Olesen, Nagy, Westerberg, & Klingberg, 2003; Pennington, 1994; Thomas et al., 1999). For example, Thomas et al. (1999) compared activation patterns in children ages 8 to 10 years, and adults, during performance of a spatial *n*-back task. In this task, subjects were required to watch four boxes for a stimulus that would appear in one of the boxes. They were then asked to recall in which box the stimulus had appeared one or two trials back from the current one. MRI analyses were performed to link brain activation patterns with behavioral trials to obtain functional imaging maps. The authors found that adults showed activation in the right dorsolateral prefrontal, right cingulate gyrus, and right temporal and parietal cortices during the memory task. Children also showed activation in right prefrontal and parietal areas, but in addition, showed activation in left precuneus cortex and left and right inferior parietal lobules. Both children and adults showed more lateral prefrontal activation in this spatial paradigm than in previous studies of nonspatial working memory from the same group (e.g., Casey et al., 1995), suggesting differences in the activation patterns of spatial and nonspatial information by this point in childhood. Studies using structural MRI have also found relationships between working memory development and structural age differences. For example, Nagy et al. (2004) found, using diffusion tensor MRI, that in children age 8 to 18 years performance on a working memory measure was correlated with measures of white matter maturation in areas of the left frontal lobe. A recent longitudinal study of white matter development using DTI techniques (Bava et al., 2010) in adolescents demonstrated a direct correlation between working memory measures and increases in fractional anisotropy between the first and second time points, suggesting that enhanced white matter coherence or stability contributes to better efficiency in working memory.

Working Memory in Early Focal Brain Damage

The literature on working memory development suggests an integral role of working memory in mediating the accomplishment of more complex language (see Baddeley, 2003), problem-solving, and other executive functioning tasks in childhood. In adults, working memory deficits have been linked to PFC damage, as noted above (see review by Engle et al., 1999), and the imaging literature reviewed above suggests roles of both dorsal and ventral PFC, parietal areas, and fiber tracts connecting these areas in working memory functioning. Studies of children with traumatic brain injury have found impairments in working memory (letter *n*-back tasks) that are related to left frontal lesions (Levin et al., 2004) and to performance on more complex language tasks (Chapman et al., 2006). There have been very few studies of working memory after early focal brain injury, and the few that have been reported have conflicting results. Daniela et al. (2010) found no deficits in working memory in children with frontal or temporal lobe lesional epilepsy prior to surgery. In contrast, using an fMRI task, Everts et al. (2010) found verbal working memory deficits in children with focal epilepsy. However, these deficits were linked with language lateralization, such that children with "atypical" language lateralization (bilateral or right hemisphere lateralization) had more preserved verbal working memory than those with left hemisphere lateralization. They hypothesize that the "transfer" of language to atypical language areas is more advantageous for verbal memory function. Thus, their study emphasizes the plasticity of the developing brain rather than indicating a "hard-wired" approach to working memory during development. Westmacott et al. (2010) found slightly lower working memory index scores (using the Wechsler Intelligence Scale index measures) in children who had suffered perinatal unilateral strokes compared with those who had suffered a stroke at a later age (beyond 1 month of life). However, they found no effect of lesion site or side on working memory index scores in these children. In contrast to the study by Everts et al. (2010), they interpret their findings to suggest selective vulnerability of the brain at early stages of development, rather than enhanced plasticity. Nichols et al. (2004) used the California Verbal Learning Test—Children's Version (CVLT-C) to study verbal learning and memory in children with perinatal stroke as well as three other groups of children with neurodevelopmental disorders—specific language impairment, Williams syndrome, and Down syndrome. The CVLT is a list-learning task in which a list of 15 words from three semantic categories (fruits, clothing, and toys) is given. After the list is read, the child is asked to repeat as many words as he or she can remember. The list is then read four more times, and after each trial the child is again asked to repeat as many words as he or she can. After the fifth trial there is a separate interference list of 15 words presented and the child is asked to recall those words. He or she is then asked to recall the first series of words. The examiner then cues the child by asking for the words by semantic category (tell me all of the fruits you can remember from the first list). This is the immediate recall trial. There is then a 20-minute gap during which the child is asked to do some other activity, such as draw a picture. After 20 minutes, he or she is again asked to recall as many of the words from the first list as possible, first from free recall and then cued by semantic category. Finally, the child is presented with a series of words and asked if each word was on the first list or not (recognition memory). In the Nichols study, 14 children with perinatal stroke ages 6 to 14 years were tested. An assessment of language was also documented in order to compare verbal learning with language ability. Children with perinatal stroke had normal receptive language scores, and performed as well as typically developing controls on the first learning trial. However, as the trials continued, the stroke group had increasing difficulty with verbal memory, and by the fifth trial and the delayed trials, they were performing at a significantly lower level than controls. There were no clear differences related to the side of the lesion.

Studies to date on working memory after perinatal brain injury suggest subtle working memory deficits. However, there remains a paucity of information on working memory after early focal brain damage, and this precludes speculation about the similarities and differences in neural correlates of working memory during human development, and highlights the need for such studies in the future.

EXECUTIVE FUNCTION

Adult Models

Executive functions (EFs) are a complex set of separate but integrated cognitive abilities that allow individuals to carry out goal-directed behaviors and include organization, planning, and execution of behaviors that are in their best interests and allow independent functioning in daily living and in social interactions. As described by Miyake et al. (2000), EFs are "general purpose control mechanisms that modulate the operation of various cognitive subprocesses and thereby regulate the dynamics of human cognition." Although EFs are generally discussed as though they are a series of separate functions, they all are part of a single construct. Miyake et al. (2000) have defined three core functions that underlie all EF abilities. They studied 137 undergraduates using several tasks to tap different aspects of EF and extracted commonalities and differences in responses. They were able to identify three basic EF components that they believe underlie all EF skills: inhibition (the ability to inhibit a response when necessary), working memory (the ability to retain information in short-term storage and to be able to use it to complete a task), and shifting attention (the ability to move one's attention to a different topic/locale when necessary to obtain relevant information). Executive functions have been thought to be largely subserved by the PFC, which has rich cortical and subcortical connections throughout the brain (Damasio & Anderson, 1993). Response inhibition is associated with activity in the right inferior frontal gyrus in fMRI studies (Xue, Aron, & Poldrack, 2008). Medial prefrontal areas have been implicated in response inhibition (Chevrier, Noseworthy, & Schachar, 2007). However, numerous studies have shown a more widespread neural network subserving EF and cognitive flexibility. For example, the rostrolateral PFC is thought to support the selection and manipulation of self-generated thoughts (Christoff & Gabrielli, 2000); the temporo-parietal junction has been linked to stimulus-driven orienting and attention (Kincade et al., 2005), and the subthalamic nucleus to response inhibition (Kenner et al., 2010). Thus, the earlier concept of frontal lobe control of EF may require modification to include more distributed networks for control of these complex skills.

There is significant overlap between attention, working memory, and EF, so that this discussion will be brief and will cover only specific aspects of executive function. Table 6.1 summarizes what is known about the neural substrates of these interrelated cognitive processes.

One commonly used test of executive function is the Stroop test, which involves inhibition of an automatic response in favor of a voluntary response. In this task, the subject is

TABLE 6.1 SUMMARY OF NEURAL SUBSTRATES OF SPATIAL ATTENTION, WORKING MEMORY, AND EXECUTIVE FUNCTION

Spatial Attention	Posterior parietal cortex (right and bilateral)
	Inferior frontal gyrus (right)
	Anterior cingulate
	Temporo-parietal junction
	Frontal eye fields (in the visual modality)
	Subcortical fronto-striato-thalamo-cortical network
Working Memory	Dorsolateral prefrontal cortex
	Ventrolateral prefrontal cortex
	Parietal cortex
	Cingulate cortex
	Medial premotor cortex
Executive Function	Anterior cingulate
	Bilateral lateral prefrontal cortex
	Anterior insula
	Parietal lobes

presented with conflicting information. The most commonly used form of the task involves the presentation of color names (e.g., the word "red") but the font is in a different color (e.g., blue font). The person is asked to name the color of the word rather than the color the word says (so the response would be blue for the above example). An auditory version of the Stroop task has been developed in which a male or female voice says a word that is typically associated with the opposite gender (e.g., a male voice says the word "princess"). The subject is asked to identify the gender of the word the voice is saying, rather than the gender of the voice itself. As can be seen from the description of these tasks, anyone taking such a test has to attend to the information, has to maintain the instructions in working memory, and has to inhibit the urge to name the obvious response (e.g., red for the color, male for the voice). This is the type of complex activity that is typical of what is considered EF. In fMRI studies using Stroop-like tasks, not surprisingly the same neural structures activated for attention and working memory paradigms are also activated. These include primarily a frontal-parietal network, with some additional structures involved depending on the specific task. For conflict-related activities such as occur with a Stroop decision, anterior cingulate, bilateral lateral PFC, anterior insula, and parietal lobes are most reliably implicated using fMRI techniques. In the auditory task described above, lateral PFC, anterior cingulate cortex, and left anterior insular cortex were activated. Another recent study by Roberts and Hall (2009) used both visual and auditory Stroop tasks and found activation in anterior cingulate cortex, bilateral PFC, and left superior parietal lobe with right anterior insula in the visual task only. Thus, converging evidence from multiple laboratories using different variations on EF paradigms shows similar neural networks for EF tasks.

Damage to the frontal lobes in adults has been associated with deficits in multiple aspects of EF, including planning, working memory, impulse control, and attention. Although PFC is important for many aspects of EF in adults, there is a more distributed network that includes frontal and posterior/subcortical brain regions. fMRI studies have demonstrated activation in both frontal and posterior brain regions during various EF tasks. Lesion studies in adults also demonstrate different structure–function patterns depending on the specific EF task studied. For example, right or bilateral prefrontal damage may cause deficits in selective attention, whereas right or left prefrontal and right posterior insults result in difficulty inhibiting responses to spatial locations, and left prefrontal damage causes deficits in inhibiting motor responses. Thus, a combination of data both from normal adults and from those with focal brain damage lends support to the idea that both frontal and extrafrontal brain regions may be involved in EF, and that each brain region may be responsible for different aspects of EF.

Executive Functions in Typical Development

EFs have a more protracted developmental course than any other cognitive ability. These skills are not fully mature until late adolescence or even early adult life. The brain is undergoing dramatic structural changes during the first two decades of life. During brain development, the PFC is late to mature, with continued changes in gray and white matter volume well into adolescence (Gogtay et al., 2004). It has been assumed in the past that this brain structure is responsible for EF during development, based on adult studies as well as the observation that EF skills emerge relatively late as well. Areas of PFC have been found to correspond to the ability to select and manipulate self-generated information (Dumontheil, Burgess, & Blakemore, 2008). More recent studies, however, have suggested that it is not frontal lobe development, but more global brain maturation, that is responsible for the acquisition of EFs and for the protracted developmental course of these skills. fMRI studies comparing performance on EF tasks in adults and adolescents show different patterns of brain activation between the two groups, with adults showing activation in task-relevant specific brain regions but adolescents showing more diffuse and different activation patterns in brain regions not previously known to be correlated with those particular tasks (Casey et al., 2000; Rubia et al., 2006). Other fMRI studies show that adolescents have increased activation in lateral prefrontal, parietal, and medial PFC on EF tasks (Bunge & Wright, 2007). Measures of cortical thickness in brains of children and adolescents using morphometric MRI analyses (Tamnes et al., 2010) found that the cortical thickness of posterior structures (parietal and occipital gray matter) was inversely related to performance on certain measures of EF. Cortical thickness is known to become smaller as the brain matures during adolescence (Sowell et al., 2003); thus, normal maturation of the cortical layers appears to be associated with acquisition of EF skills, rather than maturation of particular lobes of the brain. Recent studies of typically developing children using fMRI indicate that there is less frontal activation in children than in adults during EF tasks, and that overall brain maturation, rather than PFC specifically, is necessary for EF to develop (Rubia et al., 2006).

Executive Functions in Early Focal Brain Damage

Children with frontal lobe epilepsy demonstrate problems with planning and impulse control, suggesting that there may be a similar pattern of frontal lobe mediation of EF during brain development (Hernandez et al., 2002). Right frontal damage appears to have a particularly negative impact on self-regulation and adherence to rules (Jacobs & Anderson, 2002). In a study of 79 children with brain damage (Jacobs, Harvey, & Anderson, 2011) compared with typically developing controls, the brain-damaged individuals performed significantly more poorly on cognitive and EF tasks in all EF tasks, including problem-solving and cognitive flexibility, than did controls, regardless of the site of the lesion. The study suggested that total brain integrity, rather than a specific brain structure, is necessary for EF to develop (Jacobs & Anderson, 2002; Jacobs, Harvey, & Anderson, 2011). The group studied was quite diverse in terms of time of lesion onset, unilateral versus bilateral versus global brain damage, and etiology of the damage, making it somewhat difficult to interpret the significance of the results and their relevance for children with perinatal stroke. Interestingly, some studies suggest that there may be "critical periods" during brain development when damage to frontal regions may result in worse outcomes with respect to EFs. Any brain damage before age 3 may result in more severe outcomes than damage sustained after that age (Anderson et al., 2010). In a recent study comparing the cognitive and psychiatric consequences of early- versus later-onset stroke, Max, Bruce, Keatley, and Delis (2010) tested 17 children with early-onset stroke (age at occurrence less than 12 months) and 12 children with later-onset stroke (mean age at stroke 7.8 years). They administered tests of intelligence, language, memory, visual spatial skills, academic achievement, and executive functioning, as well as a psychiatric interview. Tests of EF focused on cognitive flexibility, constructional abilities, and working memory. A group of children with orthopedic problems was used as a control population. The authors found that the children with early-onset stroke performed significantly more poorly in all areas tested than the children with later-onset stroke, with the exception of the domain of EF. On EF tasks, children with early-onset stroke performed significantly better than those with late-onset stroke. The authors interpret their data to indicate early vulnerability of the brain, in which damage during a critical time in development will disrupt cognitive processes that would normally be developing during that time. Thus, since EFs develop later in childhood and adolescence, they might be spared by early damage but more susceptible to disruption by later injury. Unfortunately, since the groups studied were very heterogeneous in terms of both the etiology of the brain damage and the timing of the lesion, and the group sizes were small, it is difficult to determine the significance of the findings with relation to isolated perinatal stroke.

The above work suggests that the timing of the brain injury may be more important than the location of the damage in determining EF abilities. It is possible that during peak periods of synaptogenesis (2 to 4 years of age) the brain has more ability to reorganize, but that before and after that period there is less flexibility in setting up alternate pathways in the face of damage to one part of the brain.

Summary

As can be seen from the studies related above, spatial attention, spatial working memory, and EFs are closely related cognitive processes that allow an individual to carry out crucial goal-directed behaviors to support independent social and emotional functioning. These cognitive processes have been demonstrated to share some of the same neural substrates in studies of healthy adults as well as those with localized brain damage. In children, however, there are important differences. Although similar brain regions may underlie some aspects of these functions, the developing brain utilizes different strategies from those of the fully formed adult brain. When the developing brain is damaged, it is able to turn to new compensatory strategies that allow it to develop these crucial skills, although there may be limitations to how much reorganization is able to take place. Particularly with areas of the brain that mature slowly over many years, such as the frontal lobes, long-term outcome after early brain damage may not be clear until adult life. However, given the awareness that early focal brain damage may result in less-than-complete development of spatial attention, working memory, and EFs, early and perhaps prolonged therapeutic interventions (see Diamond & Lee, 2011, for recent review of interventions for EF development) and tracking of progress may help to improve the ultimate level of functioning of such individuals.

REFERENCES

Allen G, Buxton RB, Wong EC, Courchesne E (1997). Attentional activation of the cerebellum independent of motor involvement. *Science* 275(5308):1940–1943.

Anderson V, Spencer-Smith M, Coleman L, Anderson P, Williams J, Greenham M, Leventer RJ, Jacobs R (2010). Children's executive functions: are they poorer after very early brain insult. *Neuropsychologia* 48(7):2041–2050.

Awh E, Vogel EK, Oh SH (2006). Interactions between attention and working memory. *Neuroscience* 139(1):201–228.

Baddeley A (1992) Working memory. *Science* 255(5044):556–559.

Baddeley A (2003). Working memory and language: An overview. *J Comm Disorders* 36:189–208.

Baier B, Karnath H-O, Dietrrich M, Birklein F, Heinze C, Muller NG (2010). Keeping memory clear and stable—The contribution of human basal ganglia and prefrontal cortex to working memory. *J Neurosci* 30:9788–9792.

Ballantyne AO, Spilkin A, Hesselink J, Trauner DA (2008). Plasticity in the developing brain: intellectual, language and academic functions in children with ischaemic perinatal stroke. *Brain* 131(Pt 11):2975–2985.

Barrouillet P, Bernardin S, Camos V (2004). Time constraints and resource sharing in adults' working memory spans. *J Exp Psychol Gen* 133(1):83–100.

Barrouillet P, Camos V (2001). Developmental increase in working memory span: Resource sharing or temporal decay? *J Memory Language* 45:1–20.

Bates E, Reilly J, Wulfeck B, Dronkers N, Opie M, Fenson J, Kriz S, Jeffries R, Miller L, Herbst K (2001). Differential effects of unilateral lesions on language production in children and adults. *Brain Language* 79(2):223–265.

Bava S, Thayer R, Jacobus J, Ward M, Jernigan TL, Tapert SF (2010). Longitudinal characterization of white matter maturation during adolescence. *Brain Res* 23(1327):38–46.

Bava S, Theilmann RJ, Sach M, May SJ, Frank L, Hesselink J, Vu D, Trauner DA (2010). Developmental changes in cerebral white matter microstructure in a disorder of lysosomal storage. *Cortex* 46(2):206–216.

Bayliss DM, Jarrold C, Baddeley AD, Gunn DM, Leigh E (2005). Mapping the developmental constraints on working memory span performance. *Dev Psychol* 41:579–597.

Brocki KC, Bohlin G (2004). Executive functions in children aged 6 to 13: a dimensional and developmental study. *Dev Neuropsychol* 26(2):571–593.

Buchsbaum BR, Ye D, D'Esposito M (2011). Recency effects in the inferior parietal lobe during verbal recognition memory. *Front Hum Neurosci* 5:59.

Bunge SA, Wright SB (2007). Neurodevelopmental changes in working memory and cognitive control. *Curr Opinion Neurobiol* 17(2):243–250.

Casey BJ, Cohen JD, Jezzard P, Turner R, Noll DC, Trainor RJ, et al. (1995). Activation of prefrontal cortex in children during a nonspatial working memory task with functional MRI. *NeuroImage* 2(3):221–229.

Casey BJ, Giedd JN, Thomas KM (2000). Structural and functional brain development and its relation to cognitive development. *Biol Psychol* 54:241–257.

Chapman SB, Gamino JF, Cook LG, Hanten G, Li X, Levin HS (2006). Impaired discourse gist and working memory in children after brain injury. *Brain Language* 97(2):178–188.

Chevrier AD, Noseworthy MD, Schachar R (2007). Dissociation of response inhibition and performance monitoring in the stop signal task using event-related fMRI. *Human Brain Mapping* 28:1347–1358.

Christoff K, Gabrielli JDE (2000). The frontopolar cortex and human cognition: Evidence for a rostrocaudal hierarchical organization within the human prefrontal cortex. *Psychobiology* 28:168–186.

Chugani HT (1998). A critical period of brain development: studies of cerebral glucose utilization with PET. *Prev Med* 27(2):184–188.

Chugani HT, Phelps ME, Mazziotta JC (1987). Positron emission tomography study of human brain functional development. *Ann Neurol* 22(4):487–497.

Conlin JA, Gathercole SE, Adams JW (2005). Children's working memory: Investigating performance limitations in complex span tasks. *J Exp Child Psychol* 90:303–317.

Corbetta M, Kincade JM, Shulman GL (2002). Neural systems for visual orienting and their relationships to spatial working memory. *J Cogn Neurosci* 14(3):508–523.

Corbetta M, Miezin FM, Shulman GL, Petersen SE (1993). A PET study of visuospatial attention. *J Neurosci* 13(3):1202–1226.

Corbetta M, Shulman GL, Miezin FM, Petersen SE (1995). Superior parietal cortex activation during spatial attention shifts and visual feature conjunction [published erratum appears in Science 1995 Dec 1; 270(5241):1423]. *Science* 270(5237):802–805.

Coull JT, Frith CD (1998). Differential activation of right superior parietal cortex and intraparietal sulcus by spatial and nonspatial attention. *NeuroImage* 8(2):176–187.

Coull JT, Nobre AC (1998). Where and when to pay attention: the neural systems for directing attention to spatial locations and to time intervals as revealed by both PET and fMRI. *J Neurosci* 18(18):7426–7435.

Crone EA, Wendelken C, Donohue S, van Leijenhorst L, Bunge SA (2006). Neurocognitive development of the ability to manipulate information in working memory. *Proc Natl Acad Sci U S A* 103(24):9315–9320.

D'Esposito M, Aguirre GK, Zarahn E, Ballard D, Shin RK, Lease J (1998). Functional MRI studies of spatial and nonspatial working memory. *Brain Research. Cogn Brain Res* 7(1):1–13.

D'Esposito M, Postle BR, Ballard D, Lease J (1999). Maintenance versus manipulation of in formation held in working memory: an event-related fMRI study. *Brain Cognition* 41(1): 66–86.

D'Esposito M, Postle BR, Rypma B (2000) Prefrontal cortical contributions to working memory: evidence from event-related fMRI studies. *Exp Brain Res* 133:3–11.

Damasio AR, Anderson SW (1993). The frontal lobes. In K. M. Heilman & E. Valenstein (Eds.), Clinical Neuropsychology (3rd ed., pp. 409–460). New York: Oxford University Press.

Daniela C, Donatella L, Ilaria C, Francesca P, Alessandra G, Concetta P, Antonio M, Giampiero T, Domenica B, Concezio DR, Francesco G (2010). Surgery of children with frontal lobe lesional epilepsy: Neuropsychological study. *Brain & Development* 2010; epub ahead of print.

Delis D, Kaplan E, Kramer J (2001). Delis-Kaplan Executive Functioning System: Examiner's Manual. San Antonio: The Psychological Corporation.

Diamond A, Lee K (2011). Interventions shown to aid executive function development in children 4 to 12 years old. *Science* 333(6045):959–964.

Diwadkar VA, Carpenter PA, Just MA (2000). Collaborative activity between parietal and dorsolateral prefrontal cortex in dynamic spatial working memory revealed by fMRI. *NeuroImage* 12(1):85–99.

Downar J, Crawley AP, Mikulis DJ, Davis KD (2000). A multimodal cortical network for the detection of changes in the sensory environment. *Nature Neurosci* 3(3):277–283.

Driver J, Spence C (1998). Crossmodal attention. *Curr Opinion Neurobiol* 8(2):245–253.

Dumontheil I, Burgess PW, Blakemore SJ (2008). Development of rostral prefrontal cortex and cognitive and behavioral disorders. *Dev Med Child Neurol* 50:168–181.

Engle RW, Tuholski SW, Laughling JE, Conway ARA (1999). Working memory, short-term memory, and general fluid intelligence: A latent-variable approach. *J Exp Psychol Gen* 128:309–331.

Enns JT, Brodeur DA (1989). A developmental study of covert orienting to peripheral visual cues. *J Exp Child Psychol* 48(2):171–189.

Enns JT, Girgus JS (1985). Developmental changes in selective and integrative visual attention. *J Exp Child Psychol* 40(2):319–337.

Eriksen CW, Yeh YY (1985). Allocation of attention in the visual field. *J Exp Psychol Hum Perception Performance* 11(5):583–597.

Everts R, Harvey AS, Lillywhite L, Wrennall J, Abbott DF, Gonzalez L, Kean M, Jackson GD, Anderson V (2010). Language lateralization correlates with verbal memory performance in children with focal epilepsy. *Epilepsia* 51(4):627–638.

Farah MJ, Wong AB, Monheit MA, Morrow LA (1989). Parietal lobe mechanisms of spatial attention: modality-specific or supramodal? *Neuropsychologia* 27(4):461–470.

Fry AF, Hale S (1996). Processing speed, working memory, and fluid intelligence: Evidence for a developmental cascade. *Psychol Sci* 7:237–241.

Garon N, Bryson SE, Smith IM (2008). Executive function in preschoolers: a review using an integrative framework. *Psychol Bull* 134(1):31–60.

Gavens N, Barrouillet P (2004). Delays of retention, processing efficiency, and attentional resources in working memory span development. *J Memory Language* 51:644–657.

Gogtay N, Giedd JN, Lusk L, Hayashi KM, Greenstein D, Vaituzis AC, Nugent TF 3rd, Herman DH, Clasen LS, Toga AW, Rapoport JL, Thompson PM (2004). Dynamic mapping of human cortical development during childhood through early adulthood. *Proc Natl Acad Sci U S A* 202:8174–8179.

Goldman-Rakic PS (1987). Circuitry of primate prefrontal cortex and regulation of behavior by representational memory. In: Handbook of Physiology. The Nervous System. Higher Functions of the Brain. Bethesda, MD: American Physiological Society, pp. 373–417.

Heilman KM, Van Den Abell T (1980). Right hemisphere dominance for attention: the mechanism underlying hemispheric asymmetries of inattention (neglect). *Neurology* 30(3):327–330.

Hernandez MT, Sauerwein HC, Jambaque I, De Guise E, Lussier F, Lortie A, et al. (2002). Deficits in executive functions andmotor coordination in children with frontal lobe epilepsy. *Neuropsychologia* 40:384–400.

Hillyard SA, Vogel EK, Luck SJ (1998). Sensory gain control (amplification) as a mechanism of selective attention: electrophysiological and neuroimaging evidence. *Phil Trans Royal Soc London Ser B Biol Sci* 353(1373):1257–1270.

Huttenlocher PR (1979). Synaptic density in human frontal cortex—developmental changes and effects of aging. *Brain Res* 163(2):195–205.

Huttenlocher PR, et al. (1982). Synaptogenesis in human visual cortex—evidence for synapse elimination during normal development. *Neurosci Letters* 33(3):247–252.

Jack AI, et al. (2006). Separate modulations of human V1 associated with spatial attention and task structure. *Neuron* 51(1):135–147.

Jacobs R, Anderson V (2002). Planning and problem solving skills following focal frontal brain lesions in childhood: Analysis using the Tower of London. *Child Neuropsychol* 8:93–106.

Jacobs R, Harvey AS, Anderson V. (2011) Are executive skills primarily mediated by the prefrontal cortex in childhood? *Examination of focal brain lesions in childhood. Cortex* 47(7):808–824.

Johnson MH (1996). From cortex to cognition: cognitive neuroscience studies of infant attention and perception. In Rovee-Collier C, Lipsitt LP (Eds.), Advances in Infancy Research. Stamford, CT: Ablex, pp. 161–217.

Johnson MH (2001). Functional brain development in humans. *Nature Rev Neurosci* 2(7): 475–483.

Johnson MH (2003). Development of human brain functions. *Biol Psychiatry* 54(12):1312–1336.

Johnson MH, Tucker L, Stiles J, Trauner D (1998). Visual attention in infants with perinatal brain damage: Evidence of the importance of anterior lesions. *Developmental Science* 1(1):53–58.

Jonides J, Nee DE (2006). Brain mechanisms of proactive interference in working memory. *Neuroscience* 139(1):181–193.

Just MA, Carpenter PA (1992). A capacity theory of comprehension: Individual differences in working memory. *Psychol Rev* 99:122–149.

Just MA, Carpenter PA (1999). A capacity theory for comprehension. *Psychol Rev* 99:122–149.

Kenner NM, Mumford JA, Hommer RE, Skup M, Leibenluft E, Poldrack RA (2010). Inhibitory motor control in response stopping and response switching. *J Neurosci* 30:8512–8518.

Kincade JM, Abrams RA, Astafiev SV, Shulman GL, Corbetta M (2005). An event-related functional magnetic resonance imaging study of voluntary and stimulus-driven orienting of attention. *J Neurosci* 25:4593–4604.

Klingberg T, Forssberg H, Westerberg H (2002). Increased brain activity in frontal and parietal cortex underlies the development of visuospatial working memory capacity during childhood. *J Cognitive Neurosci* 14(1):1–10.

Konrad K, et al. (2005). Development of attentional networks: an fMRI study with children and adults. *NeuroImage* 28(2):429–439.

Korkmaz B (2011). Theory of mind and neurodevelopmental disorders of childhood. *Pediatr Res* 69(5 Pt 2):101R–8R.

Kwon H, Reiss AL, Menon V (2002). Neural basis of protracted developmental changes in visuospatial working memory. *Proc Natl Acad Sci U S A* 99(20):13336–13341.

Laurent-Vannier A, Chevignard M, Pradat-Diehl P, Abada G, De Agostini M (2003). Spatial and motor neglect in children. *Neurology* 60(2):202–227.

Levin HS, Hanten G, Zhang L, Swank PR, Ewing-Cobbs L, Dennis M, et al. (2004). Changes in working memory after traumatic brain injury in children. *Neuropsychology* 18(2):240–247.

Luck SJ, Chelazzi L, Hillyard SA, Desimone R (1997). Neural mechanisms of spatial selective attention in areas V1, V2, and V4 of macaque visual cortex. *J Neurophysiol* 77(1):24–42.

Luna B (2009). Developmental changes in cognitive control through adolescence. *Advances in Child Development & Behavior* 9(37):233–278.

Macaluso E, Driver J, Frith CD (2003). Multimodal spatial representations engaged in human parietal cortex during both saccadic and manual spatial orienting. *Curr Biol* 13(12):990–999.

Macaluso E, Frith CD, Driver J (2002). Supramodal effects of covert spatial orienting triggered by visual or tactile events. *J Cognitive Neurosci* 14(3):389–401.

Mangun GR, Hillyard SA (1991). Modulations of sensory-evoked brain potentials indicate changes in perceptual processing during visual-spatial priming. *J Exp Psycho Hum Perception Performance* 17(4):1057–1074.

Martinez A, Anllo-Vento L, Sereno MI, Frank LR, Buxton RB, Dubowitz DJ, et al. (1999). Involvement of striate and extrastriate visual cortical areas in spatial attention. *Nature Neurosci* 2(4):364–369.

Martinez A, DiRusso F, Anllo-Vento L, Sereno MI, Buxton RB, Hillyard SA (2001). Putting spatial attention on the map: timing and localization of stimulus selection processes in striate and extrastriate visual areas. *Vision Res* 41(10–11):1437–1457.

Martínez A, Teder-Salejarvi W, Hillyard SA (2007). Spatial attention facilitates selection of illusory objects: evidence from event-related brain potentials. *Brain Res* 1139:143–152.

Martínez-Trujillo J, Treue S (2002). Attentional modulation strength in cortical area MT depends on stimulus contrast. *Neuron 18*;35(2):365–70.

Max JE, Bruce M, Keatley E, Delis D (2010). Pediatric stroke: plasticity, vulnerability, and age of lesion onset. *J Neuropsychiatry Clin Neurosci* 22(1):30–39.

Mayer AR, Harrington D, Adair JC, Lee R. (2006). The neural networks underlying endogenous auditory covert orienting and reorienting. *NeuroImage* 30(3):938–949.

McNab F, Klingberg T (2008) Prefrontal cortex and basal ganglia control access to working memory. *Nature Neurosci* 11:103–107.

Mesulam MM (1981). A cortical network for directed attention and unilateral neglect. *Ann Neurol* 10(4):309–325.

Miyake A, Friedman NP, Emerson MJ, Witzki AH, Howerter A, Wager TD (2000). The unity and diversity of executive functions and their contributions to complex "Frontal Lobe" tasks: a latent variable analysis. *Cognitive Psychol* 41(1):49–100.

Mohr HM, Goebel R, Linden DE (2006). Content- and task-specific dissociations of frontal activity during maintenance and manipulation in visual working memory. *J Neurosci* 26(17):4465–4471.

Mondor TA, Zatorre RJ (1995). Shifting and focusing auditory spatial attention. *J Exp Psychol Hum Percept Perform* 21(2):387–409.

Nagy Z, Westerberg H, Klingberg T (2004). Maturation of white matter is associated with the development of cognitive functions during childhood. *J Cogn Neurosci* 16(7):1227–1233.

Newman SD, Just MA, Carpenter PA (2002). The synchronization of the human cortical working memory network. *Neuroimage* 15(4):810–22.

Nichols S, Jones W, Roman MJ, Wulfeck B, Delis DC, Reilly J, Bellugi U (2004). Mechanisms of verbal memory impairment in four neurodevelopmental disorders. *Brain Lang* 88(2):180–9.

Nobre AC, Sebestyen GN, Gitelman DR, Mesulam MM, Frackowiak RS, Frith CD (1997). Functional localization of the system for visuospatial attention using positron emission tomography. *Brain* 120(Pt 3)(2):515–533.

Oakes LM, Hurley KB, Ross-Sheehy S, Luck SJ (2010). Developmental changes in infants' visual short-term memory for location. *Cognition* Dec 17. [Epub ahead of print]

Oakes LM, Messenger IM, Ross-Sheehy S, Luck SJ (2009). New evidence for rapid development of color-location binding in infants' visual short-term memory. *Vis Cogn* 17(1–2):67–82.

Olesen PJ, Macoveanu J, Tegner J, Klingberg T. (2007). Brain activity related to working memory and distraction in children and adults. *Cereb Cortex* 17(5):1047–1054.

Olesen PJ, Nagy Z, Westerberg H, Klingberg T (2003). Combined analysis of DTI and fMRI data reveals a joint maturation of white and grey matter in a fronto-parietal network. *Brain Res Cogn Brain Res* 18(1):48–57.

Owen AM, McMillan KM, Laird AR, Bullmore E (2005). N-back working memory paradigm: a meta-analysis of normative functional neuroimaging studies. *Hum Brain Mapping* 25(1): 46–59.

Pasto L, Burack JA (1997). A developmental study of visual attention: issues of filtering efficiency and focus. *Cogn Developmental Neuropsychol* 12(4):427–439.

Paus T, Collins DL, Evans AC, Leonard G, Pike B, Zijdenbos A (2001). Maturation of white matter in the human brain: a review of magnetic resonance studies. *Brain Res Bull* 54(3):255–266.

Pennington BF (1994). The working memory function of the prefrontal cortices: Implications for development and individual differences in cognition. In Haith MM, Benson JB, Roberts RJ, Pennington BF (Eds.), The Development of Future-Oriented Processes. Chicago: University of Chicago Press, pp. 243–289.

Pennington BF, Bennetto L, McAleer O, Roberts RJJ (1996). Executive functions and working memory: Theoretical and measurement issues. In Lyon GR, Krasnegor NA (Eds.), Attention, Memory, and Executive Function. Baltimore: Paul H. Brookes Publishing Co., pp. 327–348.

Petersen SE, Corbetta M, Miezin FM, Shulman GL (1994). PET studies of parietal involvement in spatial attention: comparison of different task types. *Can J Exp Psychol* 48(2):319–38

Petersen SE, Robinson DL, Currie JN (1989). Influences of lesions of parietal cortex on visual spatial attention in humans. *Exp Brain Res* 76(2):267–280.

Posner MI, Rothbart MK (1998). Attention, self-regulation and consciousness. *Philos Trans R Soc Lond B Biol Sci*. 29;353(1377):1915–27

Posner MI, Snyder CR, Davidson BJ (1980). Attention and the detection of signals. *J Exp Psychol* 109(2):160–174.

Posner MI, Walker JA, Friedrich FJ, Rafal RD (1984). Effects of parietal injury on covert orienting of attention. *J Neurosci* 4(7):1863–1874.

Posner MI, Walker JA, Friedrich FA, Rafal RD (1987). How do the parietal lobes direct covert attention? *Neuropsychologia* 25(1A):135–145.

Posner MI, et al. (1988). The development of orienting to locations and objects. In Wright RD (Ed.), Visual Attention. Oxford: Oxford University Press, pp. 269–288.

Postle BR, Awh E, Jonides J, Smith EE, D'Esposito M (2004). The where and how of attention-based rehearsal in spatial working memory. *Brain Res Cogn Brain Res* 20(2):194–205.

Powell KB, Voeller KKS (2004). Prefrontal executive function syndromes in children. *J Child Neurol* 19(10):785–797.

Reid VM, Striano T, Kaufman J, Johnson MH (2004). Eye gaze cueing facilitates neural processing of objects in 4-month-old infants. *Neuroreport* 15;15(16):2553–5.

Rhodes G (1987). Auditory attention and the representation of spatial information. *Perception and Psychophysics* 42:1–14.

Ridderinkhof KR, van der Stelt O (2000). Attention and selection in the growing child: views derived from developmental psychophysiology. *Biol Psychol* 54(1–3):55–106.

Roberts, KL, Hall DA (2008). Examining a supramodal network for conflict processing: a systematic review and novel functional magnetic resonance imaging data for related visual and auditory Stroop tasks. *J. Cogn. Neurosci.* 20:1063–1078.

Roberts RJ Jr, Pennington BR (1996). Special executive functions in children. *Developmental Neuropsychology* 12(1):105–126.

Ross-Sheehy S, Oakes LM, Luck SJ (2003). The development of visual short-term memory capacity in infants. *Child Dev* 74(6):1807–1822.

Rubia K, Smith AB, Woolley J, Nosarti C, Heyman I, Taylor E, Brammer M (2006). Progressive increase of frontostriatal brain activation from childhood to adulthood during event-related tasks of cognitive control. *Hum Brain Mapping* 27(12):973–993.

Schmithorst VJ, Wilke M, Dardzinski BJ, Holland SK (2002). Correlation of white matter diffusivity and anisotropy with age during childhood and adolescence: a cross-sectional diffusion-tensor MR imaging study. *Radiology* 222(1):212–228.

Schmithorst VJ, Wilke M, Dardzinski BJ, Holland SK (2005). Cognitive functions correlate with white matter architecture in a normal pediatric population: a diffusion tensor MRI study. *Hum Brain Mapping* 26(2):139–147.

Schmitt M, Postma A, De Haan E (2000). Interactions between exogenous auditory and visual spatial attention. *Q J Exp Psychol A* 53(1):105–130.

Schul R, Townsend J, Stiles J (2003). Development of attention orienting during the school-age years. *Developmental Sci* 6(3):262–272.

Shomstein S, Yantis S. (2004). Control of attention shifts between vision and audition in human cortex. *J Neurosci* 24(47):10702–10706.

Sowell ER, Trauner DA, Gamst A, Jernigan TL. (2002). Development of cortical and subcortical brain structures in childhood and adolescence: a structural MRI study. *Dev Med Child Neurol* 44(1):4–16.

Spence CJ, Driver J (1994). Covert spatial orienting in audition: Exogenous and endogenous mechanisms. *J Exp Psychol Perception Performance* 20:555–574.

Strauss E, Sherman E, Spreen O (2006). A Compendium of Neuropsychological Tests: Administration, Norms, and Commentary (3rd ed.). New York: Oxford University Press.

Talib TL, Pongonis SJ, Williams LS, Garg BP, Sokol DK, Saha C, Golomb MR (2008). Neuropsychologic outcomes in a case series of twins discordant for perinatal stroke. *Pediatr Neurol* 38:118–125.

Tamnes CK, Østby Y, Walhovd KB, Westlye LT, Due-Tønnessen P, Fjell AM (2010a). Neuroanatomical correlates of executive functions in children and adolescents: a magnetic resonance imaging (MRI) study of cortical thickness. *Neuropsychologia* 48(9):2496–2508.

Thiel CM, Zilles K, Fink GR (2004). Cerebral correlates of alerting, orienting and reorienting of visuospatial attention: an event-related fMRI study. *NeuroImage* 21(1):318–328.

Thomas KM, King SW, Franzen PL, Welsh TF, Berkowitz AL, Noll DC, et al. (1999). A developmental functional MRI study of spatial working memory. *NeuroImage* 10(3 Pt 1):327–338.

Toga AW, Thompson PM, Sowell ER (2006). Mapping brain maturation. *Trends Neurosci* 29(3):148–159.

Townsend J, Haist F, Adamo M, Stiles J (2003). Developmental changes in the brain substrate for spatial attention [Abstract]. Society for Neuroscience Abstracts.

Towse JN, Hitch GJ (1995). Is there a relationship between task demand and storage space in tests of working memory capacity? *Q J Exp Psychol A* 48:108–124.

Trauner DA (2003). Hemispatial neglect in young children with early unilateral brain damage. *Dev Med Child Neurol* 45(3):160–166.

Trauner DA, Nass R, Ballantyne AO (2001). Behavioral profiles of children and adolescents after pre- or peri-natal stroke. *Brain* 124:995–1002.

Tuch DS, Salat DH, Wisco JJ, Zaleta AK, Hevelone ND, Rosas HD (2005). Choice reaction time performance correlates with diffusion anisotropy in white matter pathways supporting visuospatial attention. *Proc Natl Acad Sci U S A* 102(34):1212–1227.

Westmacott R, Askalan R, MacGregor D, Anderson P, Deveber G (2010). Cognitive outcome following unilateral arterial ischaemic stroke in childhood: effects of age at stroke and lesion location. *Dev Med Child Neurol* 52(4):386–393.

Womelsdorf T, Anton-Erxleben K, Pieper F, Treue S (2006). Dynamic shifts of visual receptive fields in cortical area MT by spatial attention. *Nat Neurosci* 9(9):1156–1160.

Xue G, Aron AR, Poldrack RA (2008). Common neural substrates for inhibition of spoken and manual responses. *Cerebral Cortex* 18:1923–1932.

7

Early Communicative Development to First Words

AS ADULTS, WE consider language to be our principal communicative system, and other communicative behaviors (e.g., gesture and emotional facial expression) are viewed as supplementary. This is not the case for infants. Long before infants utter their first words, they are effective communicators: they can initiate and maintain an interaction, they can request a desired object, and they can vociferously disagree with a proposal (as in refusing to take the suggested nap). To successfully interact and communicate, infants and toddlers recruit a diverse repertoire of non-linguistic communicative behaviors; these include gestures, eye gaze, vocalizations, facial expression, as well as locomotion.

From a theoretical perspective, it was the writings of Piaget and Vygotsky that inspired the studies of these behavioral precursors to language. Following Piaget's proposal of common sensorimotor bases for language and non-linguistic symbols, as in gesture and symbolic play, an impressive body of literature has developed concerning the relations between gesture and language development in typical development (Bates, 1976; Oster, 1978; Oszcaliskan & Goldin Meadow, 2005; Volterra, Caselli, Capirci, & Pizzuto, 2005). And these studies have found consistent relations between a child's pre-linguistic gesturing and his or her later lexical development.

Whereas Piaget focused primarily on the child's cognitive development (in this case the development of language as a symbolic system), Vygotsky proposed a social-constructivist perspective in which learning is socially mediated and occurs in a social context. Thus, with the introduction of Vygotsky's ideas to the Western developmental community, the question of precursors to language broadened to encompass social aspects of early communicative interaction (Bruner, 1975; Snow, 1972). These studies began to investigate the structure of interactions between infant and adults and how they change with age. They also began to document the role of the parent or adult in the child's communicative development.

Given the tight relations between pre-linguistic communicative behaviors (e.g., gesture) and early language, and the importance of social interaction for language development, this chapter includes a discussion of the early communicative precursors to language as well as the comprehension and production of first words. The first section includes a brief overview of these behaviors in typical development; this section is followed by a discussion of the neural substrates for these abilities in adults and the nascent literature on how these neural structures develop in children. The last and largest section of this chapter is devoted to studies on early communicative development and the onset of language—that is, comprehension and production of first words—in children with perinatal stroke.

EARLY COMMUNICATIVE DEVELOPMENT IN TYPICALLY DEVELOPING INFANTS AND TODDLERS

In *The First Relationship* (1977) Stern characterizes the behavioral "dance" of mothers and their infants as they negotiate early interactions. For example, he describes the particular intonation contours and raised brows that mothers use to invite an infant to play and the steady gaze and the relaxed open-handed pose of the infant, signaling a readiness to engage. In the ensuing 35 years, much has been written on the development of the component skills necessary for successful social interactions, with particular attention to their role in the emergence of language and its subsequent development. The following is an overview of the early development of facial expression, vocalizations and babbling, and gesture in typical development, the infant's early tools for social interaction.

THE EMERGENCE AND USE OF EMOTIONAL FACIAL EXPRESSION

In the early 1970s, cross-cultural research by Paul Ekman (1972) and Carol Izard (1971) on the universality of specific emotional facial expressions (joy, sadness, surprise, disgust, anger, and fear) inspired a raft of studies on the emergence and development of facial expression in infants. Although newborns can and do contract various muscles required to produce emotional facial expressions (Oster, 1978), these early expressions appear to be endogenous—that is, produced in response to some internal stimulus. For example, when a newborn is sleeping, a variety of expressions flit across his or her face. Whereas these expressions have similar configurations to later-emerging emotional expressions (e.g., a smile or frown), it is not clear that these early facial behaviors are associated with an emotional "feeling." However, newborns will broadly imitate facial gestures (Meltzoff & Moore, 1977) and respond to different tastes with specific facial behaviors, such as pursing the lips in response to citric acid (Steiner, 1973). At about 6 weeks infants widen their eyes and fixate on the parent's face, and parents respond to their infants' direct gaze with comments such as, "My baby knows me!" Soon thereafter, the first social smile appears (smiles in response to others' smiles and to other people). Combined, the direct eye contact and smile represent a powerful tool for social interaction. By 3 to 4 months babies can use smiles and cries instrumentally—that is, they can use these behaviors to effect their goals. For example, 4- and 5-month-olds frequently smile to elicit a smile or comment from a caregiver, and they also cry to solicit a response from a caregiver in another room. Beginning at about 7 months, infants respond with a canonical angry face to frustrating situations (e.g., having a cookie removed from their hand; Stenberg & Campos, 1990) and several months later also show surprise (widened eyes and raised brows) at incongruities, such as a giraffe disappearing behind a screen, apparently to emerge as an elephant (Gratch, 1982). In sum, before the child's first words, he or she has access to a number of communicative tools and is an effective emotional communicator.

Little work has been conducted on the spontaneous use of facial expression in interactions after infancy. The few studies that exist show that adults use facial expression when reporting others' emotions or when recounting a story and taking on one of the character's roles (Bavelas & Chovil, 1997). Specifically, Bavelas and Chovil's work has shown that adults use an angry facial expression when telling about an event that angered them, or recounting a story in which a character is angry. In both cases, the use of facial expression enhances the storytelling. Ekman (Ekman, 1979) has also shown that people often furrow their brows when they ask questions. With respect to adult–child interactions, parents talking to infants and toddlers frequently recruit facial expressions to gain and maintain the infant's attention (Stern, 1977).

In a study of preschool and school-age children engaged in spontaneous interactions, preschoolers produce canonical emotional facial expressions (e.g., smiles for pleasure, raised brows for surprise, and furrowed brows for anger, puzzlement, or frustration; Reilly, Salamanca, Meza, Littlewort, & Barlett, in preparation). Reilly et al. also investigated how children integrate emotion and language by looking at how they use facial expression when they are speaking. They found that when the children (ages 3–4 and 7–8) are talking about personal events, they use facial expression about 45% of the time (55% of the time their faces were neutral), and when recounting positive stories, the expressions they use are overwhelmingly positive (i.e., smiles). Similarly, when 3- and 4-year-olds recount a negative experience, they show distress (anger, fear, or sadness). Overall, their facial expression is congruent with the emotional valence (positive/negative) of their language. In contrast, when older children (ages 7–8 years) recount a negative event, they are more likely to use a positive rather than a negative facial expression (i.e., incongruent with the content of the story). Different cultures have different social conventions for expressing emotions (so-called "display rules"), and these data suggest that by ages 7 to 8 years, children begin to acquire display rules, and they begin to "mask" their emotions. Such masking suggests the development of cognitive control for emotion (see Chapter 6) and the emergence of top-down processing of emotional expression. It should also be noted that there is significant variability in how often individual children use facial expressions in spontaneous interaction: some children produce very few expressions and others are very expressive.

With respect to perception and discrimination of facial expressions, infant studies from the 1970s and the early 1980s appeared to support the early differentiation of specific facial configurations. In fact, some early habituation studies from the 1970s and 1980s showed that infants as young as 3 months discriminated adults' expressions of happiness, anger, fear, surprise, sadness, and disgust (Barrera & Maurer, 1981; Hyson & Izard, 1985; Labarbera, Izard, Vietze, & Parisi, 1976; Young-Browne, Rosenfeld, & Horowitz, 1977). These studies suggested that very early in life, infants could discriminate a wide range of the basic emotions.

However, more recent studies have called these findings into question. After careful evaluation, they have shown that early discrimination abilities are limited. In fact, most studies suggest only a rudimentary distinction between positive and negative emotion through much of the first year, with a protracted period of refinement, particularly of negative affective categories (see Nelson, 1987, for a discussion). For example, it is not until 6 to 7 months that infants can discriminate negative and positive facial expressions (Caron, Caron, & Myers, 1982; Ludemann & Nelson, 1988; Nelson, 1987). And at 10 months they were still not discriminating non-prototypical positive and negative expressions—for example, a closed-mouth smile without the accompanying "eye crinkle." The picture that emerges is that infants are first able to make positive/negative distinctions: discrimination abilities for happy versus negative emotions are in place early on, whereas discrimination of different negative emotions emerges slowly and extends well into the school years (De Sonneville et al., 2002; Herba & Phillips, 2004; Vicari, Albertoni, et al., 2000; Vicari, Reilly, et al., 2000). For example, in a careful study of facial recognition using various intensities of expressions, Gao and Maurer (2010) report that by age 5, children's responses to happy faces are comparable to adults'; however, sensitivity to surprise, disgust, and fear continues to improve until age 10, and recognizing the subtleties of sad and angry expressions continues to develop well into adolescence.

VOCALIZATIONS

Although most healthy newborns greet the world with a lusty cry, these are not thought to be social-affective vocalizations. Rather, these first cries are in response to endogenous cues, and they signal the initial functioning of the respiratory system. However, young infants also produce positive vocalizations, such as gurgling and cooing, in the first few months of life, and these are responsive to affective vocalizations. In his seminal work *A First Language*, Roger Brown (1973) noted that affective expression played an important role in adults' talk to infants and toddlers (dubbed "motherese"). Subsequent studies of "motherese" and child-directed speech (CDS) have shown that the contours of motherese consistently reflect meaningful affective patterns, such as approval or prohibition (Fernald, 1990, 1993); moreover, infants as young as 4 months of age respond accordingly (Fernald, 1993). Such affective vocalizations constitute another channel of meaningful social interaction for the infant and adult to add to the repertoire of communicative tools.

Significantly more attention has been devoted to prosody and vocalizations as precursors to speech than to affective vocalizations. Given that speech is a continuous stream of sound, one of the infant's first tasks in language learning is to parse the ongoing speech stream—that is, to discover the boundaries of phrases and words. Studies by Jusczyk (1997) and Morgan (1996) have shown that infants use prosodic cues to segment the speech stream into both word and phrasal units using pitch, stress, and syllable length.

Every language has both consonants and vowels, and infants must learn those that are meaningful in their language. With respect to vocal production, babies coo at about 3 months; these are positive vocalic sounds (without consonants). The first consonants appear in canonical babbling that emerges between 6 and 8 months in typically developing children. Canonical babbling entails the repeated production of consonant–vowel syllables (CVCV) such as *baba* and *mama* (Oller et al., 2010). Babbling may occur as "language play" in the crib when the child is alone and talking to himself or herself (e.g., Weir, 1962). It also may constitute a turn in an interactive sequence, as when the mother holds out a toy and says, "Look at this!" and the baby says, "dada" as he or she reaches for it. In this instance, along with the reaching, the utterance "dada" represents the infant's turn in the interaction. Some researchers have found that rhythmic hand clapping or banging is associated with babbling and typically emerges during the same time frame as canonical babbling (Locke, Bekken, McMinn-Larson, & Wein, 1995; Iverson, 2010), suggesting that the emergence of babbling is indicative of a more global development of fine motor coordination. Delays of 2 to 3 months in canonical babbling as well as in rhythmic motor movements have been associated with language and speech delays later in development (Oller et al., 2010). In addition, the quality of babbling can be critical; deficits or anomalies in the syllabic quality of canonical babbling have been associated with later-developing autism (Oller et al., 2010).

Gesture

Adults gesture as they speak, and these co-speech gestures that are temporally integrated with speech often supplement the meaning of the linguistic message (McNeill, 1992). In contrast, babies use gestures as a primary means to communicate well before they talk. Moreover, these early gestures, unlike co-speech gestures, are the primary communicative message itself. The child's first gestures emerge at about 6 to 8 months of age and are those that are embedded in the action itself—for example, a child lifting her hands to be picked up, or holding out a hand to receive a treat. At about 8 to 10 months of age, deictic gestures (e.g., pointing, reaching for a desired object, showing) begin to occur frequently. And at about 12 months of age, researchers have identified symbolic or recognitory gesture use (e.g., picking up a block and using it as a telephone). Such use of recognitory or symbolic gestures has been described as a type of categorization and non-linguistic "naming" (see Bates & Dick, 2002, for a review; Goldin-Meadow & Iverson, 2010).

Studies show that recognitory gestures, which are sometimes referred to as iconic gestures because of their resemblance to features or actions of objects (e.g., flapping arms to indicate a bird) for some children, precede their use of words. Goodwyn and Acredolo (1988) compared the age of onset of these gestures to the age of onset of words and found that 9 of 22 children used these gestures prior to words, whereas the other 13 used these gestures and words at the same time. Importantly, no child used words prior to using recognitory gestures. Similarly, the use of deictic gestures not only precedes vocabulary development but also predicts vocabulary production and comprehension (Goldin-Meadow & Butcher, 2003; Iverson & Goldin-Meadow, 2005; O'Reilly, Painter, & Bornstein, 1997; Rowe, Özçaliskan, & Goldin-Meadow, 2008). Broadly, early deictic gestures are correlated with later word comprehension (Rowe et al., 2008), while the emergence of recognitory gestures is associated with the production of first words (e.g. Bates, 1979; Thal & Bates, 1988). Further, between 13 and 20 months there is a positive correlation between the number of recognitory gestures and the number of object names the child produces (Laudanna, Caselli, & Volterra, 1983). It has also been found that early parent gesture predicts child gesture. A recent study (Rowe & Goldin-Meadow, 2009) shows that socioeconomic status (SES) differences in vocabulary at 4.5 years of age can be explained by differences in earlier parental gesture use. A mediation analysis shows that the relation between early parent gesture and later child PPVT (Peabody Picture Vocabulary; Dunn & Dunn, 1981) scores is mediated by early child gesture. Thus, SES variations in parent gesture when the child is 14 months old predict differences in child gesture at 14 months, which in turn predicts vocabulary differences at age 4.5, even controlling for differences in child vocabulary at 14 months (Rowe et al., 2009).

Studies of clinical populations also report a relation between early gesture and language. For example, children with specific language impairment also have gesture deficits (Hill, Bishop, & Nimmo-Smith, 1998). Further, Thal and Tobias (1992) observed the late talkers (children below the tenth percentile for productive vocabulary at 20 months of age) from the Thal and Bates (1988) study at a 1-year follow-up. About 60% of the late talkers had caught up to typical peers within about a year and they were considered to be "late bloomers," while the remaining children had persistent language problems. In comparing early communicative gesture production in the two subgroups of late talkers, Thal and Tobias found that the "late bloomers," late talkers whose language had normalized at the 1-year follow-up, had used more communicative gesture at the earlier observation than those late talkers whose language deficits persisted at the 1-year follow-up. As is discussed below, the same relation holds true for the gesture and language development of children with perinatal lesions (PL).

FIRST WORDS: COMPREHENSION AND PRODUCTION

The first signs of language comprehension occur in social interactions at about 8 to 10 months of age. For example, the child turns and looks when his or her name is called or searches for the dog when someone asks, "Where's the dog?" The use of deictic gestures (e.g., points) appears to co-occur with the first indications of word comprehension. The child's receptive vocabulary continues to expand for several months before first words are produced. In fact, throughout language development, comprehension precedes and exceeds production in typically developing children. It is not until about 12 to 16 months, when children are thought to discover reference (i.e., that objects have names), that they begin to systematically produce words to label and request objects; these single-word utterances are often accompanied by deictic gestures (e.g., pointing, showing). For the next several months, productive vocabulary grows slowly and comprehension advances more rapidly. Thus, mean productive vocabulary size at 16 months is 31 words for girls and 20 words for boys (Fenson et al., 1993). In contrast, the 50th percentile of comprehension at 16 months is 143 words for boys and 191 words for girls. At about 16 to 20 months, researchers have noted a vocabulary burst in many different languages (Bleses et al., 2008a; Caselli et al., 1995) such that the number of productive words grows exponentially. Moreover, vocabulary composition changes to include more verbs and adjectives, in addition to the earlier-emerging nouns and names. Figure 7.1 (Fenson et al., 1993) shows the growth of productive vocabulary in typically developing children from age 8 to 30 months. The study included more than 1,200 typically developing children from three geographic regions of the United States and used the MacArthur Bates Communicative Developmental Inventory (MBCDI), a parental report instrument (1993).

Although there is a clear developmental increase in the number of words produced over the 8- to 30-month period, it is important to note the wide variability in these early stages of language development in typically developing children: whereas 24-month-old children at the 50th percentile have vocabularies of 297 words, those at the 75th percentile have 441, and those at the 25th percentile have only 156. The MBCDI has now been adapted into more than 60 different languages; what is impressive is that the growth profile for productive vocabulary is virtually identical across the languages, although the timing may vary by as much as several months (Bleses et al., 2008b).

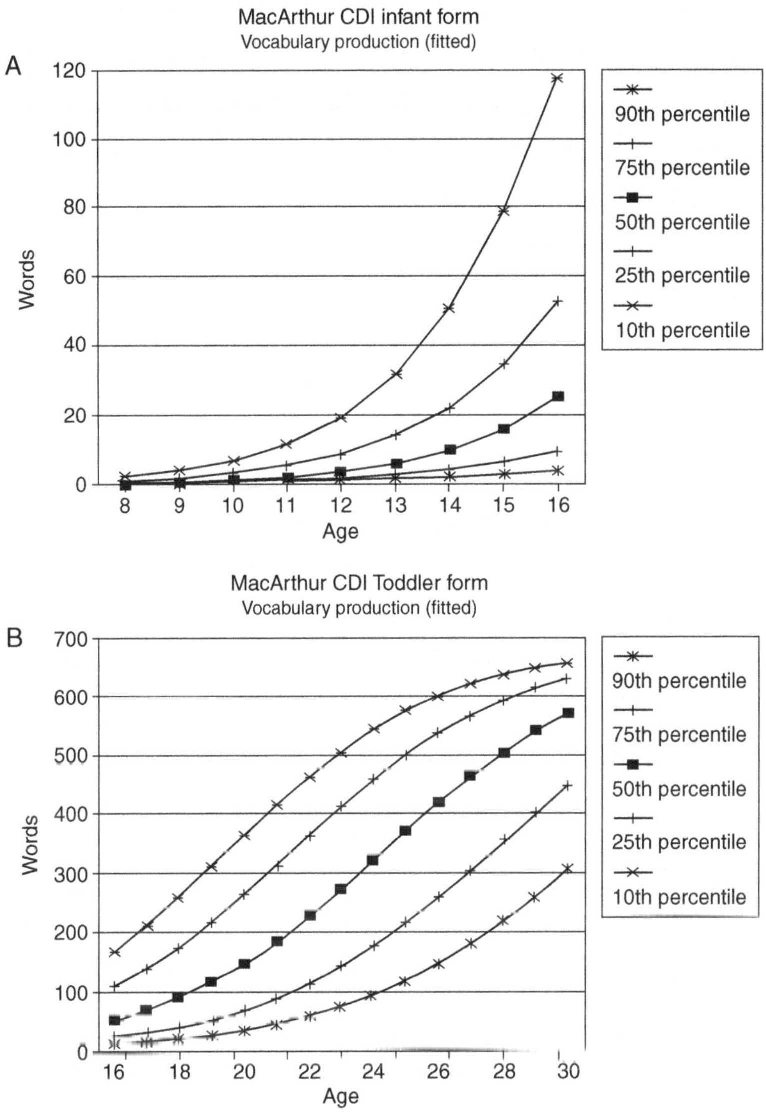

FIGURE 7.1 Productive vocabulary of typically developing infants and toddlers from the English MacArthur Communicative Inventory (CDI). Figures show the median, 25th, and 75th as well as the 10th and 90th percentiles for children at each month of age. (A) Children's productive vocabulary from 8 to 16 months of age. This period includes the onset of first words and a slow increase in total productive vocabulary. As children's vocabulary grows, individual variability also increases. (B) Vocabulary growth from 16 to 30 months of age. (Reprinted with permission from Fenson et al., 1993.)

NEURAL SUBSTRATES FOR NON-LINGUISTIC COMMUNICATION AND FIRST WORDS

With this broad outline of typical social communicative development and the emergence of first words, the following section considers the neural underpinnings for these component skills. This section begins with an overview of what is known about the neural systems for processing affect and gesture in adults. For facial affect, the discussion includes both studies on recognition and production of emotional facial expressions. Understanding the adult neural architecture is important, as it provides a context and endpoint to evaluate the developmental data. The discussion then turns to a consideration of the development of the neural systems for these communicative behavioral systems, and the last section presents the neural substrates of language. While comparatively little developmental work has been done on these issues, the small available body of data provides a guide for considering the effects of early injury on the developing neural systems for affective, communicative, and linguistic processing.

NEURAL UNDERPINNINGS OF NON-LINGUISTIC COMMUNICATION IN ADULTS

Neural Bases of Facial Affect Processing in Adults

Understanding the neural underpinnings of emotion processing in adults is relevant to developmental investigations as these underpinnings provide information about the endpoint of brain organization. The study of the neural correlates of facial affect processing in adults has been an active area of investigation within cognitive neuroscience for many decades and has yielded important information (Barton, 2003; Posamentier & Abdi, 2003) (see Chapter 5 for a more comprehensive discussion). Studies of adults with brain lesions resulting in impaired face processing abilities, known as prosopagnosia, established an important role for the right hemisphere across a range of face processing tasks (De Renzi & Perani, 1994; Stone & Valentine, 2003). Further, the models that arose from these studies posited dissociations between processing the identity of a face and other aspects of face processing, such as labeling and recognizing facial affect (Bruce & Young, 1986). These models suggest that independent brain systems are responsible for various aspects of face processing. Studies of both healthy adults and stroke patients, using both structural and functional neuroimaging, have largely confirmed this suggestion (Adolphs, 2001; Haxby et al., 2001). For example, many studies using functional imaging (PET and fMRI) have shown that face identification is linked to activity in the right fusiform gyrus region, the right posterior superior temporal sulcus, and possibly the right lateral frontal cortex (Adolphs, 2001; Haxby, Hoffman, & Gobbini, 2002). Right hemisphere fusiform gyrus activity is so ubiquitous in face identification tasks that some have dubbed this region the "fusiform face area" (FFA) (Grill-Spector, Knouf, & Kanwisher, 2004). Current debates in the field center on whether the FFA is a face-specific module (Kanwisher, 1997, 2000) or whether it is better characterized as a visual expertise area that is involved in the individuation of exemplars of any category for which one becomes an expert (Gauthier, Skudlarski, Gore, & Anderson, 2000; Haist, Lee, & Stiles, 2010; Haxby et al., 2001).

Beyond face identity processing, a distributed network of brain structures has been implicated in various aspects of emotional facial expression processing. For example, drawing on findings from both lesion studies and those of other clinical groups, Adolphs (2001) proposed a distributed and dynamic model of facial emotion recognition, which includes occiptotemporal cortices, the amygdala and orbitofrontal cortices, as well as the right frontoparietal cortices and basal ganglia. More recently, two meta-analyses of imaging studies of affect recognition (Fusar-Poli et al., 2009; Sabatinelli, Bradley, & Lang, 2001) have broadly confirmed such a network. Within such a model, right fusiform gyrus activity is associated with processing the static and invariant characteristics of the face (critical for face identity), and superior temporal sulcal and gyral activity is associated with processing movement or the changing aspects of facial expressions, including eye gaze (Haxby, Hoffman, & Gobbini, 2000; Haxby et al., 2002). The functional role of the latter regions in processing eye gaze may account for their reported activation while attending to facial emotion (Narumoto, Okadab, Sadatob, Fukuia, & Yonekurac, 2001), as the eyes serve as a highly salient cue for differentiating among specific emotional expressions. Further, many lesion and functional neuroimaging studies have found that the amygdala shows robust activation when the task involves evaluating emotional content or ambiguous stimuli, specifically in the context of evaluating facial affect. Patients with lesions to the amygdala show impaired recognition, especially to fear (Adolphs et al., 2005). Another study used function–lesion mapping to assess the regions involved in processing facial emotions; the study includes lesion maps from structural MRIs of 108 adults with focal brain lesions (Adolphs, Damasio, Tranel, Cooper, & Damasio, 2000). Findings showed regions in right hemisphere somatosensory cortex, anterior supramarginal gyrus, and insula to be critical components for the recognition of facial emotion, but not face identity. Moreover, additional analyses demonstrated that separate brain regions, including bilateral frontal lobe areas, superior temporal regions, and the left frontal operculum, were associated with labeling facial affect. Thus, in adults, partially separate brain systems appear to underlie the recognition and verbal labeling of emotional facial expression (Adolphs, Tranel, & Demasio, 2003). In summary, the preponderance of evidence from lesion and neuroimaging studies of adults suggests that the endpoint of development is marked by dynamic and distributed brain networks that make distinct contributions to face identity processing, facial affect recognition, and facial affect labeling. It is interesting to note a parallel in the developmental behavioral studies of facial expression recognition in typically developing children. Vicari et al. (2000) report partially dissociable trajectories for visual processing (discrimination/recognition) of facial expression and labeling of facial affect in school-age children.

In contrast to the extensive literature on emotion recognition, there are few recent studies examining the neural substrates mediating the production of facial expression. However, earlier clinical studies have documented "flattened" affect in adults with right hemisphere injury (Blonder, Burns, Bowers, Moore, & Heilman, 1993; Borod, 2000; Borod, Koff, Perlman Lorch, & Nicholas, 1985; Buck & Duffy, 1980). Consistent with these findings, a series of case studies of adolescents with presumed right hemisphere injury (Weintraub & Mesulam, 1983) reported that all 14 participants suffered social problems, specifically showing deficits in nonverbal communicative abilities. A study by Blonder et al. (2005) reported on a group of adult patients with right hemisphere focal injury with aprosodia (deficits in producing and understanding emotional prosody) compared to a group of patients with left hemisphere focal injury and aphasia. Consonant with earlier reports, those with right hemisphere injury smiled and laughed less frequently throughout the interview than those with left hemisphere injury, confirming a significant role for the right hemisphere in emotion expression as well as recognition.

Neural Underpinnings of Gesture in Adults

Most current research on the neural underpinnings of gesture has focused on adults and the use of pantomime or co-speech gesture—that is, gestures that accompany speech. Similar to the study of emotion, this research is important for gaining a developmental picture as it provides a description of the endpoint. This research may be pertinent in the study of the development of language, as recent research has shown that children's early pre-linguistic gestures precede and also predict the onset of language in typically developing children and in children with PL (Iverson & Goldin-Meadow, 2005; Sauer, Levine, & Goldin-Meadow, 2010). However, as noted above, pre-linguistic gestures often constitute the substance of a toddler's interaction; as such, they differ from adult gestures that accompany speech. For infants, gestures are the principal communicative message, unlike adults, for whom language is primary and gestures reinforce or supplement the linguistic content. As such, the adult imaging studies that investigate the neural underpinnings of co-speech gesture may not reflect the neural underpinnings of children's early pre-linguistic use of gesture.

Studies of adults with late-onset lesions have broadly supported the notion that gesture deficits after stroke follow a similar course to the patient's language deficits (e.g., McNeill & Pedelty, 1995). Consistent with the patient literature, more recent research using imaging techniques has focused on whether those brain regions that have long been associated with language processing—that is, the left inferior frontal gyrus (Broca's area) and the left superior temporal region (Wernicke's area)—are also activated in the processing of gestures, which could be considered the symbolic antecedents of language. Such a finding would be in line with the recent hypothesis dubbed "neural recycling" (Dehaene, 2005. See discussion of neural reuse theories, Chapter 11, this volume.), which suggests that new functional capacities are built on neural circuits that had subserved established and related functions. In fact, a recent fMRI study by Xu et al. (2009) compared activation patterns in response to two kinds of gestures (pantomimes that mimic actions, such as unscrewing the lid of a jar, and emblems that use gesture in culturally specific ways to convey a message, such as a finger to the lips to indicate "be quiet") to activation patterns in response to these same messages expressed in words. Findings showed nearly identical patterns of activation, consistent with the neural recycling hypothesis and the idea that the regions of the brain involved in language functions are more broadly specialized for interpreting symbolic messages.

Other studies have examined brain activation patterns for the interpretation of co-speech gestures. Although co-speech gesture is important in communicative interactions and contributes to language comprehension in children and adults (e.g., Kelly, Barr, Church, & Lynch, 1999; McNeill, 1992; McNeill, Alibali, & Evans, 2000), only a few studies have examined the brain regions involved in processing these gestures. Several studies have shown that the brain regions that activate in response to tasks involving action comprehension (e.g., premotor cortex, inferior parietal lobule [IPL], posterior superior temporal sulcus [STSp], and posterior superior temporal gyrus [STGp]) also activate more strongly when speech is accompanied by gesture than to speech alone (e.g., Holle, Gunter, Ruschemeyer, Hennelotter, & Iacoboni, 2008; Hubbard et al., 2009; Willems, Ozyurek, & Hagoort, 2007).

Other fMRI studies have examined the regions that are specifically involved in the integration of gesture and speech, but the results of these studies have been contradictory. For example, Willems et al. (2007) found that a portion of Broca's area (IFGTr), the pars triangularis, and the premotor cortex are more activated when a gesture is incompatible with a sentence (e.g., more activation when the word "wrote" in the sentence "He should not forget the items he wrote on the shopping list" is accompanied by the gesture for "hit" than when accompanied by the gesture for "wrote"). In contrast to Willems et al. (2007), Holle et al. (2008) reported no differential activation of the left IFG for an unrelated gesture. However, the unrelated gesture used in the Holle et al. study was a grooming gesture rather than an iconic gesture with a different semantic meaning, potentially explaining this discrepancy. Holle et al. also reported that the left STSp responds more to congruent iconic gestures than to unrelated grooming gestures. Although these studies are not in perfect agreement, they implicate specific regions of the left frontal lobe (IFG) and the temporal lobe bilaterally (STSp) in gesture–speech integration.

Following up on the findings of these studies, Dick, Goldin-Meadow, Hasson, Skipper, and Small (2009) specifically focused on the role of IFG and STSp in integrating gesture and speech. In this study, participants listened to a videotaped storyteller telling fables in four conditions: (a) accompanied by co-speech gestures that were mainly iconic and metaphoric in nature, (b) accompanied by non-gestural self-grooming hand movements, (c) accompanied by no gesture—the speaker's hands remained in her lap, and (d) no visual input—fables were presented in the auditory modality while the participant stared at a fixation cross. Dick et al. found more activation of STSp in conditions (a) and (b), both of which included hand movements, than in conditions (c) and (d), which did not include hand movements, implicating this region in processing biological motion (see also, e.g., Beauchamp, Lee, Haxby, & Martin, 2003; Bonda, Petrides, Ostry, & Evans, 1996; Puce & Perrett, 2003; Saygin, Wilxon, Hagler, Bates, & Sereno, 2004) but not a special role in processing gesture. Dick et al. (2009) also found that right IFG activated more in response to speech accompanied by self-grooming hand movements than to speech accompanied by co-speech gesture, whereas left IFG activated more to speech with gesture than in the condition with audio-only stories. There was also some hint, taking the signal-to-noise ratio into account, that left anterior IFG activated more in the gesture condition than in the self-grooming condition, which also involved hand movements. Thus, this study provides some evidence that STSp plays a role in processing hand movements, with no differential role for gesture, and that left and right IFG play differential roles in integrating speech and gesture, with left IFG activating more for co-speech gestures and right IFG activating more for self-grooming hand movements.

Skipper et al. (Skipper, Goldin-Meadow, Nusbaum, & Small, 2009) used the same story stimuli described above to identify the network of brain regions involved in processing language accompanied with co-speech gesture compared to the processing of language where the listener has access to the speaker's facial movements but where there are no hand movements. Using structural equation modeling, the researchers found different patterns of connection weights in the gesture and no-gesture conditions, suggesting that the networks supporting narrative comprehension vary dynamically depending on the kinds of information that are available to the listener—only speech versus speech and the face of the speaker versus speech, the face of the speaker, and co-speech gestures. Interestingly, Skipper et al.'s model indicates that the connection strengths of Broca's area to other cortical areas involved in language processing are weakest in the gesture condition, consistent with the possibility that semantic selection and retrieval demands are reduced by the information provided by co-speech gesture (Skipper, Goldin-Meadow, Nusbaum, & Small, 2007). This model may help explain some of the discrepancies in the studies described above. For example, grooming gestures might not help or hurt semantic selection and retrieval whereas co-speech gestures that are consistent with the spoken message might help with these demands, and co-speech gestures that are inconsistent with the spoken message might disrupt or slow down semantic selection and retrieval.

As research on the integration of speech and gesture proceeds, more attention to the nature of the speech–gesture relationship may help elucidate contradictory findings and shed light on the roles of particular neural networks in processing the rich communicative information that characterizes human language interactions. For example, there are a variety of kinds of gesture—conventional, deictic, iconic, and metaphoric—and these gestures may serve to reinforce the message conveyed in speech or add information to what is conveyed in speech. Studies to date have mainly examined reinforcing gestures and compared them either to congruent or incongruent gesture–speech relations ("hit" gesture when "write" is spoken or to self-grooming hand movements). Differences in the kinds of co-speech gestures that are examined as well as the contrasting conditions may all have an impact on the brain regions involved. Moreover, existing work has focused on the neural networks involved in integrating speech and gesture in adults, at the endpoint of development, rather than in children. Imaging studies of typically developing children combined with the study of gesture–speech integration in children with PL will help to elucidate how gesture and speech are integrated over the course of development, and the brain mechanisms that support this integration.

NEURAL UNDERPINNINGS OF NON-LINGUISTIC COMMUNICATION IN CHILDREN

Relative to the available body of literature on the neural underpinnings of non-linguistic communication in adults, studies of development have been much more limited. There is a small literature on the development of the neural systems for facial processing, but virtually no research on early gestural processing. This section will review the small set of existing studies.

With respect to children and the development of neural systems for processing emotion, de Schonen and Mathivet (1989) have shown a right hemisphere bias for face processing as early as 4 months of age. Studies using event-related potentials (ERPs) have confirmed a dimensional account of emotion development and have provided brain-based evidence for the gradual differentiation of emotion categories. At 7 months of age, infants showed contrasting patterns of neural responsiveness for negative and positive emotions (Nelson & de Haan, 1997). However, differentiated neural responses for individual negative emotional expressions did not begin to emerge until after about 12 months of age (de Haan & Nelson, 1998; Nelson, 1993; Nelson & de Haan, 1996).

With respect to the development of the ability to recognize faces, a study (Taylor, Batty, & Itier, 2004) of 5- to 14-year-old children using ERP demonstrated that face recognition does not mirror adult patterns until well into adolescence. Specifically, in their review of cognitive electrophysiological (ERP) studies in children, adolescents, and adults using face identification paradigms, Taylor et al. concluded that while early sensory-perceptual brain waves (e.g., P100, a positive voltage inflection observed approximately 100 ms after stimulus presentation) are present in children as young as 4 years of age, protracted development is observed in later components known to be particularly sensitive to face identity processing (e.g., N170, a negative voltage inflection occurring approximately 170 ms after face stimulus onset). Indeed, the N170 component can only begin to be reliably detected in mid-childhood, around 8 years of age, with adult-like patterns not reliably observed until adolescence (Taylor et al., 2004). This pattern of electrophysiological response is consistent with behavioral findings showing that face recognition has a protracted developmental time course (see Chapter 5 for an extensive discussion). Similar developmental differences have been observed in studies examining emotion and the processing of emotional facial expressions (Batty & Taylor, 2006).

While neuroimaging holds promise for understanding the development of the neural networks supporting behavioral development, pediatric functional imaging studies of facial expression of emotion are few and have produced conflicting results. For example, an fMRI study reported by Thomas et al. (2001) found that children (mean age = 11) showed greater activation bilaterally in the amygdala in response to neutral face probes than to fear face probes, the converse of what they observed in their adult sample. In contrast, an fMRI study similar to Thomas et al.'s 2001 study (Monk, 2008; Monk et al., 2003) found that adolescents (mean age = 13 years) exhibited greater activity in the right amygdala to passively viewing faces with fear expressions than to neutral expressions. Such differences may be due to differences in methodology (e.g., using a block vs. event-related design). Interestingly, Monk et al. also found that adults showed greater recruitment than children of orbitofrontal cortex in response to fear faces when explicitly required to direct attention to the emotional attributes of the facial expressions. Such findings suggest a transition to increased reliance on frontal regions for the processing of emotion with development. In sum, whereas both the behavioral and neurophysiological data suggest that recognizing emotion is an extended developmental process, investigations of their neural underpinnings are just beginning.

NEURAL UNDERPINNINGS OF LANGUAGE

Neural Substrates for Language in Adults

Building on the work of Paul Broca and Carl Wernicke 160 years ago, numerous studies of adult stroke patients speaking a variety of languages (Goodglass, 1993; Menn & Obler, 1990; Poizner, Klima, & Bellugi, 1990) have confirmed their original findings: for right-handed, and many left-handed, adults, perisylvian regions of the left hemisphere mediate multiple aspects of language. Recent imaging studies of healthy adults have begun to reveal functional networks underlying language processing with different aspects of language recruiting distinct neural systems (Binder, Desai, Graves, & Conant, 2009; Bookheimer, 2002; Brauer, Anwander, & Friederici, 2011; Hickok & Poeppel, 2007; Price, 2010). Since this chapter is focused on the initial stages of communication and language acquisition, the present discussion will be limited to adult and child studies for single words and their meanings. Once again, the adult profile is informative as it represents the developmental endpoint.

Distributed networks involving anterior and posterior regions of both hemispheres are involved in processing words and their underlying concepts. Numerous studies have found that the left inferior frontal gyrus (LIFG), especially anterior portions, plays a critical role in lexical processing and that concepts are organized in the temporal lobe according to broad categorical criteria (e.g., animacy). With respect to the role of the LIFG in lexico-semantic processing, Thompson-Schill et al. (1997, 1999) have proposed that anterior regions are implicated in retrieval, and Wagner et al. (2001) and Poldrack et al. (1999) have suggested that superior and posterior regions of the LIFG are recruited in lexical selection. These processes appear to be dissociated from content and modality. As such, one might conclude that the LIFG plays an integrative role in lexical selection and retrieval. In fact, numerous imaging studies (e.g., Brown et al., 2005) have now confirmed the earlier PET study by Petersen et al. (1988) demonstrating that the LIFG is critical in word production in adults. The common task known as verb generation entails the covert (or overt, see Brown et al., 2005) production of an associated verb when the participant hears or sees a noun. For example, given the word *dog*, one might silently produce *bark* or *fetch*. The verb generation paradigm has now been used successfully with a larger sample of adults as well as with children (e.g., Brown et al., 2005; Holland et al., 2001), as we will discuss below and in the following chapter.

Imaging studies examining semantics and the storage of conceptual information have found that a word's function plays a significant role in its storage and that this information is spatially distributed within the temporal lobe (for a review, see Bookheimer, 2002). For example, objects that are manipulable, such as a hammer or a screwdriver, activate intraparietal sulcus and ventral premotor cortex, areas that are associated with reaching/grasping and visual motion (Chao & Martin, 2000). In contrast, animals and other animate beings activate visual areas, suggesting that visual imagery plays a strong role in storing information about concepts and words. Together, such studies suggest that semantic information is stored based on both perceptual and functional information.

In contrast to the strong left hemisphere bias for generating words, prosody and intonation, as in the melodies that distinguish questions from statements (for example, "you're eating the last cookie" vs. "you're eating the last cookie?"), activate areas in the right hemisphere (Frederici & Alter, 2004; Jung-Beeman, 2005). Nonetheless, there is an ongoing debate regarding syntactic versus affective prosody (Pell, 2006; Wildgruber, Ackermann, Kreifelts, & Ethofer, 2006).

In sum, while we have learned a great deal about how the adult brain is organized for language, an outstanding question is how this end state develops. The following section begins a discussion of this topic.

The Neural Substrates of Language in Children

Jules Cotard, a colleague of Broca, made the following observation about language in children with early brain injury: "Intelligence may be normal when a hemisphere is destroyed during infancy... in these cases one never encounters aphasia" (Ritti, 1894). Moreover, from recent studies (Bates et al., 1997, 2001; Reilly, Bates, & Marchman, 1998; Reilly, Wasserman, & Appelbaum, submitted; Reilly & Wulfeck, 2004), as well as the earlier reports of

Alajouanine and Lhermitte (1965), Lenneberg (1967), and Basser (1962), it is clear that language deficits in children with unilateral brain injury, even those with left hemispherectomies, are much more subtle than those in their adult counterparts, who commonly experience persistent and debilitating aphasias. In line with such findings, Lenneberg (1967) proposed the notion of equipotentiality, that either hemisphere is capable of assuming language functions up until puberty. Such a position stood in stark contrast to a nativist view that posited that the left hemisphere was specialized for language from the start of life. However, the developmental data are mixed with regard to Lenneberg's proposal. Some studies provide evidence for an early left hemisphere advantage for speech sounds and single words. For example, an EEG study of premature newborns found a left hemisphere advantage for speech sounds (Molfese, 1980), and similar results come from an fMRI study of 3-month-olds (Dehaene-Lambertz et al., 2002). Furthermore, a recent magnetoencephalography (MEG) study (Travis et al., 2011) found that the semantic processes indexed by the adult N400 event-related component are already functional in 12- to 18-month-old toddlers; they also found that similar to adults, left fronto-temporal brain regions are recruited in a picture–word matching task. These results suggest that already by toddlerhood, single word comprehension/labeling activates left hemisphere regions. Others have used picture matching tasks in fMRI studies with older school-age children, and have also found left lateralization, in this case by age 7 (e.g., Gaillard et al., 2003). In contrast, ERP studies have revealed more distributed, bilateral patterns of activation in young children, findings more in line with Lenneberg's (1967) notion of initial hemispheric equipotentiality for language. For example, Mills, Coffey-Corina, and Neville (1997) report an ERP lexical study of toddlers and found early bilateral patterns of activation (at 13 months); left lateralization increased with age (20 months) and language learning. Specifically, those toddlers with larger vocabularies showed increased left hemisphere activity compared to age mates with smaller vocabularies. Consonant with Mills' findings, recent studies have tested verb and phoneme generation using fMRI and MEG. In large groups of typically developing children, ranging in age from 5 years through adolescence, researchers have shown no changes in the processing of phonemes. However, the activation for verb generation is initially bilateral, but lateralization to the left hemisphere increases with age (Brown et al., 2005; Holland et al., 2001; Ressel, Wilke, Lidzba, Lutzenberger, & Krageloh-Mann, 2008). It appears that lateralization for word production is indeed a developmental process. Just as different aspects of language are acquired over childhood and well into adolescence (Berman & Verhoeven, 2002; Reilly, Jisa, Baruch, & Berman, 2002; Reilly, Zamora, & McGivern, 2005), it appears that the development of the neural organization for these processes is also a protracted process.

COMMUNICATIVE DEVELOPMENT IN CHILDREN WITH PERINATAL STROKE

With a background of typical development as well as some notion of the neural substrates underlying both communicative skills and single word production in adults and typically developing children, we are now in a position to address how these behaviors develop in children with early brain injury. Such data will inform our understanding of both early brain development and the nature and extent of neural plasticity for these different communicative skills. In discussing these data, our presentation will be guided by the following questions:

1. Does the process of early communicative development and language learning in children with PL look similar to that of typically developing children?
2. And are the intermodal relations the same as in typically developing children (e.g., between gesture and speech)?
3. If there are deficits, how do they compare with those of adults with homologous lesions?
4. Do such deficits change with development?

AFFECTIVE EXPRESSION IN INFANTS AND TODDLERS WITH PERINATAL STROKE

In infant–maternal communication, eye contact and facial expression are critical tools for negotiating a successful interaction. To understand how the PL group uses facial expression, an early naturalistic study included infants from 6 to 22 months of age (Reilly, Stiles, Larsen, & Trauner, 1995). Mothers were instructed to "play with your baby as you do at home," and the mother–infant pairs were videotaped as they played on the floor. Reilly et al. used Ekman and Friesen's Facial Action Coding System (Ekman & Friesen, 1978) to measure facial expression, and they looked at the response of the baby to the mother's bids for attention. Though all the babies looked at their mothers, and all the babies smiled, the typically developing infants and those with left posterior injury smiled easily and frequently, whereas those with right posterior injury smiled much less often (Fig. 7.2). The proportions in the figure reflect the number of times the child smiled in response to his or her mother's bid for attention over all bids for attention in which the child was attending to the mother. Further, those with right PL produced proportionally more negative behaviors than controls or those children with left PL.

Longitudinal case studies were consistent with this profile; together these findings suggest that, similar to adults with late-onset strokes, the right hemisphere plays a critical role in the spontaneous production of emotional facial expression from the first year of life.

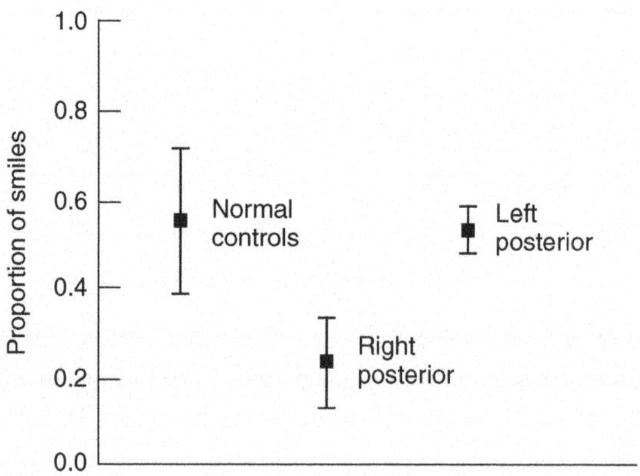

FIGURE 7.2 Proportions of smiles elicited in free play. (Reprinted with permission of the publisher from Reilly, Stiles, Larsen, & Trauner, 1995.)

Interestingly, for proportion of smiles, the children with left PL and right PL show less variability than the typically developing group. As predicted from the temperament literature (e.g., Kagan, Snidman, Arcus, & Reznick, 1994) in a group of 12 typically developing babies, there was marked heterogeneity in expressiveness, with some rather serious infants at the non-expressive extreme of the continuum (0.3) and some very smiley babies at the expressive extreme (0.8). In contrast to this wide variability, those in the PL group show more homogeneity. Although the sample was small (six children with right PL and six with left PL), their profiles with respect to positive emotional expression are strikingly clear, with the left PL group clustering tightly at the mean for controls and the right PL group falling at the low end and below the range of typically developing children.

To ascertain whether this profile is unique to facial expression or whether it reflects a broader deficit in emotional expression or a problem with visuospatial processing (see Chapter 5), a complementary study was conducted on children's pre-linguistic affective vocalizations (Reilly, Martinez, & Anderson, in preparation). Independent judges assessed the emotional quality of 2,200 vocalizations from a larger group of pre-linguistic infants with PL and typically developing infants ages 9 to 22 months. A similar profile emerged: typically developing infants and those with left PL vocalized often and 90% of their vocalizations were positive; those with right PL vocalized with comparable frequency, but produced a higher proportion of negative vocalizations and a lower proportion of positive vocalizations than either typically developing children or children with left hemisphere injury. A parental report study of temperament in the PL group shows a similar profile: infants and toddlers with right PL expressed more negativity than typically developing children or children with left PL (Nass & Koch, 1987). Together these studies suggest that the right hemisphere plays a critical role in the expression of positive emotion, both facial and vocal, from the middle of the first year of life, and that valence (i.e., positive or negative) is a significant parameter in the neural organization of emotion and temperament.

Whereas few adult studies have examined the expression of emotion in brain-injured patients in the context of naturalistic interactions, a set of studies by Blonder et al. (1991, 1993, 2005) has investigated nonverbal communicative behavior in adult stroke patients during the course of a structured interview (a comparable quasi-naturalistic setting). Her findings match those of the toddlers with PL: adults with right hemisphere injury use more negative expression than those with left hemisphere injury or non–brain-injured controls. The results from the Reilly et al. and Nass and Koch studies suggest that this aspect of brain organization is established early in life. An outstanding question concerns the plasticity of these functions when lesions occur early in development. For example, we currently do not know whether the emotional difficulties that were identified in pre-linguistic infants and toddlers with right hemisphere injury persist. Further, given the intrinsic relations between language and emotional expression, with the onset of language, how will emotional and linguistic expression be affected in this group?

An early experimental study of affective prosody in the PL group was conducted by Trauner et al. (1996). Using a battery to test comprehension, production, and imitation of both affective and linguistic prosody, they tested 31 participants with PL and control children (ages 5–20 years). To assess affective prosody, participants were asked to identify the affective tone of sentences that were neutral in content—for example, "That's a tomato" (in a sad voice); they were asked to discriminate sentences of differing or similar affective prosody; to imitate affective sentences; and to participate in a story completion task, speaking for a protagonist who displayed a certain emotion. The tasks to assess linguistic prosody were comparable and designed to measure both production and comprehension: an identification task (question vs. statement) and a discrimination task (subject vs. object stress and question vs. statement). For production, children were asked to imitate various stress patterns and to complete a story requiring different stress patterns. Children with right PL had difficulty with both affective and linguistic prosody, both receptively and productively. However, they performed similarly to controls in identifying vocal emotion and in spontaneously producing appropriate stress patterns. The performance of those with left PL matched controls for receptive affective prosody but fell below for affective productive measures; for linguistic prosody, they performed below controls for all measures except spontaneous production of stress patterns. Overall, the findings for the affective measures differ from comparable studies of adults with acquired strokes in which those with right hemisphere injury, but not left hemisphere injury, show affective deficits (Borod, 2000; Ross, 1981). With respect to linguistic prosody, the adult findings are mixed, and in the adult literature there is an ongoing debate regarding the neural underpinnings of prosody (e.g., Pell, 2006). In considering the results of Trauner et al.'s 1996 study, it should be noted that the one productive linguistic prosody task on which the children with PL performed in the range of control children was a task that involved a naturalistic behavior (i.e., answering a question). The only other task on which the children with PL performed comparably to control children required a conscious level of processing and active judgments about prosody rather than its spontaneous use. The next steps will be to assess children's use and understanding of affective and linguistic prosody in more naturalistic situations in order to evaluate their prosodic abilities in situations that are closer to those they will confront in real-world interactions.

GESTURE IN CHILDREN WITH PL

As noted previously, early gesture in typically developing infants and toddlers is highly correlated with later vocabulary development, raising questions regarding the relations of nonlinguistic behaviors to the emergence of language in the PL group. The earlier studies of gesture in children with PL used the MBCDI, a parental report, to assess gesture (Bates et al., 1997; Marchman, Miller, & Bates, 1991). In a longitudinal study of six infants, Marchman et al. (1991) found delay in both gesture and early lexical development for both comprehension and production. In a larger cross-sectional study, Bates et al. (1997) found that between the ages of 10 and 17 months, infants with right hemisphere injury, especially those with right parietal damage, were behind in both gesture and vocabulary comprehension compared to those with left hemisphere injury and controls. In a set of six longitudinal case studies of Italian children with PL, Dall'Oglio et al. (1994) also tracked gesture, and although they reported six different developmental trajectories, for each child, gestures preceded meaningful first words. And finally, a recent study from the Chicago group (Sauer, Levine & Goldin-Meadow, 2010) directly addressed the relation of gesture use and early words in children with PL. Using the MBCDI and PPVT-3 to assess vocabulary comprehension as well as spontaneous interaction at home to measure production of language and gesture, they followed 11 children from 18 to 30 months of age. Children were divided into two groups according to the number of gesture types they produced at 18 months (e.g., a point to a ball was one type and a point to a shoe was a second type). The HIGH gesture PL group was above the 25th percentile for typically developing children at 18 months, and the LOW gesture PL group was below the 25th percentile for typically developing children at 18 months. Those children with PL in the HIGH gesture group had productive vocabularies in the normal range at 22 and 26 months and receptive vocabularies in the normal range at 30 months. In contrast, those in the LOW gesture group (below the 25th percentile at 18 months) showed delay in productive vocabulary at 22 and 26 months, as well as delay in comprehension at 30 months. Importantly, early gesture predicted subsequent language trajectories at an earlier age than these language trajectories could be predicted by language itself. Although neither developmental profile was associated with lesion laterality, all the children with periventricular injury were in the high gesture group, while only two of the seven with cerebrovascular infarcts were in this group. With respect to lesion size, one of the five children with small lesions and four of the six with large lesions fell into the LOW gesture group. Together these studies suggest that gesture has a similar developmental relation to the emergence of language for children with PL as for the typically developing group; that is, gesture production at 18 months predicts later lexical production and comprehension. Biological factors that are implicated in low amounts of gesturing at 18 months of age are lesion size and location: large (often a cerebrovascular infarct) rather than a small lesion size (often a periventricular lesion). Another factor that could make a difference, based on Rowe and Goldin-Meadow's study of typically developing children (2009), is the amount of gesture that children with PL are exposed to by their caregivers. This hypothesis, of course, is in need of investigation.

EARLY LANGUAGE MILESTONES IN CHILDREN WITH PL: BABBLING

One small longitudinal study of five infants with PL (Marchman et al., 1991) included a detailed analysis of early babbling from audio- and videotaped free play sessions. Data were collected after 10 months of age when the child was already babbling but not yet producing any words. Subsequent sessions occurred after the parents reported a productive vocabulary of 10 words. On average, the children with brain injury reached these milestones several months after the typically developing group. Although there was substantial individual variability both within and across groups, there were no differences between the PL and typically developing groups in the frequency of interactions or in the total number of vocalizations. With respect to the quality of the vocalizations, those in the brain-injured group broadly mapped onto those of the controls but were delayed. There were some differences in consonant quality, such that the PL group used fewer "true consonants" than controls. However, similar to controls, consonant production was linked to word production. Moreover, the pattern of development for place and manner of articulation followed that of the control sample, but at a somewhat delayed developmental pace.

THE EMERGENCE OF FIRST WORDS

Early Comprehension

Evaluating what a toddler understands is a challenging task. The studies of infants and toddlers with PL have often used the MBCDI (a parental report with an infant and toddler version; for the younger children, from 8–16 months, there is a section that measures comprehension), experimental comprehension books, following verbal instructions, and standardized measures, such as the PPVT when children are 30 months of age and beyond. As we noted above, typically developing infants and toddlers show substantial individual variation in both early receptive and productive vocabulary. Several groups have used the MBCDI for children with early stroke; all confirm that, as a group, children with PL are delayed in the comprehension of first words (Bates et al., 1997; Dall'Oglio et al., 1994; Feldman, 1994; Feldman, Holland, Kemp, & Janosky, 1992; Marchman et al., 1991; Thal, Marchman, Stiles, & Aram, 1991; Vicari et al., 2000). Moreover, all studies note substantial variability in the group, with some children in the normal range but more children than would be expected based on norms falling into the lower percentiles. While Bates et al. found that children with right posterior lesions scored the lowest on comprehension measures between 8 and 16 months of age, other studies have not found lesion-specific laterality effects for comprehension of first words.

In a longitudinal study following a group of 22 Italian children with PL, Chilosi et al. (2005) used a comprehension task in which the child was asked to perform particular actions in response to 20 comprehension items. At the first session, when children were about 24 months of age, the group performed in the low average range, but 7 of the 11 with left PL and 2 of the 11 with right PL performed more than one standard deviation below the mean of typically developing children; at the second session, about 1 year later, all children had improved, but five children (four with left PL and one with right PL) showed persistent delay.

Looking at the continuing development of word comprehension, Sauer et al. (2010) tested their longitudinal cohort at 30 months using the PPVT-3. As a group, the children with PL had an average standard score of 84.64, one standard deviation below the mean for typically developing children, for whom the mean is 100. Again, however, they noted marked variability in the group, with the highest standard score at 113 and the lowest at 45. So again, some of the children in the PL group were clearly performing in the normal range whereas others were significantly behind. As noted above, those who were in the LOW gesture group at 18 months (with fewer gesture types) scored significantly lower than those in the HIGH gesture group on the PPVT-3.

Early Word Production

In contrast to the profile of overall delay but no lesion laterality effects for the development of receptive vocabulary in children with PL, a number of studies of early word production in the PL group have reported delay for the group overall, and in addition, have identified a more pronounced deficit in those with left hemisphere injury. Studies with larger samples of children learning both English (Bates et al., 1997) and Italian (Chilosi et al., 2005; Vicari et al., 2000) have reported greater delay in the onset and initial development of productive vocabulary in those toddlers with left hemisphere injury compared to typically developing controls and those toddlers with right hemisphere lesions (Figure 7.3). All these studies had relatively large groups of children and they all used the MBCDI, a parental report measure that has been shown to have high reliability and validity (Dale, Bates, Reznick, & Morisset, 1989).

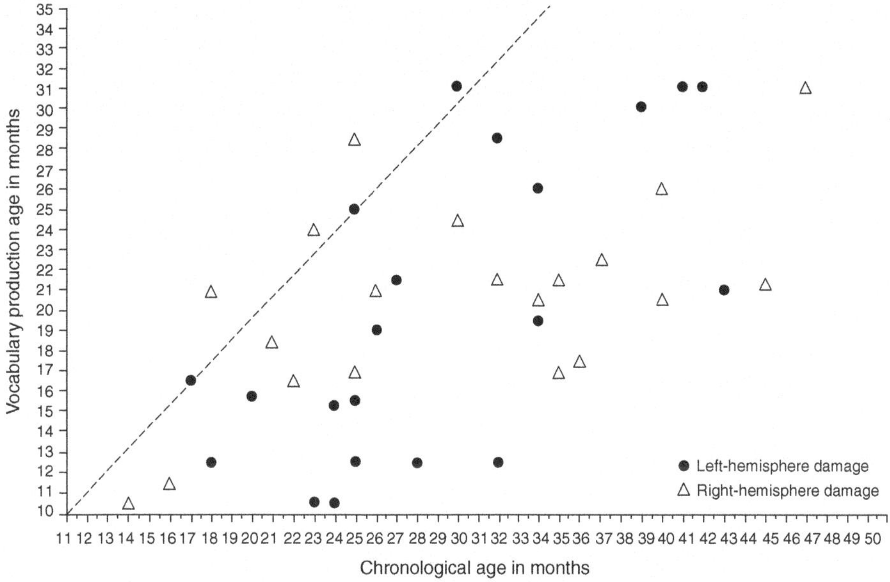

FIGURE 7.3 Productive vocabulary from Italian-speaking children with PL. Data were collected using the Italian CDI (*Il primo vocabolario del bambino: guida all'uso del questionario MacArthur per la valutazione della comunicazione e del linguaggio nei primi anni di vita*). Each child's productive vocabulary scores are compared to the Italian norms for children at that age (in months). The dotted line represents the norm. Overall the left PL group falls slightly below those with right PL. (Reprinted with permission of the publisher from Vicari, Albertoni, Chilosi, et al., 2000.)

In the largest of these studies by Vicari et al., 36 of the 42 PL children fell below the expected productive vocabulary level for their age, with an average delay of 8.26 months. Among those children who were producing only one-word utterances, those with left hemisphere injury had significantly smaller productive vocabularies than those with right hemisphere injury. However, among the children who had begun to combine words, there was no longer a site-specific difference, although overall the group of children with PL was still delayed. The longitudinal study by Chilosi et al. (2005) showed a similar pattern: lexical development was delayed at both time points (24 and 36 months) for the left PL group, whereas the right PL group performed in the typical range at both time points. In addition to language and cognitive measures, at a later time point, Chilosi et al. also performed a dichotic listening test to derive a language lateralization index. They reported a significant difference in language processing between the left PL and right PL groups: all the children with right hemisphere lesions showed the typical right ear advantage, while all those children with left hemisphere injury showed a left ear advantage, suggesting that for those with left hemisphere injury, the right hemisphere is participating in language processing to a greater degree than in children with right hemisphere injury or in typically developing children.

SUMMARY

Returning to our initial questions, the first concerned the developmental trajectory of the PL group compared to typically developing children. The results from the studies reviewed show that for the onset of language, there is delay for the PL group as a whole, regardless of lesion site. Moreover, there is delay for the group at each step in the developmental process: canonical babbling, word comprehension, early word production, and the onset of first word combinations. Nonetheless, the sequence of linguistic milestones maps onto the typical developmental profile.

Question 2 addressed the relations between communicative systems. Surveying the results of the gesture studies permits the examination of cross-modal relations in communication (e.g., gesture–language relations). For gesture, Bates et al. (1997) used parental report and found a smaller gestural repertoire in the right PL group. However, looking at the use of gesture, specifically the relation of pre-linguistic gesture to early language production in naturalistic contexts, early gesture use predicts later vocabulary in the PL group, just as it does with the typically developing group. Together the studies of language and of gesture show that, in spite of early brain injury, and regardless of lesion site, children with PL follow similar developmental trajectories to their typically developing peers. Moreover, the relation between these two communicative systems, language and gesture, appears to be similar across the groups as well.

The third question relates to similarities and differences of the children with PL to adults with homologous acquired lesions. The widespread developmental delay for early language milestones suggests that unlike the adult left-lateralized profile for single word comprehension and production, both hemispheres play a significant role in early language acquisition. Such a hypothesis is in line with functional imaging data from older typically developing children. For language skills that are in the process of developing (e.g., lexical semantic associations), typically developing children recruit both the right and left hemispheres of the brain. It is only with development, in this case later adolescence, that the adult profile of strong left lateralization emerges for such skills (Brown et al., 2005; Holland et al., 2001). As such, the PL group appears to be relying on a similar bilateral strategy to acquire new linguistic skills at each step in the process of language acquisition. Again, it is important to note that the children's profile is unlike that of adults with homologous lesions acquired later in life. However, while the acquisition picture might suggest equipotentiality of both hemispheres to mediate language functioning, recall that within the broad context of delay in the PL group for the development of early language milestones, many studies have noted a more pronounced deficit or delay in those with left hemisphere lesions. Such findings may reflect a "soft" left hemisphere bias for linguistic skills. While the left hemisphere may ultimately be optimal for mature language, it is clear that the right hemisphere plays a critical role in its acquisition and development.

The Contrasting Case of Emotion

The few studies from the PL group on the emergence of affective expression, facial and vocal, paint a somewhat different picture. From as early as 6 months of age, children with left hemisphere injury reflect affective profiles that map onto those of typically developing infants and toddlers. Those with right hemisphere lesions, however, show a qualitatively different profile: they smile less, produce significantly fewer positive vocalizations, and express more negative affect. Unlike language, where there are delays across the PL group, regardless of lesion laterality or site, the affective profile shows differential responses according to lesion site from the earliest observations. Moreover, the profile of deficits after a right pre-perinatal stroke maps onto that of adults with acquired right hemisphere lesions. Looking at these different communicative systems, it appears that the evolutionarily early and subcortically mediated system of affect is in place by at least 6 months of age. In contrast, the evolutionarily late and predominantly cortical system of language seems to be initially distributed over both hemispheres.

Our final question pertains to whether there are changes in the nature of the children's early deficits. The studies of language most clearly begin to address this question. Children with PL follow the same developmental trajectory as their typically developing peers. They approach early linguistic milestones (babbling, early word comprehension, word production) in turn, just more slowly. These young children are just beginning their linguistic journey; in the next chapter we will follow them into school age and adolescence so that we can see how language and communication evolve in older children with perinatal stroke.

REFERENCES

Adolphs R. (2001). The neurobiology of social cognition. *Curr Opinion Neurobiol* 11(2): 231–239.

Adolphs R, Damasio AR, Tranel D, Cooper G, Damasio AR. (2000). A role for somatosensory cortices in the visual recognition of emotion as revealed by three-dimensional lesion mapping. *J Neurosci* 20(7):2683–2690.

Adolphs R, Gosselin F, Buchanan TW, Tranel D, Schyns P, Damasio AR. (2005). A mechanism for impaired fear recognition after amygdala damage. *Nature* 433(7021):68–72.

Adolphs R, Tranel D, Demasio AR. (2003). Dissociable neural systems for recognizing emotions. *Brain Cognition* 52:61–69.

Alajouanine T, Lhermitte F. (1965). Acquired aphasia in children. *Brain* 88:553–562.

Barrera ME, Maurer D. (1981). Recognition of mother's photographed face by the three-month-old infant. *Child Dev* 52:714–716.

Barton JJ. (2003). Disorders of face perception and recognition. *Neurol Clin* 21(2):521–548.

Basser LS. (1962). Hemiplegia of early onset and the faculty of speech with special reference to the effects of hemispherectomy. *Brain* 85.

Bates E. (1976). Language and Context: The Acquisition of Pragmatics. New York: Academic Press.

Bates E. (1979). The Emergence of Symbols: Cognition and Communication in Infancy. New York: Academic Press.

Bates E, Dick F. (2002). Language, gesture, and the developing brain. *Dev Psychobiol* 40(3): 293–310.

Bates E, Reilly J, Wulfeck B, Dronkers N, Opie N, Fenson J. (2001). Differential effects of unilateral lesions on language production in children and adult. *Brain Language* 79(2):223–265.

Bates E, Thal D, Trauner D, Fenson J, Aram D, Eisele J, Nass R. (1997). From first words to grammar in children with focal brain injury. *Special Issue on Origins of Communication Disorders. Dev Neurol* 13(3):275–343.

Batty M, Taylor MJ. (2006). The development of emotional face processing during childhood. *Dev Sci* 9:207–220.

Bavelas JB, Chovil N. (1997). Faces in dialogue. In Russell JA, Fernandez-Dols JM (Eds.), The Psychology of Facial Expression (pp. 334–346). New York: Cambridge University Press.

Beauchamp MS, Lee KE, Haxby JV, Martin A. (2003). fMRI responses to video and point-light displays of moving humans and manipulable objects. *J Cogn Neurosci* 15:991–1001.

Berman RA, Verhoeven L. (2002). Crosslinguistic perspectives on developing text production abilities in speech and writing. *Written Language and Literacy* 5:1–44.

Binder JR, Desai RH, Graves W, Conant LL. (2009). Where is the semantic system? A critical review and meta analysis of 120 functional neuroimaging studies. *Cerebral Cortex [e-pub March 27].*

Bleses D, Vach W, Slott M, Wehberg S, Thomsen P, Madsen TO, Basboll H. (2008a). Communicative developmental inventories: Validity and main developmental trends. *J Child Language* 35(3):651–669.

Bleses D, Vach W, Slott M, Wehberg S, Thomsen P, Madsen TO, Basboll H. (2008b). Early vocabulary development in Danish and other languages: A CDI-based comparison. *J Child Language* 35(3):619–650.

Blonder L, Bowers D, Heilman KM. (1991). The role of the right hemisphere in emotional communication. *Brain* 114:1115–1127.

Blonder L, Burns AF, Bowers D, Moore RW, Heilman K. (1993). Right hemisphere facial expressivity during natural conversation. *Brain Cognition* 21(1):44–56.

Blonder L, Heilman KM, Ketterson T, Rosenbek J, Raymer A, Crosson B, . . . Rothi L. (2005). Affective facial and lexical expression in aprosodic versus aphasic stroke patients. *J Intl Neuropsychol Soc* 11(6):677–685.

Bonda E, Petrides M, Ostry D, Evans A. (1996). Specific involvement of human parietal systems and the amygdala in the perception of biological motion. *J Neurosci* 16:3737–3744.

Bookheimer S. (2002). Functional MRI of language: new approaches to understanding the cortical organization of semantic processing. *Annu Rev Neurosci* 25:151–188. doi: 10.1146/annurev.neuro.25.112701.142946

Borod J. (2000). The Neuropsychology of Emotion. New York: Oxford University Press.

Borod J, Koff E, Perlman Lorch M, Nicholas M. (1985). Channels of emotional expression in patients with unilateral brain damage. *Arch Neurol* 42(4):345–348.

Brauer J, Anwander A, Friederici AD. (2011). Neuroanatomical prerequisites for language functions in the maturing brain. *Cerebral Cortex* 21(2):459–466. doi: 10.1093/cercor/bhq108

Brown R. (1973). A First Language: The Early Stages. Cambridge, MA: Harvard University Press.

Brown TT, Lugar HM, Coalson RS, Miezin FM, Petersen SE, Schlaggar BL. (2005). Developmental changes in human cerebral functional organization for word generation. *Cerebral Cortex* 15(3):275–290. doi: 10.1093/cercor/bhh129

Bruce V, Young A. (1986). Understanding face recognition. *Br J Psychol* 77:305–327.

Bruner JS. (1975). The ontogenesis of speech acts. *J Child Language* 2:1–19.

Buck R, Duffy RJ. (1980). Nonverbal communication of affect in brain damaged patients. *Cortex* 16(3):351–362.

Caron RF, Caron AJ, Myers RS. (1982). Abstraction of invariant face expressions in infancy. *Child Dev* 53(4):1009–1015.

Caselli MC, Bates C, Casadio P, Fenson LD, Sanderl L, Weir J. (1995). A crosslinguistic study of early lexical development. *Cogn Dev* 10:159–199.

Chao LL, Martin A. (2000). Representation of manipulable man-made objects in the dorsal stream. *NeuroImage* 12:478–484.

Chilosi AM, Cipriani P, Brovedani P, Brizzolara D, Ferretti G, Pfanner PL. (2005). Atypical language lateralization and early linguistic development in children with focal brain lesions. *Dev Med Child Neurol* 47:725–730.

Dale PS, Bates E, Reznick JS, Morisset C. (1989). The validity of a parent report instrument of child language at twenty months. *J Child Language* 16:239–249.

Dall'Oglio AM, Bates E, Volterra V, Di Capua M, Pezzini G. (1994). Early cognition, communication and language in children with focal brain injury. *Dev Med Child Neurol* 36: 1076–1098.

de Haan M, Nelson CA. (1998). Discrimination and categorisation of facial expressions of emotion during infancy. In Slater A (Ed), Perceptual Development (pp. 287–309). Hove, UK: Psychology Press.

Gratch, G. (1982). Responses to hidden persons and things by 5-, 9-, and 16-month-old infants in a visual tracking situation. *Developmental Psychology*, 18: 232–237.

De Renzi E, Perani D. (1994). Prosopagnosia can be associated with damage confined to the right hemisphere: An MRI and PET study and a review of the literature. *Neuropsychologia* 32(8): 893–902.

de Schonen S, Mathviet E. (1989). First come, first served: A scenario about the development of hemispheric specialization in face recognition during infancy. *Cahiers de Psychologie Cognitive/ Current Psychology of Cognition* 9(1):3–44.

De Sonneville LM, Verschoor CA, Nijiokiktjien C, Op het Veld V, Toorenaar N, Vranken M. (2002). Facial identity and facial emotions: Speed, accuracy, and processing strategies in children and adults. *J Clin Exp Neuropsychol* 24(2):200–213.

Dehaene, S. (2005) Evolution of human cortical circuits for reading and arithmetic: The "neuronal recycling" hypothesis. In: *From monkey brain to human brain*, ed. S. Dehaene, J.-R. Duhamel, M. D. Hauser & G. Rizolatti, pp. 133–57. MITPress.

Dehaene-Lambertz G, Dehaene S, Hertz-Pannier L. (2002). Functional neuroimaging of speech perception in infants. *Science* 298(5600):2013–2015.

Dick AS, Goldin-Meadow S, Hasson U, Skipper J, Small SL. (2009). Co-speech gestures influence neural activity in brain regions associated with processing semantic information. *Hum Brain Mapp* 30:3509–3526.

Dunn LM, Dunn LM. (1981). Peabody Picture Vocabulary Test (Rev. ed.). Circle Pines, MN: American Guidance Service.

Ekman P. (1972). Universal and cultural differences in facial expressions of emotion. In Cole JK (Ed), Nebraska Symposium on Motivation. Lincoln, NE: University of Nebraska Press.

Ekman P. (1979). About Brows: Emotional and Conversational Signals.

Ekman P, Friesen W. (1978). The Facial Action Coding System. Palo Alto, CA: Consulting Psychologists Press.

Feldman HM. (1994). Language development after early brain injury: A replication study. In Tager-Flusberg H (Ed), Constraints on Language Acquisition: Studies of Atypical Children (pp. 75–90). Hillsdale, NJ: Lawrence Erlbaum.

Feldman HM, Holland AL, Kemp SS, Janosky JE. (1992). Language development after unilateral brain injury. *Brain and Language* 42:89–102.

Fenson LD, Dale P, Reznick JS, Thal D, Bates E, Hartung J, . . . Reilly J. (1993). MacArthur–Bates Communicative Development Inventories: User's Guide and Technical Manual. San Diego, CA: Singular.

Fernald A. (1990). From preference to reference: Affective and linguistic functions of prosody in speech to infants. *Infant Behavior and Development* 13:50.

Fernald A. (1993). Approval and disapproval: Infant responsiveness to vocal affect in familiar and unfamiliar languages. *Child Dev* 64(3):657–674.

Frederici A, Alter K. (2004). Lateralization of auditory language functions: A dynamic dual pathway model. *Brain Language* 89(2):267–276.

Fusar-Poli P, Placentino A, Carletti F, Allen P, Landi P, Abbamonte M, . . . Politi PL. (2009). Laterality effect on emotional faces processing. *Neurosci Lett* 452(3):262–267.

Gaillard W, Sachs BC, Whitnah J R, Ahmad Z., Balsamo L M, Petrella, J R, et al.

Developmental Aspects of Language Processing: fMRI of Verbal Fluency in Children and Adults. *Human Brain Mapping* 18:176–185(2003)

Gao X, Maurer D. (2010). A happy story: Developmental changes in children's sensitivity to facial expressions of varying intensities. *J Exp Child Psychol* 107(2):67–86.

Gauthier I, Skudlarski P, Gore JC, Anderson AW. (2000). Expertise for cars and birds recruits brain areas involved in face recognition. *Nature Neurosci* 3:191–197.

Goldin-Meadow S, Butcher C. (2003). Pointing toward two-word speech in young children. In Kita S (Ed), Pointing: Where Language, Culture, and Cognition Meet. Mahwah, NJ: Lawrence Erlbaum Associates.

Goldin-Meadow S, Iverson JM. (2010). Gesturing across the life span. In Overton WF (Ed), Cognition, Biology, and Methods across the Lifespan (Vol. 1, pp. 36–55). Hoboken, NJ: Wiley.

Goodglass H. (1993). Understanding Aphasia. San Diego: Academic Press.

Goodwyn SW, Acredolo LP. (1988). Symbolic gesturing in normal infants. *Child Dev* 59(2): 450–466.

Grill-Spector K, Knouf N, Kanwisher N. (2004). The fusiform face area subserves face perception, not generic within-category identification. *Nature Neurosci* 7(5):555–562.

Haist F, Lee K, Stiles J. (2010). Individuating faces and common objects produces equal responses in the putative face processing areas in the ventral occipitotemporal cortex. *Frontiers Neurosci* 4:1–15.

Haxby JV, Gobbini MI, Furey ML, Ishai A, Schouten JL, Pietrini P. (2001). Distributed and overlapping representation of faces and objects in ventral temporal cortex. *Science* 293(5539):2425–2430.

Haxby JV, Hoffman EA, Gobbini MI. (2000). The distributed human neural system for face perception. *Trends Cogn Sci* 4(6):59–67.

Haxby JV, Hoffman EA, Gobbini MI. (2002). Human neural systems for face recognition and social ommunication. *Biol Psychiatry* 51(1):59–67.

Herba C, Phillips M. (2004). Development of facial expression recognition from childhood to adolescence: Behavioural and neurological perspectives. *J Child Psychol Psychiatry* 45:207–220.

Hickok G, Poeppel D. (2007). The cortical organization of speech processing. *Nature Rev Neurosci* 8(5):393–402.

Hill EL, Bishiop DVM, Nimmo-Smith I. (1998). Representational gestures in developmental coordination disorder and specific language impairment: Error-types and the reliability of ratings. *Human Movement Sci* 17(4–5):655–678.

Holland SK, Plante E, Weber Byars A, Strawsburg RH, Schmithorst VJ, Ball WS, Jr. (2001). Normal fMRI brain activation patterns in children performing a verb generation task. *NeuroImage* 14(4):837–843. doi: 10.1006/nimg.2001.0875

Holle H, Gunter TC, Ruschemeyer SA, Hennelotter A, Iacoboni M. (2008). Neural correlates of the processing of co-speech gestures. *NeuroImage* 39:2010–2024.

Hubbard AL,Wilson SM,Callan DE, & Dapretto, M. (2009). *Giving speech a hand: Gesture modulates activity in auditory cortex during speech perception. Hum Brain Mapp*, 30: 1028–1037.

Hyson MC, Izard CE. (1985). Continuities and changes in emotion expressions during brief separation at 13 and 18 months. *Dev Psychol* 21(6):1165–1170.

Iverson, J.M. (2010). Developing language in a developing body: The relationship between motor development and language development. *Journal of Child Language*, 37: 229–261.

Iverson JM, Goldin-Meadow S. (2005). Gesture paves the way for language development. *Psychol Sci* 16(5):367–371.

Izard CR. (1971). The Face of Emotion. New York: Appleton Century Crofts.

Jung-Beeman M. (2005). Bilateral brain processes for comprehending natural language. *Trends Cogn Sci* 9(11):512–518. doi: 10.1016/j.tics.2005.09.009

Jusczyk P. (1997). How attention to sound properties may facilitate learning other elements of linguistic organization. In Jusczyk P (Ed), The Discovery of Spoken Language. Cambridge, MA: MIT Press.

Kagan J, Snidman N, Arcus D, Reznick JS. (1994). Galen's prophecy: Temperament in Human Nature. New York: Basic Books.

Kanwisher N. (1997). The fusiform face area: A module in human extrastriate cortex specialized for face perception. *J Neurosci* 17:4302–4311.

Kanwisher N. (2000). Domain specificity in face perception. *Nature Neurosci* 3:759–763.

Kelly SD, Barr DJ, Church RB, Lynch K. (1999). Offering a hand to pragmatic understanding: The role of speech and gesture in comprehension and memory. *J Memory Language* 40: 577–592.

Labarbera JD, Izard CE, Vietze P, Parisi SA. (1976). Four- and six-month-old infants' visual responses to joy, anger, and neutral expressions. *Child Dev* 47:535–538.

Laudanna A, Caselli C, Volterra V. (1983). Comprensione verbale e imitazione gestualein bambini di 20 mesi/Verbal comprehension and gestural imitation in 20-month-old infants. *Giornali Italiano di Psicologia* 10(2):271–287.

Lenneberg EH. (1967). Biological Foundations of Language. New York: John Wiley and Sons, Inc.

Locke JL, Bekken KE, McMinn-Larson L, Wein D. (1995). Emergent control of manual and vocal-motor activity in relation to the development of speech. *Brain and Language* 51(3):489–508.

Ludemann PM, Nelson CA. (1988). Categorical representation of facial expressions by 7-month-old infants. *Dev Psychol* 24(4):492–501.

Marchman VA, Miller R, Bates E. (1991). Babble and first words in children with focal brain injury. *Applied Psycholinguistics* 12:1–22.

McNeill D. (1992). Hand and Mind: What Gestures Reveal about Thought. Chicago: University of Chicago Press.

McNeill D, Alibali MW, Evans JL. (2000). The role of gesture in children's spoken language: Now they need it, now they don't. *J Nonverbal Behavior* 24:131–150.

McNeill D, Pedelty L. (1995). Right brain and gesture. In Reilly J, Emmorey K (Eds), Language, Space and Gesture. Hillsdale, NJ: Lawrence Erlbaum and Associates.

Meltzoff AN, Moore K. (1977). Imitation of facial and manual gestures by human neonates quick view. *Science New Series* 198(4312):75–78.

Menn L, Obler LK. (Eds). (1990). Agrammatic Aphasia: Cross-Language Narrative Sourcebook. Amsterdam/Philadelphia: John Benjamins.

Mills DL, Coffey-Corina S, Neville HJ. (1997). Language comprehension specialization from 13 to 20 months. *Dev Neuropsychol* 13(3):397–445.

Molfese D. (1980). Hemispheric specialization for temporal information: Implications for the perception of voicing cues during speech perception. *Brain and Language* 22(2):285–299.

Monk CS. (2008). The development of emotion-related neural circuitry in health and psychopathology. *Dev Psychopathol* 20(4):1231–1250.

Monk CS, McClure EB, Nelson EE, Zarahn E, Bilder RM, Leibenluft E, . . . Pine DS. (2003). Adolescent immaturity in attention-related brain engagement to emotional facial expressions. *NeuroImage* 20(1):420–428.

Morgan J. (1996). Signal to Syntax: Bootstrapping from Speech to Grammar in Early Acquisition. Mahwah, NJ: Lawrence Erlbaum and Associates.

Narumoto J, Okadab T, Sadatob N, Fukuia K, Yonekurac Y. (2001). Attention to emotion modulates fMRI activity in human right superior temporal sulcus. *Cogn Brain Res* 12(2):225–231.

Nass R, Koch D. (1987). Temperament differences in toddlers with early unilateral right- and left-brain damage. *Dev Neuropsychol* 3(2):93–99.

Nelson CA. (1987). The recognition of facial expressions in the first two years of life: Mechanisms of development. *Child Dev* 58(4):889–909.

Nelson CA. (1993). The recognition of facial expressions in infancy: Behavioral and electrophysiological correlates. In de Boysson-Bardies B, de Schonen S, Jusczyk P, MacNeilage P, Morton J (Eds), Developmental Neurocognition: Speech and Face Processing in the First Year of Life (pp. 187–193). The Netherlands: Kluwer Academic Press.

Nelson CA, de Haan M. (1996). Neural correlates of infants' visual responsiveness to facial expresion of emotion. *Dev Psychobiol* 29(7):577–595.

Nelson CA, de Haan M. (1997). A neurobehavioral approach to the recognition of facial expressions in infancy. In Russell JA, Fernandez-Dols JM (Eds), The Psychology of Facial Expression (pp. 176–204). New York: Cambridge University Press.

Oller DK, Niyogic P, Gray S, Richards JA, Gilkerson J, Xu D, . . . Warren SF. (2010). Automated vocal analysis of naturalistic recordings from children with autism, language delay, and typical development. *Proc Natl Acad Sci U S A* 107(30):13354–13359.

O'Reilly AW, Painter KM, Bornstein MH. (1997). Relations between language and symbolic gesture development in early childhood. *Cogn Dev* 12(2):185–197.

Oster H. (1978). Facial expression and affect development. In Lewis M, Rosenblum L (Eds), The Development of Affect. New York: Plenum.

Oszcaliskan S, Goldin-Meadow S. (2005). Gesture is at the cutting edge of early language development. *Cognition* 96:101–113.

Pell MD. (2006). Cerebral mechanisms for understanding emotional prosody in speech. *Brain Language* 96(2):221–234.

Petersen SE, Fox PT, Posner MI, Mintun M, Raichle ME. (1988). Positron emission tomographic studies of the cortical anatomy of single word processing. *Nature* 331:585–589.

Poizner H, Klima ES, Bellugi U. (1990). What the Hands Reveal about the Brain. Cambridge, MA: MIT Press.

Poldrack R, Wagner A, Prull M, Desmond J, Glover G, Gabrieli JD. (1999). Functional specialization for semantic and phonological processing in the left interior prefrontal cortex. *NeuroImage* 10:15–35.

Posamentier MT, Abdi H. (2003). Processing faces and facial expressions. *Neuropsychol Rev* 13(3):113–143.

Price CJ. (2010). The anatomy of language: a review of 100 fMRI studies published in 2009. *Ann NY Acad Sci* 1191:62–88. doi: 10.1111/j.1749-6632.2010.05444.x

Puce A, Perrett D. (2003). Electrophysiology and brain imaging of biological motion. *Philos Trans Royal Soc London Biol Sci* 258:435–445.

Reilly J, Bates E, Marchman VA. (1998). Narrative discourse in children with early focal brain injury. *Brain and Language* 61:335–375.

Reilly J, Jisa H, Baruch E, Berman RA. (2002). Propositional attitudes: the development of modality. *Written Language and Literacy* 2:183–218.

Reilly J, Martinez R, Anderson DA. (in preparation), Prelinguistic vocalizations in infants with early focal brain injury.

Reilly J, Salamanca L, Meza L, Littlewort R, Barlett M. (in preparation). A new perspective on facial expression production in children.

Reilly J, Stiles J, Larsen J, Trauner D. (1995). Affective facial expression in infants with focal brain damage. *Neuropsychologia* 33(1):83–99.

Reilly J, Wasserman G, Appelbaum M. (submitted). Later language development in narratives in children with perinatal stroke.

Reilly J, Wulfeck B. (2004). Plasticity and development: Language in atypical children. *Brain and Language* 88(2):163–166.

Reilly J, Zamora A, McGivern RF. (2005). Developing perspective in English: The acquisition of stance. *J Pragmatics* 37(2):185–208.

Ressel V, Wilke M, Lidzba K, Lutzenberger W, Krageloh-Mann I. (2008). Increases in language lateralization in normal children as observed using magnetoencephalography. *Brain and Language* 106(3):167–176. doi: 10.1016/j.bandl.2008.01.004

Ritti A. (1894). Eloge du Docteur Jules Cotard. [From a paper read at the Annual Public Lecture of the Société Médico Psychologique on 30 April 1894]. [Copy held in Rare Manuscripts Section, Library of School of Medicine, Paris 36 pages, catalog no.56613/6]. Imprimèrie de la Cour d'Appel, Paris.

Ross ED. (1981). The aprosodias: functional-anatomic organization of the affect components of language in the right hemisphere. *Arch Neurol* 38:561–569.

Rowe, ML Goldin-Meadow, S. (2009). Differences in early gesture explain SES disparities in child vocabulary size at school entry. *Science*, 323:951–953.

Rowe ML, Ozcaliskan S, Goldin-Meadow S. (2008). Learning words by hand: Gesture's role in predicting vocabulary development. *First Language* 28(2):182–199.

Sabatinelli D, Bradley MM, Lang PJ. (2001). Affective startle modulation in anticipation and perception. *Psychophysiology* 38:719–722.

Sauer E, Levine SC, Goldin-Meadow S. (2010). Early gesture predicts language delay in children with pre- or perinatal brain lesions. *Child Dev* 81(2):528–239.

Saygin AP, Wilxon SM, Hagler DJJ, Bates E, Sereno MI. (2004). Point-light biological motion perception activates human pre-motor cortex. *J Neurosci* 24:6181–6188.

Skipper, J., Goldin-Meadow, S., Nusbaum, H.C., & Small, S.L. (2007). Speech-associated gestures, Broca's area, and the human mirror system. *Brain and Language*: 101, 260–277.

Skipper J, Goldin-Meadow S, Nusbaum HC, Small SL. (2009). Gestures orchestrate brain networks for language understanding. *Curr Biol* 19:661–667.

Snow CE. (1972). Mothers' speech to children learning language. *Child Dev* 43:549–565.

Steiner JE. (1973). The gustofacial response: Observation on normal and anencephalic newborn infants. Paper presented at the Oral sensation and perception: Development in the fetus and infant, Fourth symposium.

Stenberg CR, Campos JJ. (1990). The development of anger expressions in infancy. In Stein BLN, Trabasso T (Ed), Psychological and Biological Approaches to Emotion (pp. 247–282). Hillsdale, NJ: Lawrence Erlbaum.

Stern D. (1977). The First Relationship: Infant and Mother. Cambridge: Harvard University Press.

Stone A, Valentine T. (2003). Viewpoint: Perspectives on prosopagnosia and models of face recognition. *Cortex* 39(1):31–40.

Taylor MJ, Batty M, Itier RJ. (2004). The faces of development: a review of early face processing over childhood. *J Cogn Neurosci* 16(8):1426–1442.

Thal D, Bates E. (1988). Language and gesture in late talkers. *J Speech Hearing Res* 31:115–123.

Thal D, Marchman VA, Stiles J, Aram D. (1991). Early lexical development in children with focal brain injury. *Brain and Language* 40(4):491–527.

Thal D, Tobias S. (1992). Communicative gestures in children with delayed onset of oral expressive vocabulary. *J Speech Hearing Res* 35:1281–1289.

Thomas KM, Drevets WC, Whalen PJ, Eccard CH, Dahl RE, Ryan ND, Casey BJ. (2001). Amygdala response to facial expressions in children and adults. *Biol Psychiatry* 49(4): 309–316.

Thompson-Schill S, Aguirre G, D'Esposito M, Farah M. (1999). A neural basis for category and modality specificity of semantic knowledge. *Neuropsychologia* 37:671–676.

Thompson-Schill S, D'Esposito M, Aguirre G, Farah M. (1997). Role of the left inferior prefrontal cortex in retrieval of semantic knowledge: A reevaluation. *Proc Natl Acad Sci U S A* 94:14792–14797.

Trauner D, Ballantyne A, Friedland S, Chase C. (1996). Disorders of affective and linguistic prosody in children after early unilateral brain damage. *Ann Neurol* 39(3):361–367.

Travis KE, Leonard MK, Brown TT, Hagler DJJ, Curran M, Dale AM, . . . Halgren E. (2011). Spatiotemporal neural dynamics of word understanding in 12- to 18-month-old infants. *Cerebral Cortex* 21(8):1832–1839.

Vicari S, Albertoni A, Chilosi AM, Cipriani P, Cioni G, Bates E. (2000). Plasticity and reorganization during language development in children with early brain injury. *Cortex* 36(1):31–46.

Vicari S, Reilly JS, Pasqualetti P, Vizzotto A, Caltagirone C. (2000). Recognition of facial expressions of emotions in school-age children: the intersection of perceptual and semantic categories. *Acta Paediatr 89*(7):836–845.

Volterra V, Caselli MC, Capirci O, Pizzuto E. (2005). Gesture and the emergence and development of language. In Tomasello M, Slobin D (Eds), Beyond Nature-Nurture: Essays in Honor of Elizabeth Bates. Mahwah, NJ: Lawrence Erlbaum.

Wagner A, Pare-Blagoev EJ, Clark J, Poldrack RA. (2001). Recovering meaning: Left prefrontal cortex guides controlled semantic retrieval. *Neuron* 31:329–338.

Weintraub S, Mesulam M. (1983). Developmental learning disabilities of the right hemisphere: Emotional, interpersonal, and cognitive components. *Arch Neurol* 19:5–11.

Xu, J, Gannon, PJ, Emmorey, K, Smith, JF, Brain, AR (2009). Symbolic gestures and spoken language are processed by a common neural system. *Proc Natl Adad Sci*, 106, 20664–20669.

Weir J. (1962). Language in the Crib. The Hague: Mouton.

Wildgruber D, Ackermann H, Kreifelts B, Ethofer T. (2006). Cerebral processing of linguistic and emotional prosody: fMRI studies. *Progress Brain Res* 156:249–268.

Willems RM, Ozyurek A, Hagoort P. (2007). When language meets action: The neural integration of gesture and speech. *Cerebral Cortex* 17:2322–2333.

Young-Browne G, Rosenfeld HM, Horowitz FD. (1977). Infant discrimination of facial expressions. *Child Dev* 48(2):555–562.

8

Later Language Development

SYNTAX AND DISCOURSE

THE PREVIOUS CHAPTER focused on the emergence of pre-linguistic communicative skills, including early vocalizations, facial expression, and gesture; these were followed by discussions of studies of infants' first words. Initially, productive vocabulary grows slowly, with an average of about 10 words at 12 to 14 months of age; then a burst generally occurs at about age 16 to 18 months in which the child quickly acquires a multitude of new words and often requests labels for objects. A productive vocabulary in the neighborhood of 100 to 200 words sets the stage for the onset of syntax and grammar and the child begins to produce two-word utterances. Typically, children begin to form such two-word "telegraphic" sentences (e.g., *more apple*; *go bye-bye*) between 20 and 24 months, and these first syntactic constructions generally include content words, such as nouns, verbs, and adjectives, rather than function words (e.g., determiners, prepositions). These early sentences include a variety of semantic relations, such as agent–action (*kitty ride*); action–object (*want cookie*); object–location (*shoe off*); action–location (*go out*); and possessor–object (*Mommy shoe*). From the two-word phase, children rapidly go on to construct longer sentences, generally reflecting similar semantic relations, by combining these first semantic notions (e.g., *Mommy shoe off*) or with additional elaboration (*want two cookie!*). In acquiring English, morphology emerges slowly, with *–ing* generally appearing as one of the first verb markings and tense, pronouns, and number marking slowly emerging over the following months (Brown, 1973; de Villiers & de Villiers, 1973). Complex sentences (that is, two simple sentences or propositions that can be joined by a connector) emerge around the third birthday. For English, these first complex utterances include verb complements (e.g., *I wan' go outside*) or the coordinate conjunction *and*, which is followed by semantically more complex connectors, such as *because, when, before, if, so, but* (Limber, 1973). By a child's fourth birthday, he or she has access to the majority of syntactic constructions of his or her language (Slobin, 1992). Nonetheless, language development continues with an ever-expanding vocabulary, and grammar and syntax become more fluent and sophisticated as children produce and understand increasingly complex sentential structures.

As we noted earlier, studies of adult patterns of brain organization for language have a long history, and current studies have confirmed Broca's and Wernicke's original discoveries: for 95% to 98% of adults, core aspects of language (phonology, morphology, and syntax) are primarily mediated by a left frontotemporal network (Binder, Desai, Graves, & Conant, 2009; Bookheimer, 2002; Brauer, Anwander, & Friederici, 2011; Hickok & Poeppel, 2007; Price, 2010; Rasmussen & Milner, 1977). As we discussed in the previous chapter, studies of early language acquisition in children with perinatal lesions (PL) have all noted a delay in language onset regardless of lesion site. Within this broad context of delay, one study reported an increased delay in comprehension in infants with right posterior injury (Bates et al., 1997), and several studies reported an increased delay in lexical production in children with left hemisphere lesions (Bates et al. 1997; Chilosi, Cipriani, Bertuccelli, Pfanner, & Cioni, 2001; Vicari et al., 2000). This chapter follows these children as they begin to acquire and develop morphology and syntax. The vast majority of studies involve monolingual speakers of English, but studies of children with PL who are learning other languages help us understand the generalizability of the English findings, as well as identify the possible role of language-specific features. The first section of this chapter is concerned with early word combinations and the acquisition of morphology and particular syntactic structures; the second portion of the chapter is devoted to how children with PL use these linguistic structures in two discourse genres: maintaining a conversation and narrating stories. Whereas the data from the youngest children provided information about the onset of language, examining language development in children with PL into adolescence will permit us to address issues regarding the nature of later language development (e.g., the fluent use of syntax for various discourse functions), as well as the range and scope of neuroplasticity for language.

FIRST SENTENCES: COMBINING WORDS

Toddlers' first two-word utterances herald the onset of grammar, and parents are often the first to witness this linguistic milestone. As such, parental report has proven to be an effective tool for assessing early language development (Dale, Bates, Reznick, & Morisset, 1989). Recruiting a large group of toddlers with PL, Bates et al. (1997) used the MacArthur Bates Communicative Development Inventories (MBCDI) (Fenson et al., 1993), a parental report form, to chronicle early grammatical development. They reported that at ages 19 to 31 months, the children with left posterior, temporal damage showed deficits in both lexical and grammatical production; this profile stands in contrast to typical adult findings of comprehension deficits in adult stroke patients with such lesions. To complement the parental report data from the MBCDI, Bates et al. also collected and analyzed spontaneous language samples from 30 children with PL (24 left PL; 6 right PL) ages 20 to 44 months. Their findings were consistent with the parental report data: for mean length of utterance (MLU), those children with left posterior injury had shorter utterances on average than the typically developing children and than children with injury to other brain regions. Overall, the MLU of the PL group was measurably shorter than that of controls. In fact, using *z* scores, the mean for the PL group was −0.88, almost one standard deviation below the mean for typically developing children, but the range for the PL group was broad, with *z* scores ranging −3.17 to +2.15. Considering the MLU scores from the PL group in relation to those of typically developing children, of the 30 children with PL, 16 of them (53%) fell below the 10th percentile of the typically developing age-matched young children.

For toddlers and preschoolers, as noted above, samples of spontaneous speech are a fruitful and commonly used method to evaluate productive language abilities. Feldman et al. (Feldman, 1994, 2005; Feldman et al., 1992) also used this method and followed a small group of children with PL longitudinally during the preschool years to investigate language trajectories. They too reported initial delay for the PL group overall, and to measure morphology and syntax they used the Index of Productive Syntax (IPSYN) (Scarborough, 1991) to evaluate their free speech samples. The IPSYN is a measure of emergent morphology and syntax designed to evaluate morpho-syntactic development in English up to age 4. Similar to Bates et al. (1997), they found wide variability but no site-specific profiles: half their group with left hemisphere injury fell well below the typically developing group, as did half of those with right hemisphere injury. Language development in typically developing toddlers also shows variability (Fenson et al., 1993, 1994); however, the profiles of the PL group tend to be even more variable than in the typically developing group, with a larger percentage of children falling below the 10th percentile. This increased variability in the PL group may well be a reflection of the lesioned brain adapting and recruiting alternative strategies and/or regions for language processing. Complementing the smaller longitudinal studies by Feldman et al., a cross-sectional study of free speech data from 21 36-month-old children with PL also used the IPSYN (Thal, Reilly, Siebert, Jeffries, & Fenson, 2004). They reported similar findings: delay in morphology and syntax compared to controls with no site-specific profiles. These data are consistent with a larger longitudinal study of children with PL conducted by Rowe, Levine, Fisher, and Goldin-Meadow (2009). They too reported overall delay in the onset of language and development of syntax. However, rather than lesion site, they found that lesion size modulated the developmental trajectory for both productive vocabulary and syntax. In sum, the studies focusing on the onset of syntax find overall delay in the PL group accompanied by broad variability. Both the studies by Bates et al. and Rowe et al. found delay across the PL group. However, in the Rowe et al. study, lesion size but not site was correlated with deficits, and in the Bates et al. study, lesion site, specifically left temporal injury, was related to greater lexical and syntactic deficits. This apparent conflict might be attributable to differences in the study groups. Whereas the Bates et. al study included principally children with large cortical middle cerebral artery (MCA) strokes, the Rowe et al. study included both cases of children with MCA strokes and others with smaller periventricular lesions (PVL). Thus the two studies differ in both the size and type of lesions under examination.

Complementing these studies on American English-speaking children, two groups in Italy have also been following language development in children with PL. In addition to the lexical studies noted in the previous chapter, Chilosi et al. (2005) have reported on the development of grammar in the PL group as well. Unlike English, Italian has a rich morphology, with articles and adjectives agreeing in both number and gender with the noun they modify (*la bella ragazza* [the beautiful girl], *il bel ragazzo* [the beautiful boy]) as well as verbs that obligatorily mark person and tense (*mangio* [I eat], *mangi* [you (singular) eat], *mangiamo* [we eat]). Typically developing Italian children acquire the frequent and regular morphology of Italian earlier than typically developing American children master the sparse and somewhat irregular morphology of English (Caselli & Casadio, 1995; Caselli et al., 2005). In the Chilosi et al. study, 24 children with PL were assessed for comprehension (following commands with toys) and for productive language using language samples at about age 24 months (T1) and at 3 years (T2) of age. In the comprehension task, the mean *z* score was in the low average range; however, 7 of 11 children with left hemisphere injury and 2 of 11 with right hemisphere injury were more than one standard deviation below the norm. While both groups improved with age, at T2, the left lesion group (LPL) continued to score below the level of the right lesion group (RPL). With respect to production, at the first data point, none of the children with left hemisphere lesions were combining words, whereas 5 of the 12 with right hemisphere injury were combining words. At T2, 10 of the 12 with LPL and 4 of the 12 with RPL showed a persistent delay in morphology and syntax. In addition to side of lesion, Chilosi et al. noted that the presence of seizures and lesion size also played a role in the children's performance.

Considering these data together, they suggest that early brain injury to either hemisphere results in a delay in the emergence of first words and first word combinations (i.e., the onset of syntax). Thus, it appears that launching a language and developing a grammar recruits both hemispheres of the brain. Moreover, the language trajectory of the PL group is not a one-time "catch-up," but rather the data suggest an iterative developmental process in which we observe delay at each phase of language acquisition, in this case vocabulary, morphology, and syntax. There is also a recurrent theme of children with left hemisphere injury faring somewhat worse than those with right hemisphere injury, especially on measures of productive language, both vocabulary and syntax. Moreover, larger lesion size and the presence of seizures is associated with more marked language problems. Finally, the acquisition of language in the PL group is characterized by significant variability with respect to the time course of development for individual children.

THE ROLE OF INPUT TO LANGUAGE DEVELOPMENT

Although children all over the world acquire the language of their families, one enduring question in language acquisition concerns the factors that play a role in individual differences in language development. Over the past 20 years, studies have shown the importance of input to language development. It is clear that both the frequency and quality of the language that the child hears play a crucial role in the child's language acquisition (Hart & Risley, 1992; Huttenlocher, Vasilyeva, Cymerman, & Levine, 2002). Given that the PL group is initially delayed in language acquisition, what role might input play? Does it have a comparable role to input for TD children? Rowe, Levine, Fisher, and Goldin-Meadow (2009) modeled vocabulary and syntactic production for 80 children (53 typically developing and 27 with PL) between 14 and 46 months of age: vocabulary production was measured by the number of word types produced, and syntactic production was measured by MLU extracted from spontaneous language samples. The two groups of children (PL and typically developing) differed from each other at 14 and 46 months in vocabulary production, and syntactic development differed at 38, 42, and 46 months. Caregiver input was measured by the number of word types and the MLU of the parents when children were 30 months old. Rowe et al. found that caregiver input was a significant predictor of vocabulary and syntactic growth for both groups of children, PL and typically developing; however, input was a stronger predictor of syntactic growth for children with PL than the typically developing group. Thus, in the face of early lesions, the quality of input appears to play an even more important role in language development than for typically developing children, particularly for the more complex aspects of language such as syntactic development (See Figure 9.4).

The Rowe et al. study also examined the role of lesion characteristics in the language trajectories of children with PL. Although there were no laterality differences, other lesion characteristics (lesion size, type, seizure history) affected the language trajectories of children with PL. Children with large lesions and children with cerebrovascular lesions produced fewer word types at 30 months than children with smaller lesions or periventricular lesions. With respect to the growth of vocabulary, children with large and small lesions did not differ from typically developing children, whereas those with medium lesions had smaller vocabularies than controls. With respect to MLU, children with large lesions and children with cerebrovascular lesions (in contrast with those with periventricular lesions) had shorter MLUs at 30 months than the typically developing group; moreover, their growth rate was slower than that of typically developing children. Finally, children who experienced seizures had shorter MLUs at 30 months than the typically developing group as well. Together these findings confirm previous work both on the language profiles of children with PL as well as on the significance of language input in the early phases of language acquisition. They further suggest that the quality and quantity of language input is especially important for children for whom language represents a particular challenge; these results have clear clinical implications, which will be elaborated in Chapter 10.

MORPHOLOGY AND LATER SYNTACTIC DEVELOPMENT

Studies Using Standardized Tests

Spontaneous speech data, as in the studies using language samples above, provide one perspective on a child's productive language; in this context the child is at liberty to choose the vocabulary and sentence structures he or she uses. Thus, such measures provide only a partial picture of his or her productive language skills. An alternative method of assessing language that is especially effective with older children is standardized tests. Given that these methods systematically test increasingly complex language abilities, such measures provide complementary profiles of a child's morpho-syntactic abilities to those gleaned from spontaneous discourse. Several studies report findings on the PL group from the Clinical Evaluation of Language Fundamentals (CELF) (Semel, Wiig & Secord, 1995), a widely used standardized language measure for English that includes eight subtests to yield a Total Language Score, as well as separate Receptive and Expressive scores. In a cross sectional study of a group of 28 school-age and adolescent participants with PL, Ballantyne, Spilkin, and Trauner (2007) reported no differences in performance between those with left or right hemisphere injury. However, both groups performed significantly below the level of controls, ranking below the 14th percentile on all three cumulative scores (Total, Receptive, and Expressive). Additionally, their data showed wide variability, with Total Language Standard Scores in the PL group ranging from 50 to 132 (100 is the mean score of the standardization sample; 50th percentile). In a follow-up longitudinal study, Ballantyne, Spilkin, Hesselink, and Trauner (2008) reported comparable findings. As others have noted (Chilosi et al., 2005; Dall'Oglio, Bates, Volterra, Di Capua, & Pezzini, 1994), Ballantyne et al. found that the presence of seizures profoundly affected language outcomes; in fact, mean scores were more than 20 points lower for the seizure group, moving them into the severely impaired range.

MacWhinney et al. (2000) used several subtests from the CELF with a group of 14 children with PL; they noted that the children had particular difficulty with the subtests of

Formulating Sentences (expressive) and Oral Directions (receptive), performing more than one standard deviation below the mean for their age. In Formulating Sentences, the child is given one or two words and a picture and asked to make a sentence about the picture using the specified words. In Oral Directions, children are asked to perform actions on objects according to increasingly complex directions. In addition to language, both these subtests require using language to solve a problem. The standard scores for each subtest range from 0 to 20, with a mean of 10 and a standard deviation of 3. In MacWhinney et al.'s study of children with left hemisphere injury (LPL), their mean scores for the Formulated Sentences subtest was 5.8 (SD = 4.0), and the range was 3 to 17; the mean for the Oral Directions subtest was 6.4 (SD = 2.5), and the range was 3 to 11. In addition to the CELF, they also used the Peabody Picture Vocabulary test (PPVT-R) (Dunn & Dunn, 1981), a standardized receptive vocabulary test, and the Leiter International Performance Scale (Leiter, 1979) a nonverbal IQ test. Interestingly, the PL group (12 LPL and 2 RPL) scored well within the normal range on both these tests. In sum, on cumulative standardized language measures, for both receptive and productive language, school-age children and adolescents in the PL group perform below the mean performance level of the normative sample except on receptive vocabulary and nonverbal cognition. In addition, there is significant variability, which does not correlate with IQ or lesion site, but is consistently affected by the presence of seizures. Of note, the language tasks that cause difficulties for children with PL are complex tasks that require working memory and problem-solving skills.

The following sections discuss experimental studies of English morphology and syntax with the PL group. These complement the standardized measures by examining the subtleties of performance with particular morpho-syntactic structures. Often such results reveal patterns of strengths and deficits that may be masked in standardized tests.

Mastering the Morphology of English

Roger Brown (1973) described morphology as the "ivy in the brick wall." Grammatical morphology involves those small modulations of meaning that signal, for example, number (singular/plural) or tense (past, present progressive, future, etc.). For instance, the past tense in English is marked with the suffix *–ed* for regular verbs, such as *walk/walked* or *skip/skipped*, but for many common verbs, the past tense is irregular, as in *eat/ate, sing/sang,* or *bring/brought*. Around their second birthday, many children use these forms appropriately; however, subsequently they begin to make errors, as in *"I bringeded you some flowers"* or *"we holded the baby bunny."* These over-regularizations suggest that the child is acquiring rules for forming past tense, and these errors persist well into school age. As such, the English past tense has garnered a great deal of attention in the acquisition literature. Marchman et al. (2004) compared a group of 22 young children with PL (mean age 6.8 years) to their age-matched controls and children with Language Impairment on a past tense task. For the PL group, they found no differences in performance according to lesion site; moreover, the PL and typically developing groups performed comparably and better than the children with Language Impairment. Older children in both groups (PL and typically developing) made fewer errors than their younger counterparts, and, importantly, the PL and typically developing groups made similar error types. For both the PL and typically developing groups, receptive vocabulary (as measured by the PPVT) was correlated with morphological performance. As such, at this age, the trajectory of morphological development, as well as its relation to receptive vocabulary, is comparable in the PL group to that of their typically developing peers.

Another study looking at morphological development in children with PL focused on tag questions (Weckerly, Wulfeck, & Reilly, 2004). To elicit a confirmation, English speakers often attach a short question to the end of a statement: *John wants to go to the 6 o'clock movie,* ***doesn't he?*** Although these tag questions are short, they are morphologically challenging. They require the speaker to pronomonalize the subject (*John* to *he*), supply the appropriate auxiliary verb (*does*), reverse its valence (positive to negative in this case), and make the auxiliary verb agree in number with the pronoun (third person singular). As such, tag questions are an excellent mechanism to test morphological abilities without taxing semantics or other problem-solving skills. Adapting the tag task from Dennis et al. (1982), Weckerly et al. contrasted the performance of children and adolescents with PL with their age-matched peers and with children with Language Impairment (age range was 4–16 years). Overall, for the PL group, there were no right/left differences and the PL group performed better than those with Language Impairment. Looking at the rank order for acquiring the different morphological aspects of tags (agreement, auxiliary, polarity, and pronominalization), all three groups of children acquired the various parameters in the same order. These results suggest that they all use similar strategies to acquire English morphology despite recruiting different brain structures.

In Weckerly et al.'s study, for the overall scores (Fig. 8.1A), there were no group differences at the youngest age (4–7), and all the children did relatively poorly. In the middle groups (ages 8–11), the PL group did not differ significantly from controls, and the Language Impairment group was worse than either the typically developing or PL group. In the oldest group (ages 12–16), both the Language Impairment and PL groups performed worse than the TD group, suggesting that at this point in language development, the PL group is progressing at a slower rate than the controls. As the plateau in performance of the PL group does not reflect the lack of mastering a specific component of tag questions (Fig. 8.1B), these results appear to reflect decreased resources on the part of the PL group, as the oldest PL group performs much like the middle age group. These results represent one of the first experimental indications of limited resources for morpho-syntactic acquisition in children with PL as they move into adolescence.

Learning English Syntax

In English sentences, the basic word order is Subject—Verb—Object (or agent—action—experiencer); however, in passive sentences (e.g., *John was kissed by the baby*) the thematic roles are reversed as the experiencer (*John*) is pre-verbal, and the agent (*the baby*) is post-verbal. The canonical word order can also be disrupted in certain relative clause constructions (e.g., *The boy that the dog was chasing took his toy*). Studies of adults with agrammatic, conduction, and Wernicke's aphasias have noted that patients have particular trouble interpreting complex sentences, especially those in which word or thematic order is non-canonical or there is significant embedding (Blumstein, Goodglass, Statlender, & Biber, 1983). To investigate the degree to which such interpretive complexity affects children with PL, Eisele and Aram (1994) examined comprehension (performing actions with toys) and production (using imitation) of complex sentences in a group of children with perinatal stroke.

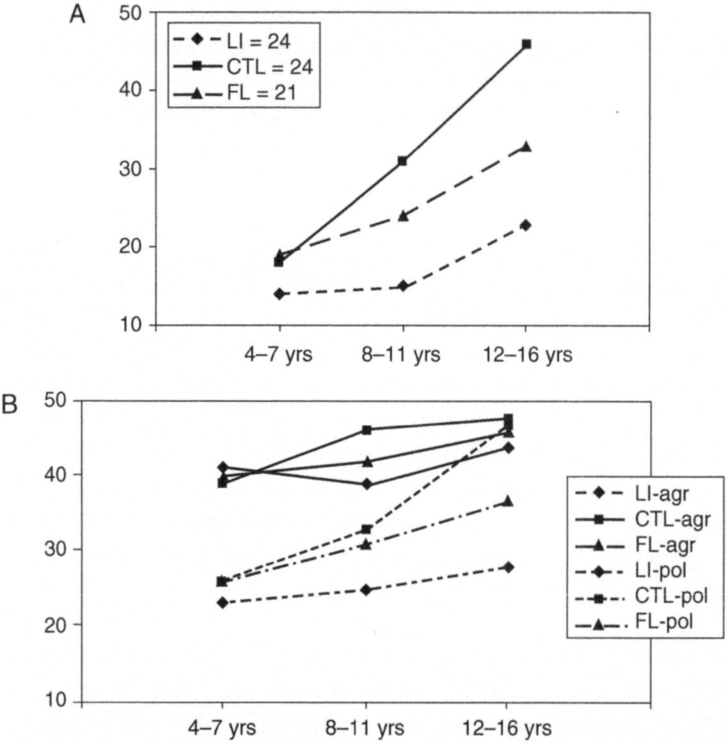

FIGURE 8.1 Tag questions. (A) Number of overall correct responses out of a total of 48 for the three groups of children and adolescents (LI, children with language impairment; CTL, controls; FL, children with perinatal lesions). Whereas those with LI are persistently below both the typically developing group and and those with PL, it is not until adolescence (age 12–16) that the PL group, as well as the LI group, is significantly below controls. (B) Correct responses for two aspects of tag questions: subject–verb agreement and polarity. Although all groups do relatively well with agreement, polarity is the last aspect of tag questions to be mastered; this profile is shared by all three groups of children. Considering the polarity findings, in the middle age group, the PL and typically developing participants are comparable; by adolescence, the oldest typically developing group is achieving 100%, but both the PL and LI older groups are significantly behind. (Reprinted with permission from Weckerly, Wulfeck, & Reilly, 2004.)

Their results provide information on the nature of later language development and deficits in children with PL. For the eight children with LPL, all were in the normal range for comprehension; that is, they could appropriately act out the sentence types comparably to age-matched peers. However, for the production task, five showed deficits in imitating the complex sentence types. There was no clear lesion site correlation. Of the three children with right hemisphere perinatal injury, one child was significantly below the norm for both comprehension and production, the second was in the normal range for comprehension but low on production, and the third performed like the control group. To summarize, overall we see variability with a tendency for a left hemisphere effect for production, but none for comprehension, and variable results for those with right hemisphere injury.

A comprehension study complementing these results was conducted by Feldman et al. (Feldman, MacWhinney, & Sacco, 2002). They gave children short sentences that varied in terms of word order and animacy, and then asked children to identify the agent of the action. For example, using canonical English word order (noun—verb—noun [NVN]), they used sentences such as, "The cow kicked the pencil" or "The pencil kicked the cow;" alternative orders included VNN or NNV, as in "The cat the bear kissed." They measured accuracy, strategy, and reaction time. They compared the performance of their PL group (12 LPL and 3 RPL) to a large control sample of children ages 5 to 10. Overall, the reaction times of the PL group were slower than controls, and all children with LPL and two of the three with RPL showed lower accuracy than the control group. They concluded that rather than a left hemisphere bias for language, their findings suggest that the deficits for both those with LPL and RPL reflect a smaller neural network for language processing in the PL group.

In addition to testing receptive and expressive language, another means of evaluating language knowledge is to ask children to make grammaticality judgments on grammatical and ungrammatical sentences. Reaction time studies can assess both grammatical sensitivity and temporal aspects of language processing. Studies of typically developing children have shown that with age, children become faster at integrating information, and reaction times decrease. Using a grammaticality judgment task, children listened to both grammatical and ungrammatical simple sentences and were asked to judge whether the sentences were "good" or "bad" grammar. The ungrammatical sentences included different types of violations (e.g., movement, omission, or substitution of both auxiliary verbs and determiners). The early study of typically developing children (Wulfeck, Bates, & Capasso, 1991) found that older children were more sensitive to violations than younger children, and that children were better at identifying word order violations than subject–verb agreement violations, unlike adults, who were sensitive to all violation types. Using the same test, Wulfeck et al. (2004) tested a group of school-age children with PL and compared them to both typically developing children and a group of children with Language Impairment. They reported no differences by side of lesion for the PL group. Like their typically developing peers, the children with PL were more sensitive to movement or word order violations than agreement violations. Further, while the grammatical sensitivity of the PL group was somewhat below the controls, their performance was well above chance and, like controls, they improved with age. With respect to reaction time, all groups improved with age, and there were no significant group differences between the PL and typically developing groups.

Using a similar approach, Dick, Wulfeck, Krupa-Kwiatkowski, and Bates (2004) tested school-age children and adults on their ability to interpret a variety of sentence types: those that maintain canonical word order (active: *The dog is biting the cat*; or subject cleft: *It is the dog that is biting the cat*) and those that do not (passive: *The cat is bitten by the dog*; or object cleft: *It is the cat that the dog is biting*). They also varied the subject–verb agreement (e.g., *It is the cat that the dogs are biting*). Children heard the sentences and saw pictures of the participating animals; they were asked to point to the agent of the action. In the above examples, the agent would be the dog(s). Similar to the majority of studies investigating morphology and syntax in the PL group, Dick et al. reported no significant differences in the RPL and LPL groups. Moreover, the overall PL performance was almost identical to that of the typically developing group on the active and subject cleft sentences. However, the PL group was significantly less accurate than the typically developing group with the non-canonical word orders, and their performance on object clefts was considerably worse than on passives. This profile was also reflected in their reaction times. A supplementary analysis comparing the PL group to the youngest controls (ages 5–7) showed no group differences. In line with others, these findings suggest that the PL group as a whole is approaching the language-learning task in a similar manner to typically developing children, but over an extended time course. Moreover, they appear to reflect the less mature profiles of younger children.

Together the behavioral studies of morpho-syntactic development indicate subtle impairments in the children with PL. Findings of a left hemisphere deficit for production in the early phases of language development appear to have resolved such that in processing complex language, the PL group overall is subtly behind their typically developing peers with no discernable hemispheric differences. However, we see development on all fronts with the older groups, as they consistently perform better than their younger counterparts, at least until adolescence, where there is some evidence of limitations on development in production. Overall, the findings suggest that language development is an extended process for typically developing children, and even more so for those with perinatal stroke. Interestingly, patterns of performance, as well as errors and error types in the PL group, are all reminiscent of younger typically developing children. These similarities imply that children with PL approach the language-learning process in a similar manner to their typically developing peers, despite differences in neural mediation. Thus, the process of language acquisition (in this case, English) is constrained: we do not see anomalous errors in the PL group or qualitatively different learning trajectories.

THE NEURAL CORRELATES OF LANGUAGE

The Neural Correlates of Language in Typically Developing Children

A logical question concerns the neural substrates of language in the PL group, and a number of studies have used functional magnetic resonance imaging (fMRI) for this purpose. fMRI provides an index of regional task-associated brain activity. It indirectly measures neural activity by detecting blood flow and blood oxygen extraction in brain regions where metabolic activity is enhanced, presumably because of engagement in the experimental task. To minimize movement artifacts, these studies typically employ tasks where the child silently generates his or her response, and the studies to date primarily include covert single word responses (but see Brown et al., 2005, for spoken responses). As such, these studies reflect lexical semantic rather than syntactic underpinnings of language; that is, they reflect a circumscribed aspect of language.

Before we review the studies from the PL group, it is important to consider the findings from typically developing children. There are now several cross-sectional and longitudinal functional imaging studies of language processing in typically developing children and adolescents. For example, Holland et al. (2001) used the verb generation task, which has shown strong left lateralization in adults (Petersen, Fox, Posner, Mintun, & Raichle, 1988). Using fMRI, 17 typically developing children and adolescents (ages 7–17 years) heard concrete nouns and were asked to covertly produce an associated verb (e.g., for the stimulus *ball*, the child would silently think of verbs such as *kick* or *throw*). Holland et al. reported that overall, the verb generation task showed left lateralized activity; however, they also found that the lateralization index (that is, the degree of left lateralization) increased with age, as did activation within Broca's area. Concurrently, they reported a complementary decrease in activation with age in the right hemisphere. As such, the younger children recruit the right hemisphere for this productive language task to a greater degree than the older adolescents, and left lateralization appears to be a developmental process. Consonant with these findings is a longitudinal study by Szaflarski et al. (2006). Also using a covert verb generation paradigm with a block design, Szaflarski et al. tested 30 typically developing children (ages 5, 6, and 7 years) at five consecutive annual data points (although not all children have the entire set). Complementing the results from Holland et al. (2001), they found increasing activation with age in the left inferior frontal gyrus (LIFG) and left middle frontal gyrus (LMFG), right lingual and inferior temporal gyri, the left medial temporal gyrus, and left angular gyrus. Concurrently, activation decreased with age in several regions: left posterior insula, left superior frontal gyrus, left thalamus, and right anterior cingulate gyrus. As children's lexical and semantic abilities develop over the school-age period, these studies show an increased recruitment of classic language areas and a concomitant decrease in recruitment of alternative areas that have been implicated in attention and task performance.

Other groups have used simpler lexical tasks. For example, Balsamo et al. (2006) used a semantic decision task that required children to decide whether the presented stimulus was a word or not. In their study of typically developing 5- to 10-year-old children, they found strong activation in the left hemisphere. Similar to the adult pattern, areas activated included the left inferior frontal gyrus, left middle temporal gyrus, and, unexpectedly, the left fusiform gyrus (LFG). Interestingly, rather than age, activation of the dorsolateral prefrontal cortex and activation of the LFG were correlated with task accuracy. Similarly, Gaillard et al. (2003) asked children (ages 7–14) and adults to silently generate exemplars of particular categories (e.g., animals, furniture, food). They found no appreciable differences in activation sites between the child and adult groups. Activation was found in the left inferior gyrus (IFG) and middle frontal gyrus (MFG) as well as medial frontal areas including sensory motor areas, thalamus, and left parietal lobe. However, the extent of activation, especially in the left IFG and MFG, was significantly greater in the adult than in the child group. Gaillard et al. suggested that producing single words by category is strongly lateralized by age 7. How might this apparent conflict regarding lateralization be resolved?

The answer may lie in development; that is, just as different aspects of language emerge at different ages, it may well be that earlier-emerging language skills lateralize to the left hemisphere earlier in development than later-developing skills. The ideal solution would be to test 2- and 3-year-olds, just as the target linguistic skills come online, and follow neural activation patterns for particular skills as they develop. However, fMRI requires children to follow directions and to lie very still, two skills absent from a toddler's repertoire. An alternative strategy would be to compare the degree of lateralization to the classic language areas (Broca's and Wernicke's areas) in tasks tapping both early-developing (e.g., labeling) and later-developing (e.g., verb generation) aspects of language in school-age children. One pertinent study is that by Schmithorst et al. (2007), who gave 283 typically developing school-age children and adolescents (ages 7–18) a picture matching task. The children saw two pictures, and as they heard a word, they pressed either a right or left button to indicate the picture with which this word was associated. Whereas activation in areas associated with processing objects (ventral visual pathway) increased with age, there was no significant change in activation patterns in those regions reflecting left hemisphere lateralization (e.g., the left inferior and middle frontal regions, left middle temporal, medial frontal, and angular gyri). Such findings are consonant with those of Gaillard and suggest that such functions as word–picture labeling are already lateralized by age 7. One additional study that sheds light on the developmental changes children's brains undergo is that by Brown et al. (2005). They conducted three lexical semantic tasks using an event-related design with 95 participants (ages 7–32 years): rhyming, verb generation, and antonym production. Subjects produced their responses aloud. The event-related design and overt responses permitted an analysis of task performance and the possibility of identifying changes associated with age, independent of performance. They found systematic changes with age even when comparing children and adults who performed comparably: left frontal regions demonstrated the greatest increases in activation (they "grew up" [i.e., progressive development]), while right frontal regions showed the most significant decreases in activation (they "grew down" [i.e., regressive development]). Outside frontal regions, developmental changes included an overall decrease in activation. Brown's findings help illustrate the developmental process of increased left lateralization for lexical association tasks, characterizing functional neural development as comprising both progressive and regressive processes. Also, by using overt verbal responses and controlling for subject performance accuracies and response times, this study was able to dissociate age-related effects in activation from those driven by differences in task performance.

Complementing the lexical tasks, a recent study by Nunez et al. (2011) used structural and functional imaging techniques to investigate the developing neural correlates of semantic and syntactic processing in typically developing children ages 7 to 15. In both tasks the children heard two sentences and were asked if the two sentences "mean the same." In the semantic condition, one word was replaced with a synonym, and in the syntactic condition, word order was varied. However, both tasks required semantic evaluations. With respect to structural changes, they found that with age, the thickness of the right pars triangularis increased with a concomitant decrease in activation of the right IFG. They also report an increased activation of the left IFG correlated with syntactic performance, independent of age; such findings suggest that children with more advanced syntactic/semantic skills show more left lateralization for these language tasks. Finally, a study by Saccumen et al. (2006) used fMRI to investigate the neural underpinnings of sentence comprehension by employing the same stimuli as the Dick et al. study above. Consistent with developmental studies of verb generation, in their typically developing group of adolescents, they found activation in both the right and left IFG and superior temporal regions as illustrated in Figure 8.2. In contrast, the adult activation is strongly left lateralized.

In summary, lexical and sentential neuroimaging studies in typically developing children show bilateral activation with increasing lateralization to the left hemisphere with age and increased language proficiency; they also show concomitant decreasing participation of the right hemisphere. This dynamic profile of development for left lateralization of language processing extends well into adolescence and reflects both progressive and regressive processes.

The Neural Correlates of Language in Children with Perinatal Stroke

This brief overview of the imaging studies of typically developing children will help in interpreting and contextualizing the findings from the children with PL. Early studies, for example by Muller et al. (1999), used PET and concluded that the right hemisphere had assumed language functions for children with left hemisphere injury. Staudt et al. (2002) used fMRI to investigate lexical skills in five young adults who had perinatal left periventricular lesions.

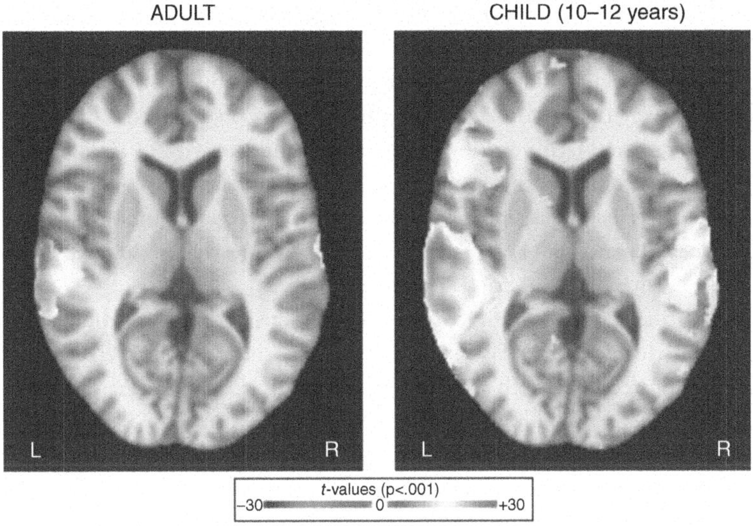

FIGURE. 8.2 Activation for adults and 10-year old children on a complex sentence comprehension task. Adults show strongly left lateralized activation in superior temporal regions typically associated with language comprehension. By contrast, children show significant bilateral activation of superior temporal regions; in addition they activate more anterior inferior frontal regions that are typically associated with productive language in adults. Thus children show activation of the extended left hemisphere language network, and in addition recruit homologous regions of the right hemisphere. (Adapted with permission from Saccumen et al. 2006.) (See color insert.)

They administered a word chain task wherein the participant silently generates a word that begins with the letter that terminated the previous word (e.g., *cat/top/pot/tape*). Overall, in the group comparisons, they found maximum activation in the left IFG (Broca's area) for controls and comparable activation in the right IFG (Broca's homologue) in the patient group. They interpreted their findings as suggesting that language had organized to the right hemisphere. However, they also reported activation in the left hemisphere for some participants in the LPL group. Other neuroimaging studies with children with perinatal left hemisphere lesions have used a verb generation task (Jacola et al., 2006; Liegeois, Connelly, Cross, Vargha-Khadem, & Baldeweg, 2004; Tillema et al., 2008). Overall, they have reported activation in the right homologue of Broca's area, as well as activation in the left hemisphere for some patients. One comparatively large study by Raja Beharelle et al. (2010) tested 25 participants with perinatal left hemisphere injury ranging in age from 7 to 29 years and their healthy siblings. Performance on a battery of standardized measures including the PPVT, Expressive Vocabulary Test (Williams, 1997), category fluency, and the CELF was correlated with brain activation on a covert category fluency task administered in the scanner. The PL group performed within the published norms on the standardized tests but below the level of their sibling controls. Lateralization indices were computed from brain areas activated during the fluency task. The typically developing siblings showed the expected left hemisphere lateralization for the fluency test both in the anterior and posterior regions. In contrast, the patient group overall showed more of a right lateralized pattern of activity in anterior regions and bilateral activity posteriorly. However, in anterior regions, increased lateralization to the left hemisphere correlated with higher global language scores in the LPL group. For posterior regions, they found a curvilinear relation, with more bilateral activation correlating with better language scores. Such findings suggest that having some residual function in the left hemisphere enhances language performance. These findings are congruent with those of Liegeois et al., Tillema et al., and Jacola et al., who also imaged children with PL during a silent verb generation task. The results of these studies suggest two alternative possibilities: (1) There is a left hemisphere bias for language, and thus, those who have access to these regions show better language performance; or (2) It may be an issue of volume; that is, language performance may be better when more tissue can be recruited.

Another pertinent study investigated right hemisphere activation in school-age children (7–12 years) with left perinatal stroke compared to a large control group (Fair et al., 2009). By using an event-related fMRI verb generation task and overt responses (similar to the study with typically developing children by Brown et al.) they were able to examine performance accuracy and individual patterns of right hemisphere activation in the children with LPL. In the group comparisons (typically developing vs. LPL) they found no statistical differences in right hemisphere activation. However, in considering correct responses and individual performance, the children with LPL recruited more areas within the right hemisphere, and interestingly, these right hemisphere regions varied by individual. This study is important as these findings enhance our understanding of how the injured brain develops alternative organizations to support language functions.

One of the few studies looking at the neural correlates of complex syntax comprehension in the PL group is that by Saccumen et al. (2006) mentioned above. Again, using the same sentential stimuli as in the Dick et al. (2004) study, Saccumen et al. had adolescents with PL perform this sentence comprehension task in the magnet. Looking at the results from this imaging study, they reported that patients with left hemisphere injury showed more right hemisphere activation, but all had some left hemisphere activity, including tissue adjacent to the lesion as is illustrated in Figure 8.3.

Similar to the findings of Staudt et al. (2002), Jacola et al. (2006), Tillema et al. (2008), and Raja Beharelle et al. (2010), these results are consistent with a "soft" left hemisphere bias for language, or the possibility that increased tissue activation enhances performance.

Examining the results from imaging studies in the PL group in the context of studies from typically developing children presents a somewhat different picture of neural organization for language than the simple right hemisphere homologue model implies. In the wake of early injury there appear to be multiple paths to developing the neural substrate for language processing. For the majority of children with LPL, bilateral organization that recruits both residual left hemisphere tissue as well as right hemisphere brain regions appears to provide the optimal outcome. Data from typically developing children provide an interesting model of how this distributed neural system might arise following early brain injury. Imaging studies of typically developing children show that early in development children recruit a more distributed, bilateral system for many language tasks. With development and mastery of different aspects of language, those systems become increasingly left lateralized and activation localizes to areas associated with mature language processing. Injury may preclude the normal progression to the left lateralized profile; rather, elements of the earlier, less mature bilateral patterns of brain organization stabilize and are retained. The result is a functional, though not ideal, neurobehavioral system for language following early brain injury.

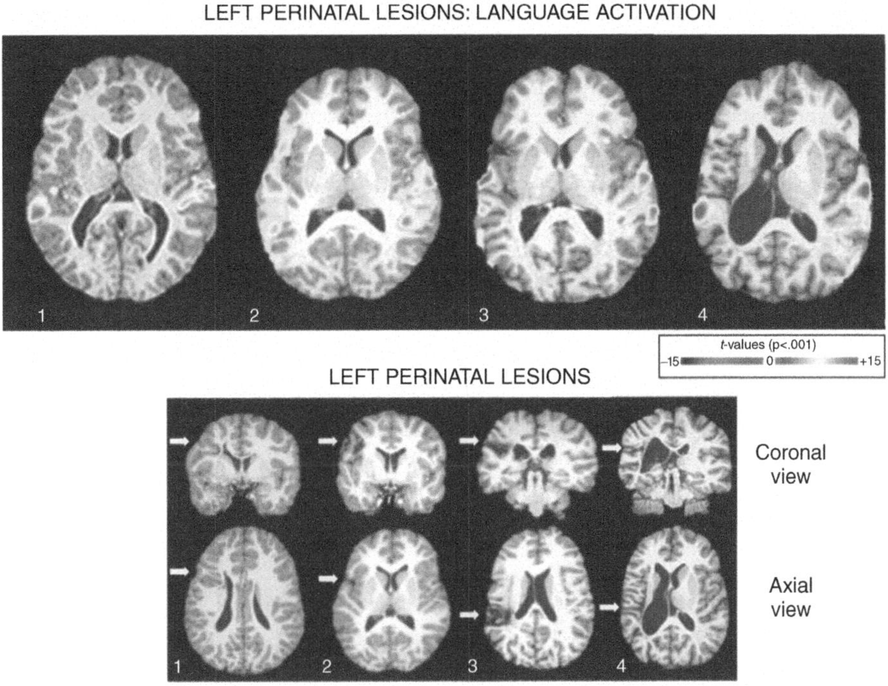

FIGURE 8.3 Activation for adolescent patients with left PL on a sentence comprehension task. Patients with left PL show strong activation in the typical left hemisphere language areas in inferior frontal and superior temporal brain regions, recruiting spared tissue in the vicinity of the lesion. They also recruit homologous regions of the right hemisphere. This pattern of activation is similar to the patterns reported for younger typically developing children. Such data suggest that following a perinatal stroke, immature, but largely typical, language networks stabilize and come to support mature language functions. (Adapted with permission from Saccumen et al. 2006.) (See color insert.)

A CAUTIONARY NOTE

While these first imaging studies of children with PL are indeed exciting, it is important to be cautious in interpreting them. As noted above, when considering the neural underpinnings of language in the PL group, especially those with LPL, the findings and interpretations are mixed. There are those who propose a "reorganization" with the right hemisphere assuming language functioning (e.g., Staudt et al., 2002) and others who have shown that language performance is best in those with left activation in the anterior regions, despite left hemisphere injury (Raja Beharelle et al., 2010), suggesting either a "soft" left hemisphere bias for language, or that the increased network that includes additional tissue (of the left hemisphere) yields better performance. We are not yet at a point where we can test these competing hypotheses. Additional limitations to the currently available studies include small sample sizes—for instance, three children (Guzzetta et al., 2008; Jacola et al., 2006) who vary widely in age (7 to adult), performing tasks that are covert and that ask for single-word responses. Especially with children, it is difficult to know whether they are complying as they lie in the magnet. Moreover, only one fMRI study with patients with PL has correlated activation during imaging with broader behavioral measures of language performance (Raja Beharelle et al., 2010); this was a cross-sectional study with participants from a broad age spectrum (ages 7–29 years). In addition, the vast majority of pediatric imaging studies require only single-word responses; thus, they are testing lexical semantics rather than morphology and syntax. Finally, because fMRI demands that children lie very still, it is not amenable for young children who are just beginning to acquire syntax. It is also important to keep in mind that the recent large-scale studies using these same paradigms (e.g., verb generation) in typically developing children (e.g., Brown et al., 2005, Holland et al., 2001; Ressel, Wilke, Lidzba, Lutzenberger, & Krageloh-Mann, 2008; Szaflarski et al., 2006) have shown a gradual lateralization of language function to the left hemisphere that reaches adult profiles only in adolescence. Thus, lateralization for language is a developmental process, and, to date, we do not yet have longitudinal imaging studies on the PL group, nor do we have sufficient studies that directly test syntactic abilities in either typically developing children or those with perinatal stroke. We are just beginning to understand the neural underpinnings of language development in typically developing children and have just scratched the surface for the PL group; there remain many important questions for future studies.

DISCOURSE: COMBINING SENTENCES FOR SPECIFIC DISCOURSE PURPOSES

By age 4-5, TD children are producing the majority of the grammatical structures of their language. Language development after age 5, in addition to an expanding vocabulary, reflects the increasingly flexible use of vocabulary and grammatical structures for different discourse genres. A conversation, where turns alternate between two speakers, is the first discourse genre in which children participate. In fact, before they even begin to talk, infants can take turns in a dyadic interaction with a partner (e.g., rolling a ball back and forth). In a conversation, however, one needs to understand that a particular topic is under discussion, that a question needs to be answered, and that the content of the answer is dictated by the semantics of the question.

Studies of adults with right hemisphere strokes have found that the right hemisphere plays a role in pragmatics, or how language is used in social contexts. Right hemisphere patients can have difficulty in certain discourse situations (e.g., Joanette & Brownell, 1989). For example, there are cases in which the responses to questions from right hemisphere patients are not relevant to the topic or question. Other studies have found a marked volubility in right hemisphere patients (Bates, Reilly, Wulfeck, Dronkers, Opie, Fenson, 2001); still others (Gardner, Brownell, Wapner, & Micheow, 1983) have shown that adults with injury to the right hemisphere often have difficulty with non-literal language (e.g., humor, metaphor, and sarcasm). Additional pragmatic impairments that characterize patients with right hemisphere injury acquired during adulthood are their difficulties with discourse cohesion and coherence (e.g., running on, failing to convey the point or "gist" of a story and using pronouns without referents).

Conversations with Children with PL

To look at conversational skills, Bates et al. (2001) used a biographical interview to compare spontaneous conversations in children with PL (ages 5–8) to those of adults with homologous lesions. The semi-structured interviews included age-appropriate questions, for example about family, friends, pets, and television preferences. Bates et al. reported that the 21 adults with acquired strokes displayed the predicted profile of lesion-specific deficit: those adults with left hemisphere injury who were severely aphasic showed low syntactic diversity, increased omissions, and a high incidence of morphological errors; lexical substitutions and neologisms characterized the Wernicke's aphasics. The three non-aphasic patients with left hemisphere lesions and those with right hemisphere lesions were garrulous and produced twice as many propositions as controls. Overall, their speech was relatively empty and disinhibited. In contrast, the spontaneous language of children with PL was comparable to typically developing children in terms of mastery of English morphology and the frequency of recruiting complex sentences (Fig. 8.4). Thus, the earlier site-specific differences reported by Bates et al. (1997) appeared to have resolved by age 5 to 8; additionally with respect to the measures of morpho-syntax, the PL group was performing comparably to their age-matched, typically developing peers in this conversational context.

One aspect of discourse that has been noted to be challenging for adults with right hemisphere injury is that of discourse cohesion, and one marker of cohesion is the successful use of pronouns. Anaphora is using a pronoun to refer to a preceding noun phrase and thus links utterances, rendering the discourse more cohesive (Halliday & Hasan, 1976). For example, in the sentence "James likes to cook and he often hosts dinner parties" the pronoun *he* in the second clause is an anaphoric reference to James. Dardier et al. (2005) used the same biographical interview data evaluated by Bates et al. (2001) to investigate the children's use of anaphora. They found that both the typically developing children and those with PL used many pronouns for which the referent was ambiguous. However, they also reported that in the younger group (ages 5 and 6) the children with RPL used significantly more ambiguous pronouns than either typically developing children or those with LPL. Looking at the older group (7 and 8 years), there were no longer differences, and both the LPL and RPL groups performed in the normal range. Together these two studies suggest that in this everyday situation of conversation, by age 7 to 8, the PL group develops a functional command of the morphology and syntax of English that is comparable to typically developing children. However, the data on anaphora suggest that, similar to adults, the right hemisphere may mediate how children learn to successfully deploy these structures for discourse purposes. Unlike adults, however, the difficulties of children with RPL appear to be transitory and resolve by 7 to 8 years of age. In the next section we look at a more challenging discourse context, the narrative, to investigate how discourse context might influence a child's spoken language abilities.

Narratives in Children with PL

To tell a story, speakers not only must have a command of the grammar, but also must organize their utterances in a logical manner to convey a coherent and meaningful narrative. Reilly et al. (Reilly, Bates, & Marchman, 1998; Reilly et al., 2004) asked children to tell a story as they looked through the wordless picture book *Frog, Where Are You?* (Mayer, 1969). This is a traditional "quest" story: a boy has caught a frog that escapes during the night. The subsequent adventures of the boy in his search for the frog make up the story. Although children as young as age 2 have some idea of a story (Appleby, 1978), it is not until age 4 to 5 that children begin to produce monologic narratives (when the child can tell the story by himself or herself), and

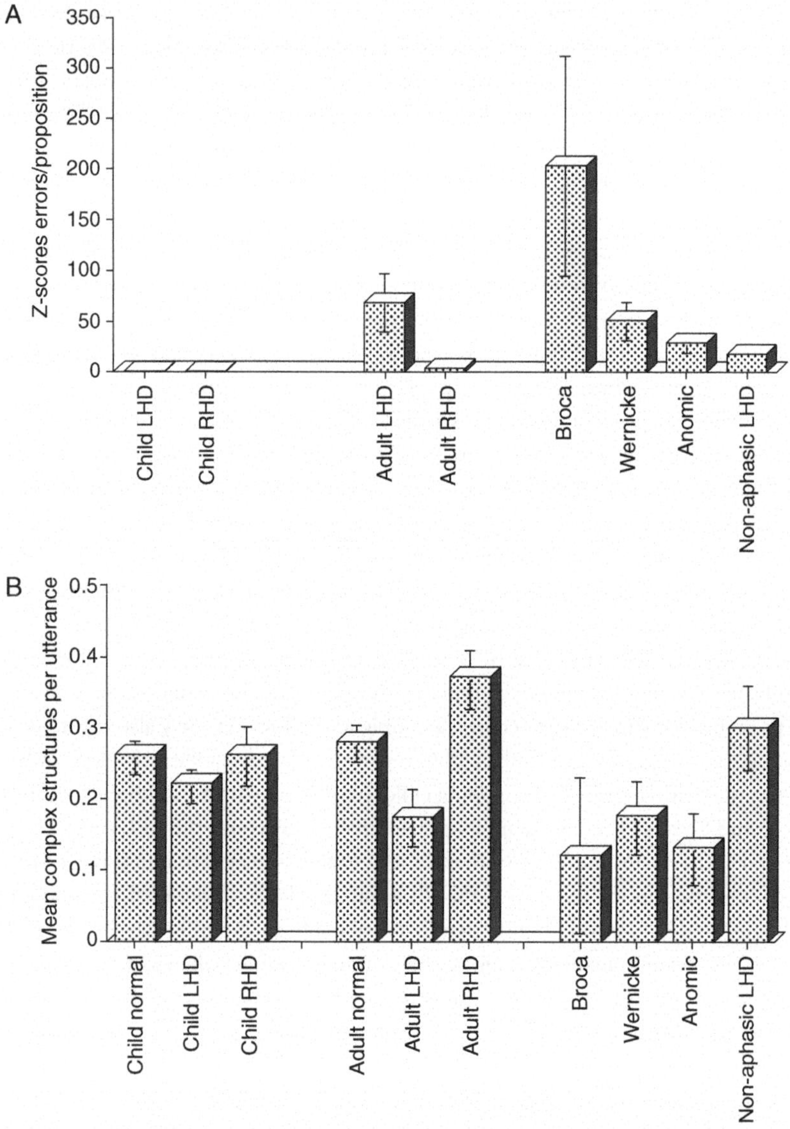

FIGURE 8.4 Grammatical performance in children and adults. (A) Z-scores for the proportion of errors by propositions. The LPL and RPL groups are comparable to typically developing age-matched children. In contrast, adults with left hemisphere injury (LHD) make more errors than either typically developing adults or those with right hemisphere injury (RHD). (B) Mean number of complex sentences over the total number of propositions. Children with PL (both left and right) use amounts comparable to the typically developing child group. Adults with left hemisphere injury use fewer than neurologically healthy adults, whereas adults with right hemisphere injury use more complex structures, reflecting their disinhibited style of conversation. (Reprinted with permission from Bates et al., 2001.)

these stories tend to reflect a horizontally linked sequence of events, using *and* or *and then,* to connect the individual actions). By age 8, typically developing children relate stories reflecting a multilevel organization, where individual episodes are linked to the overarching goal (e.g., finding the frog).

In the *Frog* narratives from the children with PL, there was no effect of lesion site, but overall, their spoken stories were shorter than those of controls. Further, in the younger group (ages 4–6 years), the PL group used proportionally fewer complex sentences and made more grammatical errors than their age-matched controls. This profile contrasts with the biographical interview data discussed above. The findings suggest that for the PL group, morphology is still vulnerable in this age range. The added cognitive demands of telling a story appear to exact a price. In examining the children's errors, Reilly et al. commented that the grammatical errors of the children with PL were similar in type to those of younger typically developing children. In line with other studies of the PL group, these data confirm the notion that although on an extended timescale, language acquisition in the PL group follows a similar path to the typically developing group. In the oldest group of children (age 10–12), the performance of the PL group was still below the level of controls, but in the low normal range for both grammatical and narrative measures (e.g., number of episodes, reiteration of the narrative theme). Further, a qualitative evaluation that categorized 20 stories as good, medium, or bad on the basis of such aspects as plot, elaboration, coherence, and theme revealed a clear separation of the groups. At age 6 and 7 years, all but one story in the top category came from controls, and all but one in the lowest category came from the PL group. Despite their continued development in morphology and syntax, this PL group fell behind their age-matched controls for both narrative and grammatical aspects of storytelling.

Although no side-specific differences were found in the morpho-syntactic measures, there was a trend reflecting less frequent use of complex sentences in those with RPL than those with LPL (Reilly et al., 1998). One function of complex sentences in a narrative is to link the episodes of the story (e.g., "*when the boy was sleeping,* the frog escaped!"), or to integrate the local event with the theme or goal of the narrative, searching for the lost frog (e.g., "he looked in the hole *to try and find his frog*"). It is likely that the decreased use of complex syntax in narratives reflects an impairment in the use of language for discourse cohesion. A follow-up longitudinal study of 16 PL children at four data points (ages 4–14) confirms that those with RPL continue to use proportionally fewer complex sentences than either those with LPL or controls (Reilly, Stiles & Appelbaum, 2009), as seen in Figure 8.5. This profile is reminiscent of that of adults with right hemisphere injury and suggests that the right hemisphere plays a significant role in discourse integration. That this profile comes to light in the narrative but not in conversational contexts (Bates et al., 2001) suggests that this particular deficit is revealed only in linguistic situations that are challenging for the child.

Another narrative study with a different group of PL children was conducted by Demir, Levine, and Goldin-Meadow (2010). They too were interested in whether the plasticity exhibited by children with PL for earlier-developing aspects of language would extend to more complex, later-developing language functions such as narrative production. They asked 5- and 6-year-olds to generate stories from story stems; they also used standardized tests to evaluate vocabulary and syntax. The results of the standardized tests showed that the PL group did not differ from controls on either vocabulary (as measured by the PPVT) or syntax (as measured by the CELF). However, in the narratives, the children with PL performed worse than the

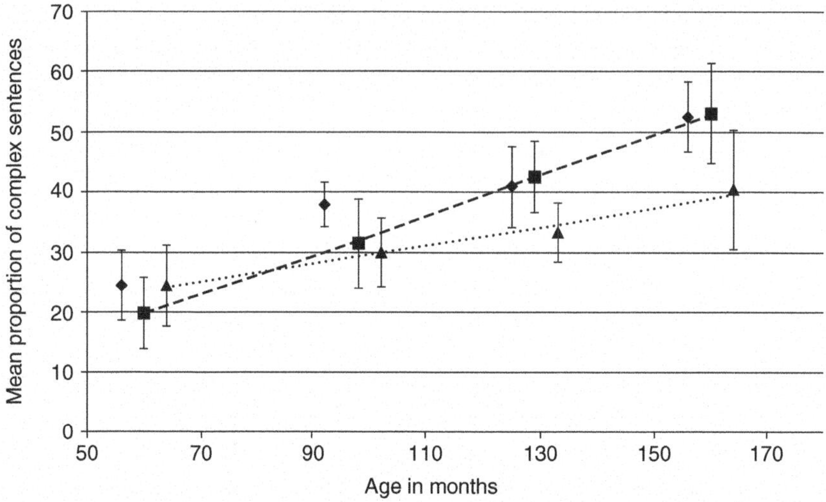

FIGURE 8.5 Frequency of complex sentences in *Frog* stories. The cross-sectional data for typically developing children (diamond shapes) suggests a not-unexpected general increase with age in the use of complex syntax. The longitudinal data of children with right and left hemisphere injury display decidedly different growth trajectories, with the growth in the use of complex syntax being much more rapid for those with LPL (squares) than for those with RPL (triangles). Further, while those with either RPL or LPL initially produce complex syntax at a level below that of typically developing children, those with left hemisphere injury are using complex sentences as frequently as the controls by the third age point, whereas those with right hemisphere injury do not. Recall that the use of complex sentences is a rhetorical choice. We can tell stories using all simple sentences and it is grammatical, but perhaps less efficient. If we think about the function of complex sentences in a narrative, they serve to linguistically integrate the events and to explicitly label the relationship between those events. As such, they are a linguistic tool to create a cohesive narrative. The less frequent recruitment of such structures by those with right hemisphere injury subtly reflects the profile reported in adults with acquired right hemisphere strokes. (Reilly, Stiles & Appelbaum, 2009.)

typically developing group on various narrative measures, including narrative length (the number of utterances), syntax (the number of subordinate clauses), vocabulary (the number of word types), and narrative complexity (as measured by a scale of story structure scores developed by Stein & Glenn, 1979). There were no effects of lesion size, type, or side. These results mirror those of the narrative studies from Reilly et al. previously mentioned in terms of language and narrative performance: children in this younger age group are still struggling with language in the narrative context as well as with telling stories with mature narrative structure, notably stories that have goals. It is important to note that in the Demir et al. study (2010) the vocabulary and syntax of the PL group was comparable to their typically developing controls on standardized tests, outside the narrative. However, measuring these same linguistic skills within the narrative, the performance of the PL group was lower than the typically developing group. These contrasting results again point to the critical role of discourse context in language performance. They also suggest that to understand the language profile of children with PL, and other children with language problems, it is important to examine their language skills in various contexts. For the PL group, it appears that the increased challenge of creating a story diminishes their linguistic performance. These results may stem from a particular vulnerability of language skills in the children with early brain injury or from a more general impact of diminished neural resources on the performance of complex, demanding tasks.

Recent work has examined the role of input in the development of children's narrative abilities. Data from the Chicago Longitudinal Language Study indicates that the narrative skills of children with PL assessed at ages 5 to 6 years are more highly related to parents' earlier talk about the past and the future at an earlier age (assessed during naturalistic interactions at 30 months) than is the case for typically developing children. Again, as for other aspects of cognition and language, robust input may be even more important for the development of the narrative skills of children with early brain injury than it is for typically developing children.

One of the most striking aspects of language development in the PL group has been the remarkable plasticity for language during the earlier stages of language learning. However, we know little regarding the extent and nature of this plasticity in the later stages of language development. To address this issue, Reilly, Wasserman, and Appelbaum (submitted) examined personal narratives of 7- to 16-year-old children with PL. In this situation, the participants were asked to tell about a time when someone had made them sad or angry. Their results differ somewhat from previous studies in that those with right hemisphere injury generally perform closer to the TD group (except for using complex sentences); however, those with left hemisphere injury use less complex syntax and fewer syntactic types, make more morphological errors, and have more impoverished story settings than controls. Similar to the findings of Demir et al. (2010), these results suggest that despite their good progress in acquiring the structures of language, as the task becomes more difficult, subtle linguistic deficits reappear. In this case, the findings suggest that those with RPL continue to show a slight integrative deficit, as indexed by their decreased use of complex syntax, and those with LPL are more challenged in both morphology and syntax, echoing the earliest linguistic profiles for these children. And finally, with the added challenge of structuring a personal story with emotional content, this more complex discourse task begins to reveal possible constraints on neuroplasticity for language.

Conclusions

In summary, children with PL do surprisingly well in acquiring the grammatical structures of their language, although there is enormous variability in their performance throughout development. Initially, there is delay in children with *either* RPL or LPL. However, once children begin to acquire language, the language structures emerge following the same patterns evident in typically developing children. Unlike adults with homologous damage, early site-specific deficits appear to resolve, and, by mid-school age, the group with PL performs in the low normal range in spontaneous speech. But language acquisition is not just a matter of "catching up"; rather, at each new level of linguistic challenge, there is initial delay and subsequent development in mastering grammatical structures. With respect to how the children with PL are acquiring language, the few imaging studies suggest that for those with LPL, patterns of activation that include the right and the left hemisphere as well are more supportive of strong language functioning. This bilateral pattern of activation shares similarities with younger typically developing children. Regarding pragmatics, or how the group with PL uses language, there is emerging evidence that the right hemisphere may play a role early on in integrating discourse; children with right hemisphere injury mirror the profile of adults with similar injury, but in a subtler manner, and those with left hemisphere injury show increased morpho-syntactic deficits as the task difficulty increases. These findings suggest that there may well be "soft" biases for particular language functions that are similar to the adult model, but they are markedly more subtle in the children with PL. Further, similar to the acquisition of linguistic structures, in pragmatic development, there is evidence of an iterative profile wherein early deficits resolve with age to again be revealed in more challenging discourse contexts. Finally, robust input may be particularly important for the development of complex language skills in children with PL as syntactic and narrative skills are more strongly related to input variations in children with perinatal stroke than is the case for typically developing children.

REFERENCES

Appleby A. (1978). The Child's Concept of Story. Chicago: University of Chicago Press.

Ballantyne AO, Spilkin AM, Trauner DA. (2007). Language outcome after perinatal stroke: Does side matter? *Child Neuropsychol* 13(6):494–509.

Ballantyne A, Spilkin AM, Hesselink J, Trauner D. (2008). Plasticity in the developing brain: Intellectual, language and academic functions in children with ischaemic perinatal stroke. *Brain* 131(11):2975–2985.

Balsamo LM, Xu B, Gaillard WD. (2006). Language lateralization and the role of the fusiform gyrus in semantic processing in young children. *NeuroImage* 31(3):1306–1314.

Bates E, Reilly J, Wulfeck B, Dronkers N, Opie N, Fenson J. (2001). Differential effects of unilateral lesions on language production in children and adult. *Brain and Language* 79(2):223–265.

Bates E, Thal D, Trauner D, Fenson J, Aram D, Eisele J, Nass R. (1997). From first words to grammar in children with focal brain injury. *Special Issue on Origins of Communication Disorders. Dev Neurol* 13(3):275–343.

Binder JR, Desai RH, Graves WW, Conant LL. (2009). Where is the semantic system? A critical review and meta analysis of 120 functional neuroimaging studies. *Cerebral Cortex [e-pub March 27].*

Blumstein SE, Goodglass H, Statlender S, Biber C. (1983). Comprehension strategies determining reference in aphasia: A study of reflexivization. *Brain and Language* 18(1):115–127.

Bookheimer S. (2002). Functional MRI of language: new approaches to understanding the cortical organization of semantic processing. *Annu Rev Neurosci* 25 151–188. doi: 10.1146/annurev.neuro.25.112701.142946

Brauer J, Anwander A, Friederici AD. (2011). Neuroanatomical prerequisites for language functions in the maturing brain. *Cerebral Cortex* 21(2):459–466. doi: 10.1093/cercor/bhq108

Brown R. (1973). A First Language: The Early Stages. Cambridge, MA: Harvard University Press.

Brown TT, Lugar HM, Coalson RS, Miezin FM, Petersen SE, Schlaggar BL. (2005). Developmental changes in human cerebral functional organization for word generation. *Cerebral Cortex* 15(3):275–290. doi: 10.1093/cercor/bhh129

Caselli MC, Casadio P. (1995). Il primo vocabolario del bambino: guida all'uso del questionario MacArthur per la valutazione della comunicazione e del linguaggio nei primi anni di vita (The child's first words: guide for the use of the MacArthur questionnaire for assessing communication and language in the first years of life). Milan: FrancoAngeli.

Caselli MC, Devescovi A, Marchione D, Pasqualetti P, Reilly J, Bates E. (2005). A cross-linguistic study of the relationship between grammar and lexical development. *J Child Language* 32:759–786.

Chilosi AM, Cipriani P, Bertuccelli B, Pfanner PL, Cioni G. (2001). Early cognitive and communication development in children with focal brain lesions. *J Child Neurol* 16:309–316.

Chilosi AM, Cipriani P, Brovedani P, Brizzolara D, Ferretti G, Pfanner PL. (2005). Atypical language lateralization and early linguistic development in children with focal brain lesions. *Dev Med Child Neurol* 47:725–730.

Dale PS, Bates E, Reznick JS, Morisset C. (1989). The validity of a parent report instrument of child language at twenty months. *J Child Language* 16:239–249.

Dall'Oglio AM, Bates E, Volterra V, Di Capua M, Pezzini G. (1994). Early cognition, communication and language in children with focal brain injury. *Dev Med Child Neurol* 36: 1076–1098.

Dardier V, Reilly J, Bates E, Delaye C, Laurent-Vannier A. (2005). La cohesion du discours de chez les enfants et les adolescents cerbroleses: Analyse de l'usage des prnoms et des connecteurs. Cashiers d'*acquisition et pathologie du Langage* 101–114.

de Villiers JG, de Villiers PA. (1973). A cross-sectional study of the acquisition of grammatical morphemes in child speech. *J Psycholinguistic Res* 2(3):267–278.

Demir OE, Levine SC, Goldin-Meadow S. (2010). Narrative skill in children with early unilateral brain injury: A possible limit to functional plasticity. *Dev Sci* 13(4):636–647.

Dennis M, Sugar J, Witaker HA. (1982). The acquisition of tag questions. *Child Dev* 53(5): 1254–1257.

Dick F, Wulfeck B, Krupa-Kwiatkowski M, Bates E. (2004). The development of complex sentence interpretation in typically developing children compared with children with specific language impairments or early unilateral focal lesions. *Dev Sci* 7(3):360–377.

Dunn LM, Dunn LM. (1981). Peabody Picture Vocabulary Test (Rev. ed.). Circle Pines, MN: American Guidance Service.

Eisele J, Aram D. (1994). Comprehension and imitation of syntax following early hemisphere damage. *Brain and Language* 46:212–231.

Fair DA, Choi AH, Dosenback YB, Coalson RS, Miezin FM, Petersen SE, Schlaggar BL. (2009). The functional organization of trial-related activity in lexical processing after early left hemispheric brain lesions: An event-related fMRI study. *Brain Language* 114(2):135–146.

Feldman HM. (1994). Language development after early brain injury: A replication study. In Tager-Flusberg H (Ed.), Constraints on Language Acquisition: Studies of Atypical Children (pp. 75–90). Hillsdale, NJ: Lawrence Erlbaum.

Feldman HM. (2005). Language learning with an injured brain. *Language Learning and Development* 1(3 4):89–102.

Feldman HM, Holland AL, Kemp SS, Janosky JE. (1992). Language development after unilateral brain injury *Brain and Language* 42:89–102.

Feldman HM, MacWhinney B, Sacco K. (2002). Sentence processing in children with early unilateral brain injury. *Brain Language* 83(2):335–352.

Fenson LD, Dale P, Reznick JS, Thal D, Bates E, Hartung J, . . . Reilly J. (1993). MacArthur–Bates Communicative Development Inventories. San Diego, CA: Singular.

Fenson LD, Dale PS, Reznick JS, Bates E, Thal D, Pethick S. (1994). Variability in early communicative development. *Monographs of the Society for Research in Child Development* 59(5):1–173.

Gaillard WD, Sachs BC, Whitnah JR. (2003). Developmental aspects of language processing: fMRI of verbal fluency in children and adults. *Hum Brain Mapp* 18:176–185.

Gardner H, Brownell H, Wapner W, Micheow D. (1983). Missing the point: The role of the right hemisphere in the processing of complex linguistic materials. In Perceman E (Ed.), Cognitive Processing in the Right Hemisphere (pp. 169–191). New York: Academic Press.

Guzzetta A, Pecini C, Biagi L, Tosetti M, Brizzolara D, Chilosi AM, . . . Cioni G. (2008). Language organisation in left perinatal stroke. *Neuropediatrics* 39(3):157–163.

Halliday MA, Hasan R. (1976). Cohesion in English. London: Longman.

Hart B, Risley TR. (1992). American parenting of language-learning children: Persisting differences in family-child interactions observed in natural home environments. *Dev Psychol* 28(6):1096–1105.

Hickok G, Poeppel D. (2007). The cortical organization of speech processing. *Nature Rev Neurosci* 8(5):393–402.

Holland SK, Plante E, Weber Byars A, Strawsburg RH, Schmithorst VJ, Ball WS Jr. (2001). Normal fMRI brain activation patterns in children performing a verb generation task. *NeuroImage* 14(4):837–843. doi: 10.1006/nimg.2001.0875

Huttenlocher J, Vasilyeva M, Cymerman E, Levine SC. (2002). Language input at home and at school: Relation to syntax. *Cognitive Psychol* 45:337–374.

Jacola LM, Schapiro MB, Schmithorst VJ, Byars AW, Strawsburg RH, Szaflarski JP, . . . Holland A. L. (2006). Functional magnetic resonance imaging reveals atypical language organization in children following perinatal left middle cerebral artery stroke. *Europediatrics* 37(1):46–52.

Joanette Y, Brownell H. (1989). Discourse Ability and Brain Damage. New York: Springer Verlag.

Leiter RG. (1979). Lieter International Performance Scale. Wood Dale, IL: Stoelting Company.

Liegeois F, Connelly A, Cross JH, Vargha-Khadem F, Baldeweg T. (2004). Language reorganization in children with early-onset lesions of the left hemisphere: an fMRI study. *Brain* 127(6): 1229–1236. doi: 10.1093/brain/awh159

Limber J. (1973). The genesis of complex sentences. In Moore T (Ed.), Cognitive Development and the Acquisition of Language. New York: Academic Press.

MacWhinney B, Feldman HM, Sacco K, Valdes-Peres R. (2000). Online measures of basic language skills in children with early focal brain lesions. *Brain and Language* 71:400–431.

Marchman VA, Saccumen C, Wulfeck B. (2004). Productive use of the English past tense in children with focal brain injury and specific language impairment. *Brain and Language* 88(2):202–214.

Mayer M. (1969). Frog Where Are You? New York: Dial Publishing.

Müller RA, Behen ME, Rothermel RD, Muzik O, Chakraborty PK, Chugani HT. (1999). Brain organization for language in children, adolescents, and adults with left hemisphere lesion: A PET study. *Progress in Neuro-Psychopharmacology and Biological Psychiatry* 23:657–668.

Nunez SC, Dapretto M, Katzir T, Starr A, Bramen J, Kan E, . . . Sowell ER. (2011). fMRI of syntactic processing in typically developing children: structural correlates in the inferior frontal gyrus. *Dev Cogn Neurosci* 1(3):313–323. doi: 10.1016/j.dcn.2011.02.004

Petersen SE, Fox PT, Posner MI, Mintun M, Raichle ME. (1988). Positron emission tomographic studies of the cortical anatomy of single word processing. *Nature* 331:585–589.

Price CJ. (2010). The anatomy of language: a review of 100 fMRI studies published in 2009. *Ann NY Acad Sci* 1191:62–88. doi: 10.1111/j.1749–6632.2010.05444.x

Raja Beharelle A, Dick AS, Josse G, Solodkin A, Huttenlocher PR, Levine SC, Small SL. (2010). Left hemisphere regions are critical for language in the face of early left focal brain injury. *Brain* 133(Pt 6):1707–1716. doi: 10.1093/brain/awq104

Rasmussen T, Milner B. (1977). The role of early left brain injury in determining lateralization of cerebral speech functions. *Ann NY Acad Sci* 299:355–369.

Reilly J, Bates E, Marchman VA. (1998). Narrative discourse in children with early focal brain injury. *Brain and Language* 61:335–375.

Reilly J, Losh M, Bellugi U, Wulfeck B. (2004). "Frog where are you?": Narratives in children with specific language impairment, early focal brain injury, and Williams syndrome. *Brain Language* 88(2):229–247.

Reilly, J Stiles J & Appelbaum M (2009). Degrees of Plasticity: Language acquisition and use in children with perinatal stroke. Paper presented at biennial meeting of SRCD, Denver, CO.

Reilly J, Wasserman S, Appelbaum M. (submitted). Later language development in narratives in children with perinatal stroke.

Ressel V, Wilke M, Lidzba K, Lutzenberger W, Krageloh-Mann I. (2008). Increases in language lateralization in normal children as observed using magnetoencephalography. *Brain and Language* 106(3):167–176. doi: 10.1016/j.bandl.2008.01.004

Rowe ML, Levine SC, Fisher J, Goldin-Meadow S. (2009). The joint effects of biology and input on the language development of brain-injured children. *Dev Psychol* 45:90–102.

Saccumen C, Dick F, Kwiatowski M, Moses P, Bates E, Perani D. (2006). Language processing in children and adolescents with early unilateral focal brain lesion: A fMRI study. Paper presented at the Meeting for the Organization for Human Brain Mapping, Florence, Italy.

Scarborough HS. (1991). Preschool literacy experience and later reading achievement. *J Learning Disabilities* 24(8):508–511.

Schmithorst VJ, Holland SK, Plante E. (2007). Object identification and lexical/semantic access in children: A functional magnetic resonance imaging study of word-picture mapping. *Hum Brain Mapp* 28(10):1060–1074.

Semel, E., Wiig, E., & Secord, W. (1995). *Clinical evaluation of language fundamentals*. San Antonio, TX: Psychological Corporation.

Slobin,D. (Ed.). (1992). The Crosslinguistic Study of Language Acquisition. Hillsdale, NJ: Lawrence Erlbaum.

Staudt M, Lidzba K, Grodd W, Wildgruber D, Erb M, Krageloh-Mann I. (2002). Right hemispheric organization of language following early left-sided brain lesions: Functional *MRI topography. NeuroImage* 16(4):954–967.

Szaflarski JP, Holland SK, Schmithorst VJ, Byars AW. (2006). fMRI study of language lateralization in children and adults. *Hum Brain Mapp* 27(3):202–212. doi: 10.1002/hbm.20177

Thal D, Reilly J, Siebert L, Jeffries R, Fenson J. (2004). Language development in children at risk for language impairment: Cross-population comparisons. *Brain and Language* 88:167–179.

Tillema JM, Byars AW, Jacola LM, Schapiro MB, Schmithorst VJ, Szaflarski JP, Holland SK. (2008). Cortical reorganization of language functioning following perinatal left MCA stroke. *Brain and Language* 105:99–111.

Vicari S, Albertoni A, Chilosi AM, Cipriani P, Cioni G, Bates E. (2000). Plasticity and reorganization during language development in children with early brain injury. *Cortex* 36(1):31–46.

Weckerly J, Wulfeck B, Reilly J. (2004). The development of morphosyntactic ability in atypical populations: The acquisition of tag questions in children with early focal lesions and children with specific-language impairment. *Brain Language* 88(2):190–201.

Williams KT. (1997). Expressive Vocabulary Test. Circle Pines, MN: American Guidance Service.

Wulfeck B, Bates E, Capasso R. (1991). A crosslinguistic study of grammaticality judgments in Broca's aphasia. *Brain and Language* 42(2):311–336.

Wulfeck B, Bates E, Krupa-Kwiatkowski M, Saltzman D. (2004). Grammaticality sensitivity in children with early focal brain injury and children with specific language impairment. *Brain and Language* 88:215–228.

9

Plasticity of Overall Intellectual Functioning

EVIDENCE FROM STANDARDIZED TESTS

THE PLASTICITY OF overall level of intellectual functioning in children with PL has been a question of interest since the earliest studies of this population. Currently, there is widespread agreement that children with PL typically display more subtle cognitive deficits in specific domains (e.g., language, spatial thinking) than is the case for individuals with seemingly similar lesions that are incurred later in life (see Chapters 5 through 8). However, it is much less clear that this early functional plasticity extends to overall level of intellectual functioning as assessed by performance on standardized IQ tests.

One possibility is that early lesions result in significant deficits in overall level of intellectual functioning, in contrast to the subtle deficits observed for specific functions. Such a finding would indicate that there is some limitation to functional plasticity following early brain lesions. Moreover, the finding of IQ deficits coupled with the finding of normality or only subtle deficits for specific functions would indicate that when a lesion is superimposed on a developing brain, functional deficits are shallower and broader in scope than is the case for lesions incurred later in life, when functional deficits tend to be deeper but narrower in scope. On the other hand, it is possible that early functional plasticity extends to overall level of intellectual functioning and that the IQ of children with PL is left relatively unscathed—that is, it does not differ significantly from that of typically developing children. As discussed below, it is also possible that the story is more complex, and that the IQ level of children with PL may vary depending on the developmental time point when they are assessed. For example, IQ levels of children with PL may fall in the fully normal range when children are assessed at early ages but are lower when they are assessed at later developmental time points because of the increased processing demands of the questions that must be answered correctly in order to maintain the same IQ level over time.

INTELLECTUAL FUNCTIONING IN CHILDREN WITH PL: IQ AND ACHIEVEMENT TESTS AS MEASURES

The question of how overall level of intellectual functioning fares after pre- or perinatal lesions has generally been addressed using standardized IQ tests. These tests provide a Full Scale IQ score, which is regarded as a reflection of general or overall level of intellectual functioning. In addition, IQ tests often provide Verbal and Performance IQ scores. The Verbal IQ score typically is a composite of performance on subtests that assess receptive and expressive language skills, verbal reasoning skills, and verbal working memory; the Performance IQ score typically is a composite of performance on subtests that assess perceptual reasoning skills, visuomotor skills, and processing speed. In addition to these measures, many IQ tests provide individual subtest scores that feed into the broader IQ scores. The most recent version of a widely used IQ test for children, the Wechsler Intelligence Scale for Children, Fourth Edition (WISC-IV), is even more refined, providing a Full Scale IQ score as well as four index scores (Verbal Comprehension, Perceptual Reasoning, Working Memory, and Processing Speed) and individual subtest scores. Because the WISC-IV (2003) is relatively new, most of the research on the IQ of children with PL has not yet used these index scores. Rather, most studies used an earlier version of the Wechsler IQ tests, which provide a Full Scale IQ Score (FIQ), a Verbal IQ score (VIQ), a Performance IQ score (PIQ), and individual scaled scores on the subtests that make up these scores.

In addition to IQ tests, a smaller number of studies have administered standardized achievement tests to children with PL to assess their school-related skills, including reading, writing, and mathematical skills. Although IQ tests are typically viewed as reflecting "intellectual potential" and achievement tests are typically viewed as reflecting more learned abilities, individuals' scores on these two types of tests are typically highly correlated (e.g., Deary, Strand, Smith, & Fernandes, 2007), and scores on both kinds of tests are clearly influenced by the kinds of supports and instructions children receive at home and at school (e.g., Ceci, 1991; Gould, 1981; Nesbitt, 2009). One notable difference between IQ tests and achievement tests is that IQ tests typically do not assess reading skills, whereas achievement tests almost always include tests that involve reading decoding and comprehension.

The use of standardized IQ tests to assess level of cognitive functioning has certain advantages and disadvantages that apply to all populations. On the plus side, these kinds of tests are psychometrically sound. In particular, they are reliable and valid and provide norm-referenced scores based on the performance of stratified samples of children that are representative of the population of the United States at each of the ages to which the test can be administered. On the minus side, these kinds of tests provide only a broad picture of intellectual functioning rather than precise information about specific cognitive processes. Even performance on individual subtests taps into multiple cognitive abilities. For example, one subtest on the WISC-III is called Picture Completion. The child is shown a series of pictures and is asked, "What is the most important thing missing in this picture?" To perform well on this test, the child must have both knowledge of objects in the world and the ability to process the visuospatial information in each picture. Questions concerning the resilience and fragility of particular processing capacities are better addressed using the kinds of tasks that cognitive psychologists employ in carefully designed experiments. Although it is not really fair to criticize IQ tests for not providing more precise information about the nature of strengths and weaknesses—they were not designed for this purpose—it is important to recognize this limitation.

In our review of research on the plasticity of intellectual functioning in children with PL, we focus on the following five questions in turn:

1. Is the plasticity of the young brain sufficient to support levels of IQ and school achievement in children with PL that are comparable to typically developing children?
2. Does the pattern of IQ scores exhibited by children with PL mirror the pattern seen in adults who have similar focal lesions?
3. Are the IQ scores of children with PL as stable over time as those of typically developing children?
4. What are the lesion characteristics that relate to IQ levels in children with PL?
5. Are the effects of input on IQ similar to those observed in typically developing children?

1. IS THE PLASTICITY OF THE YOUNG BRAIN SUFFICIENT TO SUPPORT LEVELS OF IQ AND SCHOOL ACHIEVEMENT IN CHILDREN WITH PL THAT ARE COMPARABLE TO TYPICALLY DEVELOPING CHILDREN?

IQ Levels

Several studies have examined the IQ levels of children with perinatal unilateral brain injury in relation to control children. Most of these studies have focused on whether there are group differences in IQ. Also important is the question of whether the extent of variation of IQ scores among typically developing children and children with early unilateral lesions differs.

With respect to the question of whether there are mean differences in the IQ levels of children with PL and typically developing children, some studies report no group differences (e.g., Aram & Ekelman, 1986; Bates, Vicari, & Trauner, 1999; Riva & Cazzaniga, 1986 [right-sided lesions only]; Vargha-Khadem, O'Gorman, & Watters, 1985; Woods & Carey, 1979). In contrast, other studies report that the mean IQ scores of children with early unilateral brain injury are significantly below the mean level of typically developing children (e.g., Banich, Levine, & Huttenlocher, 1990; Levine, Huttenlocher, Banich, & Duda, 1987; Perlstein & Hood, 1955; Riva & Cazzaniga, 1986 [left-sided lesions only]; St. James-Roberts, 1981; Woods, 1980). Ballantyne, Scarvie, and Trauner (1994) compared the IQ level of a group of children with PL to that of a well-matched control group and found that the mean IQ level of the children with PL was significantly lower than would be expected based on socioeconomic status (SES), albeit still in the normal range.

What factor(s) might explain the differences in these findings? One possibility is that studies reporting lower IQs in the PL group than in the typically developing group may have included a higher proportion of children with larger lesions (e.g., Levine, Kraus, Alexander, Suriyakham, & Huttenlocher, 2005) and/or a higher proportion of children with a history of seizures (e.g., Vargha-Khadem, Isaacs, van der Werf, Robb, & Wilson, 1992) than studies reporting IQ levels that do not differ from typically developing children. Such variations across individual studies are to be expected because sample sizes tend to be small. (A more detailed consideration of the relation of biological characteristics of early lesions to the IQ of children with PL is included under Questions 2 and 3, below).

Another possibility is that those studies reporting normal IQ levels (90–110 according to the Wechsler scales) or no significant difference between the IQ levels of children with PL and typically developing children assessed children at younger ages than those reporting lower IQ levels in children with PL. Supporting this possibility, one study that reported an IQ level in the "normal range" in their sample of children with unilateral perinatal lesions (Mean IQ level = 93.3) assessed the children between 3 and 9 years of age (Bates, Vicari & Trauner, 1999). Similarly, Wulfeck, Trauner, and Tallal (1991) assessed children with early lesions between 6 and 24 months of age on the Bayley Scales of Infant Development and found no deficits in global intellectual functioning. In contrast, several studies reporting somewhat lower IQ levels (mean IQ levels between 80 and 90, considered to be in the low normal range according to the Wechsler scales) assessed children at later ages (e.g., Duval, Dumont, Braun, & Montour-Proulx, 2002; Levine et al., 2005; Perlstein & Hood, 1955; St. James-Roberts, 1981). This issue is considered in more detail below (see Question 3).

A third possibility is that studies reporting average IQ levels in children with PL eliminated children with IQs below a certain level from their sample whereas studies reporting IQ levels that are below average in children with PL retained their entire sample of children with PL in the analysis in which IQ levels were compared. Vargha-Khadem, O'Gorman, and Watters (1985), for example, report that they eliminated four children with PL with IQs below 75, two with left hemisphere PL (LPL), and two with right hemisphere PL (RPL). The remaining children in their sample had mean IQs in the normal range, but eliminating the children with IQs below 75 certainly raised the reported mean.

A final factor that may influence findings is whether IQ levels of children with PL are compared to those of a well-matched control group or to the population mean. This can have an impact on reported findings and on conclusions that are reached. For example, consider the possibility that a relatively small sample of children with PL come from families with medium to high SES. This SES status would tend to elevate their IQ scores compared to a sample that is representative of the overall population in terms of SES and might lead to the conclusion that IQ is not affected byPL. In contrast, comparing the IQ level of children with PL to a control group that is matched in terms of demographic factors (e.g., both groups are from higher SES backgrounds) might lead to the conclusion that IQ level is affected by PL. A case in point emerges from the findings of Ballantyne, Scarvie, and Trauner (1994). The eight children with LPL in their study had a mean FIQ of 93.62, a mean VIQ of 94.75, and a mean PIQ of 92.75, and the nine children with RPL had a mean FIQ of 98.56, a mean VIQ of 104.78, and a mean PIQ of 91.44. While all of these scores are in the normal range of the Wechsler scale, comparison to control groups who were matched to the children with PL for SES, sex, and age revealed that the children with PL had significant IQ deficits. In particular, the control groups scored between 118.56 and 124.56 on the various IQ scales. This finding highlights the importance of using well-matched control groups in order to assess whether there are deficits in IQ functioning in children with PL. It is not enough to rely on population norms because the particular sample of children with PL being assessed may be from a demographic group that is functioning well above the mean of the normative sample.

Considered together, the data from existing studies seem most consistent with the view that the mean IQ level of children with PL is in the low normal range (IQ 80–90). But these children, like typically developing children, are individuals who do not always reflect the mean of their respective groups. In fact, studies assessing the IQ levels of children with PL clearly show that there are wide variations in the scores of individual children. For example, in Levine et al.'s (2005) study, the FIQ of the children with PL ranged from 76 to 124, or more than three standard deviations, when the children were tested between 4 and 6 years of age. Moreover, at the high end, the score of 124 falls in the superior range according to the Wechsler classification scheme (top 6.7% of the population), and at the low end the score of 76 falls in the borderline range according to the Wechsler scheme (bottom 6.7% of the population). In another study, the mean FIQ of children with PL was 87.92 when they were tested at a mean age of 13 years 11 months (SD = 1 year, 5 months), but scores of individual participants ranged from 63.86 to 97.69 (Gonzalez-Monge et al., 2009). In fact, Levine et al. (1987) report that the variation in IQ scores of children with PL is significantly greater than that in the general population, most likely reflecting the contribution of lesion characteristics to other sources of variation.

School Achievement

Only a handful of studies have examined academic achievement in children with PL. Vargha-Khadem, Frith, O'Gorman, and Watters (1983) presented a paper at the International Neuropsychological Society (cited by Aram & Ekelman, 1988) in which they reported that 13 of 17 (76%) children with LPL compared to only 5 of 15 (33%) children with RPL were below grade level in reading and significantly below the level of typically developing control children. In a later published study that included 53 children, mainly with PL (N = 38) but also 15 with postnatal unilateral lesions (age at lesion ranging from 2 months to 13.8 years), Frith and Vagha-Khadem (2001) reported significantly lower performance in boys with LPL compared to typical controls in reading decoding and spelling. There were no differences for boys with RPL, or for girls with either LPL or RPL compared to typically developing control children. Thus, in this study, LPL was only associated with reading and spelling deficits in boys. Another study implicating LPL in written language difficulties was carried out by Woods and Carey (1979), who found that children with LPL had greater spelling difficulties than children with RPL and control children, regardless of time of lesion onset.

Several other studies suggest that children with early brain lesions have difficulty with academic achievement but have not found that LPL are particularly detrimental. Aram and Ekelman (1988) found that children with LPL scored significantly lower on written language achievement than control children, whereas children with RPL scored significantly lower than control children on the reading, math, and written language sections of the Woodcock Johnson Psycho-Educational Battery: Tests of Cognitive Ability and Achievement. It should be noted, that Aram and Ekelman's participants (except for six children with prenatal lesions) consisted of children with strokes mainly sustained postnatally, after cardiac catheterization or surgery. Thus, these findings may not generalize to children with PL who do not have heart problems and concomitant chronic problems with cerebral blood perfusion. However, consistent with Aram and Ekelman's general conclusions, a recent study that assessed 18 children with PL and 24 control children in the early elementary school grades on the Wechsler Intelligence Scale for Children-Revised (WISC-R) and the Wide Range Achievement Test-Revised (WRAT-R), found that the children with PL scored significantly lower than the control group on both the IQ and achievement test measures

(Ballantyne, Spilkin, Hesselink, & Trauner, 2008). On the WRAT-R, scores of children with PL were significantly lower on all three subtests—Reading, Spelling, and Arithmetic. Within the PL group, no effects of lesion laterality were found for either WISC-R or WRAT-R scores and children with seizures scored significantly lower than those without seizures on each of the WISC-R IQ scales (FIQ, VIQ, PIQ) but not on any of the WRAT-R subtests.

New data collected as part of the longitudinal language project at the University of Chicago examined various reading and mathematics achievement scores of children with RPL and LPL and compared it to a typically developing control group. Various subtests of the Woodcock-Johnson Tests of Achievement III (Woodcock, McGrew, & Mather, 2001) were administered in the fall and spring of kindergarten and first and second grades. Reading decoding was assessed through the Letter-Word Identification (identifying letters and reading increasingly difficult words) and Word Attack (reading phonologically pronounceable non-words) subtests, reading comprehension was assessed by the Passage Comprehension subtest; mathematical calculation skills were assessed by the Calculation subtest; and mathematics word problem skills were assessed by the Applied Problems subtest. Results did not show significant differences between the PL group and the typically developing control group on the reading decoding subtests or on either of the mathematics subtests. In contrast, on the Passage Comprehension subtest, there were significant differences between the scores of the children with PL and the typically developing children at all time points from the fall of first grade through the spring of second grade. Additionally, reading comprehension and decoding grew less over the summer periods (between the spring and fall testing points) than during the school year (between the fall and spring testing points). Moreover, summer growth was less marked for the children with PL than for the TD children. The results for reading comprehension indicate that the kinds of instructional support children receive at school, at least in the early grades, may be particularly important for sustaining the learning trajectories of children with PL (Demir, Carlson, & Levine, in preparation).

Considered collectively, these studies indicate that children with PL tend to have difficulty with certain aspects of academic achievement. These school-related achievement problems may be related to the general finding that IQ levels are somewhat lower in this group as well as to behavioral problems, which have been shown to be elevated in children with PL (Trauner, Panyard-Davis, & Ballantyne, 1996). Of note, in the Trauner et al. (1996) study, parents of children with PL and control children filled out a behavioral questionnaire, the Personality Inventory for Children (PIC; Wirt, Lachar, Klinedinst, & Seat, 1984), and their responses indicated that children with PL had significant impairment on scales assessing academic and cognitive achievement, as well as on scales assessing general adjustment and social skills. The fact that parents' responses on the academic achievement and intellectual screening scales were not related to children's IQ scores on the WPPSI (Wechsler, 1967) or the WISC-R (Wechsler, 1974) is consistent with the possibility that social and behavioral factors contributed to the school achievement difficulties of the children with PL.

2. Does the Pattern of IQ Scores Exhibited by Children with Perinatal, Unilateral Brain Injury Mirror that Seen in Adults?

Typically, studies with adult patients with unilateral stroke report that VIQ/PIQ discrepancy patterns are associated with lesion laterality. In particular, in adults with acquired unilateral lesions, mainly from stroke, PIQ tends to be higher than VIQ after left hemisphere lesions and Verbal IQ tends to be higher than Performance IQ after right hemisphere lesions (e.g., Bornstein & Matarazzo, 1982; McGlone, 1978; Milner, 1975; Warrington, James, & Maciejewski, 1986). Other studies with adults, however, have reported a tendency for VIQ to be higher than PIQ regardless of lesion laterality, albeit with larger discrepancies in that direction for patients with right hemisphere lesions than for those with left hemisphere lesions (e.g., Zillmer, Waechtler, Harris, Khan, & Fowler, 1992). This discrepancy across studies may be due to variations in when the participants are tested during the recovery process and whether patients with aphasia are included or excluded from the study (Zilmer et al., 1992). Thus, Zillmer et al. (1992) noted that their patients were tested acutely (within 2–3 weeks of stroke) and that other studies reporting VIQ advantages for patients with left as well as right hemisphere lesions have also assessed patients during the acute phase, (e.g., Kaufman, 1990; Snow, Freedman & Ford, 1986; Todd, Coolidge, & Satz, 1977).

Many studies have asked whether children with PL, like adults, also show IQ patterns that correspond to the laterality of their lesions—that is, higher VIQ for those with RPL and higher PIQ for those with LPL. Given the documented plasticity of the young brain, it is possible that this is not the case for lesions of pre- or perinatal origin. Rather, after an early lesion, intact brain regions may develop to meet the cognitive demands of the environment in fairly even ways. That is, early in development, the functions of many brain regions are relatively unspecified and may proceed to develop in ways that do not create large site-specific deficits. In fact, many studies have reported that VIQ and PIQ levels are similar, showing little discrepancy, following both LPL and RPL (e.g., Ballantyne, Spilken, Hesselink & Trauner, 2008; Bates et al., 1999; Levine, Huttenlocher, Banich, & Duda, 1987; Vargha-Khadem, O'Gorman, & Watters, 1985; Vargha-Khadem et al., 1992; Woods, 1980). Bates, Vicari, and Trauner (1999) reported that VIQ and PIQ are significantly correlated in children with PL ($r = 0.65, p < 0.0001$) in their sample. Figure 9.1 shows their plot of VIQ versus PIQ for the individual children in their sample. This figure shows an approximately even distribution of children with LPL and RPL among the 16 children for whom PIQ > VIQ and the 27 children for whom VIQ > PIQ, and statistical tests show null effects for the interaction of lesion laterality and IQ scale. Other studies also report no difference in the pattern of VIQ/PIQ scores as a function of lesion laterality, but find that VIQ was higher than PIQ regardless of lesion laterality (Carlson, Uvebran, Hugdahl, Arvidsson, Wiklund & von Wendt, 1994; Goodman & Yude, 1996; Vargha-Khadem, Isaacs, Van Der Werf, Robb & Wilson, 1992; Muter, Taylor, & Vargha-Kadem, 1997). This finding is consistent with the notion that language functions may be selectively preserved when lesions are incurred early in development (Woods & Teuber, 1973).

In contrast to these findings, several studies have reported differential effects of LPL and RPL on VIQ and PIQ. Several studies have reported that both VIQ and PIQ are affected by early LPL, whereas PIQ is specifically affected by early RPL (Aram & Ekelman, 1986; Ballantyne, Scarvie, & Trauner, 1994; Riva & Cazzaniga, 1986; Woods & Teuber, 1973). In contrast, Nass, Peterson, and Koch (1989) reported that in children with LPL, VIQ is significantly higher than PIQ and that in children with RPL, VIQ and PIQ do not significantly differ. Moreover, in children with LPL, FIQ and VIQ are significantly higher than in children with RPL. Nass et al. (1989) hypothesized that the verbal sparing after early LPL is attributable to a maturational gradient in brain development such that the left hemisphere

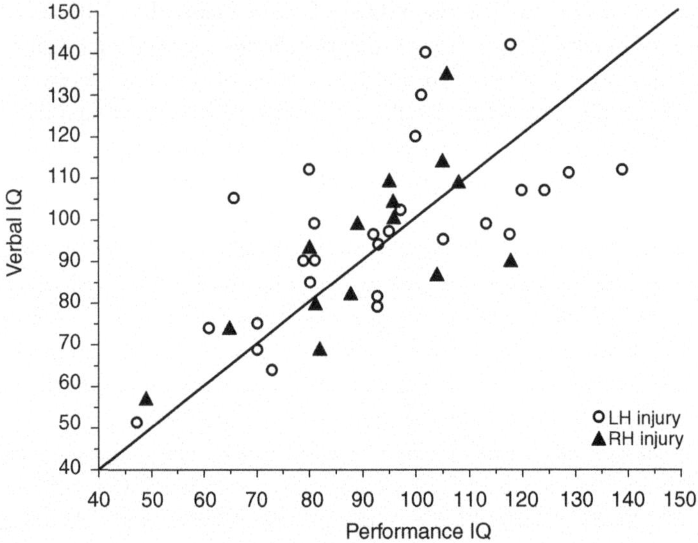

FIGURE 9.1 A plot of the PIQ (x-axis) and VIQ (y-axis) of a group of children from the San Diego study of PL children, with lesion laterality indicated (open circles: LPL; closed triangles: RPL). Note that PIQ and VIQ are significantly correlated and that there is no tendency for VIQ to be higher than PIQ in children with RPL or for PIQ to be higher than VIQ for children with LPL. (From Bates, Vicari, & Trauner, 1999.)

matures earlier than the right hemisphere (Corballis & Morgan, 1978). According to Corballis and Morgan's maturational gradient hypothesis, a hypothesis that has gained some support from a study examining brain magnetic auditory evoked fields in third-trimester fetuses (Schleussner et al., 2004), the less mature right hemisphere would be more capable of subsuming the functions of the damaged left hemisphere than the more mature left hemisphere would be at subsuming the functions of the less mature right hemisphere. Nass et al. also invoke "the crowding hypothesis," first proposed by Teuber (1975), to explain why PIQ is significantly lower than VIQ after early LPL. According to this hypothesis, when the right hemisphere becomes involved in language functions after LPL, this has a detrimental effect on the functions that would typically involve circuits within this hemisphere, notably visuospatial functions, thus "crowding" these functions. At least one part of this hypothesis appears to be correct based on fMRI data—that is, areas in the inferior frontal gyrus of the right hemisphere activate in children with LPL during a verb generation task, and these areas are homologous to the areas in the left hemisphere that activate during this task in typically developing children (Tillema, Byars, Jacola, Schapiro, Schmithorst, Szaflarski, & Holland, 2008). However, as will be detailed in Chapter 11, there are various ways in which LPL may affect visuospatial functions other than via "crowding," and the crowding hypothesis as an explanation for tradeoffs between language functions and visuospatial functions is not well grounded in neurobiological or neurobehavioral data.

None of the reported findings on IQ patterns in children with PL report the adult pattern of greater negative impact on VIQ after left hemisphere injury and greater negative impact on PIQ after right hemisphere injury. This raises several important questions. First, does this pattern emerge developmentally after PL lesions? That is, is it not apparent when assessments are given at early ages but apparent when assessments are given at later ages? To date, there is no evidence that this is the case for oral language skills but perhaps some weak support that it may be the case of written language, as reviewed above (e.g., Woods & Carey, 1979) Second, if this site-specific pattern of deficits is present after lesions that occur during adulthood but not after PL, when does the adult pattern first emerge? There is some indication that right hemisphere injury may affect PIQ more than VIQ when lesions occur after age 1 (Woods, 1980). Consistent with this finding, in a review of the literature, Hogan, Kirkham and Isaacs (2000) reported that for a group of 38 children in a study at Great Ormond Street Hospital for Children in London, the pattern of IQ scores after right hemisphere injury was consistent with the adult literature (VIQ 99.5, PIQ 91.7), but the pattern of IQ scores after left hemisphere injury was not (VIQ 91.7, PIQ 92.0), even after postnatal stroke.

3. Does the Level of IQ of Children with Early Brain Injury Show the Same Stability over Time as Has Been Observed for Typically Developing Children?

Because early brain lesions are superimposed on a rapidly developing brain, the magnitude and nature of deficits may change over time (Levine et al, 2005). That is, cognitive functioning of children with PL is affected by multiple factors, some shared by typically developing children and others unique to children with brain injury. Factors that are shared with typically developing children include the developmental status of particular brain regions at the time of the assessment. This, in turn, is affected by multiple maturational and experiential factors that interact in complex ways (e.g., Greenough, Black, & Wallace, 1987; Noble, McCandliss, & Farah, 2007; see also Chapter 11 of this book). Unique to children with PL, cognitive functioning is affected by the nature of the lesions and the capacity of the lesioned brain to develop in ways that allow it to handle increasingly demanding cognitive tasks (Feldman, 2005).

Animal studies provide evidence that there are changes in the cognitive consequences of lesions over the course of development. For example, Goldman (1971, 1974) found that monkeys whose dorsolateral frontal lobes were lesioned bilaterally during the neonatal period perform only slightly worse than a nonlesioned age-matched control group, and significantly better than a late-lesioned group, on a delayed alternation test administered when the monkeys were 12 to 18 months of age. However, the early-lesioned monkeys showed deficits compared to nonlesioned controls on the delayed alternation task when assessed later, at 2 years of age, albeit still better than late-lesioned monkeys. The emergence of a deficit at 2 years of age may reflect the maturation of the dorsolateral frontal lobes in the intact control monkeys. That is, at the earlier time point, the dorsolateral prefrontal cortex is insufficiently developed to contribute to performance on the delayed alternation task in intact control monkeys. However, by the later time point, this region had matured enough to have a positive impact on the performance of the intact monkeys, leading to the appearance of a deficit in the lesioned monkeys (also see Chapter 1 for discussion of Goldman's work). Thus, following early lesions, plasticity observed at an early developmental time point may not be observed at a later developmental time point.

Such findings have important implications for the study of cognitive functioning in children with PL. In particular, these findings suggest that a fall-off in IQ level in children with

PL may reflect the time course of development of particular brain regions. It is also possible to think about the possibility of a fall-off in IQ over time in children with PL in terms of the processing demands of tasks that children need to master to maintain the same IQ level over time. Assuming that the processing demands of items on IQ tests increase as children get older, and that early brain damage limits the brain's computational capacities, the IQ disparity between children with PL and typically developing children might be expected to widen over time. Such a widening of IQ disparities over time would not be unique to children with PL, as a growing body of longitudinal studies comparing the IQs of children with a variety of developmental disorders, genetic disorders, and neurological syndromes reveals this pattern. For example, several studies indicate that there is a decline in IQ during childhood for children with fragile X syndrome (e.g., Brun et al., 1995; Hagerman et al., 1989), and similar findings have been reported for children with Down syndrome (Carr, 1988) and autism (Fisch, Simensen, & Schroer, 2002).

Such findings indicate that it is critical to assess children with PL at multiple time points, and ideally to use longitudinal data to obtain an accurate picture of the functional consequences of early lesions, which may be different at different developmental time points. Such an approach allows for a more accurate picture of the extent and limits of functional plasticity than assessing children with PL at a single developmental time point. Unfortunately, the existing literature on the IQ of children who have sustained pre- or perinatal injury to the left or right hemisphere of the brain is mainly based on studies that have assessed children at only one time point. These studies leave us with a somewhat mixed pattern of results: some report that the average IQ of children in this population is about one standard deviation below that of control children, whereas others report that there is no significant difference in the IQs of children with PL and typically developing children (see Question 1 above). Below we review research specifically addressing the possibility that the IQ levels of children with PL change over the course of development, and that they are significantly lower when children with PL are assessed at older ages than when they are assessed at younger ages.

The first study to address the possibility that the IQ level of children with PL decreases over the course of development was a cross-sectional study carried out by Banich, Levine, Kim, and Huttenlocher (1990). In this study, the IQs of a group of children with PL who were tested at different ages were examined to determine whether the children tested at older ages had lower IQs than the children tested at younger ages. Indeed, findings showed a significant negative relation between FIQ and the age of the child at the time of assessment such that the older the child was when tested, the lower was his or her IQ. The fall-off in IQ level appeared to begin at about 6 to 8 years of age. Consistent with these cross-sectional data, several studies have reported a marginally significant negative correlation of IQ and age at the time of assessment in their studies of children with PL (Bates et al., 1999; Nass et al., 1985). However, cross-sectional findings such as these leave open the possibility that different groups were sampled at the different time points, and that group differences could account for the IQ difference. That is, it is possible that the children who were assessed at the earlier ages were less severely affected than the children assessed at older ages. This, in fact, could happen because children with larger lesions and more severe problems might have been more likely than children with smaller lesions and less severe problems to continue seeing a pediatric neurologist, the source of referrals for many research studies of the population with PL.

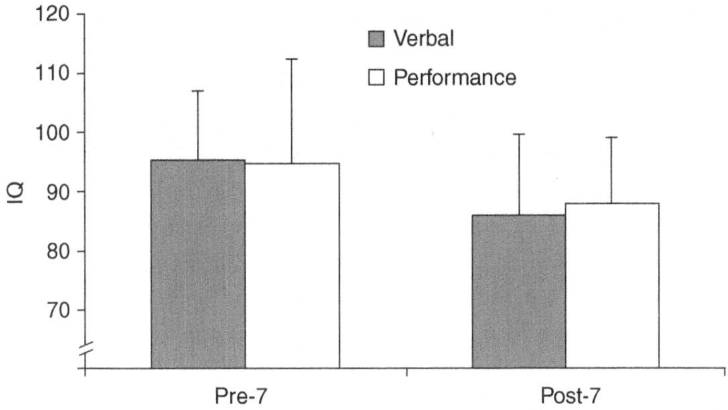

FIGURE 9.2 Mean VIQ and PIQ for children with PL when tested before age 7 and after age 7. Note that the same children had higher mean IQ scores when tested before age 7 than after age 7. (From Levine et al., 2005.)

Several studies have now obtained longitudinal data on the IQ of children with PL, which provides more definitive information about whether IQ levels decline with age. Findings of a study by Levine et al. (2005) indicate that the IQ levels of these children tend to decline over time. In this study, 15 children with PL were administered a standardized IQ test at two developmental time points. At the first time point, children ranged in age from 4 years 3 months to 6 years 10 months (mean 4 years 10 months) and at the second time point they ranged in age from 7 years 6 months to 21 years 7 months (mean age 14 years 0 months). An analysis of variance revealed a significant fall-off in IQ level over time, both for VIQ and PIQ (Fig. 9.2). Of the 15 children studied, 12 showed a decline in IQ level, 2 showed an increase, and 1 showed no change. As shown below, the FIQ of the children with PL ranged from 76 to 124 when they were tested between 4 and 6 years of age. However, when these same children were tested between 7 and 21 years of age, their FIQ ranged from 71 to 103 (Fig. 9.3).

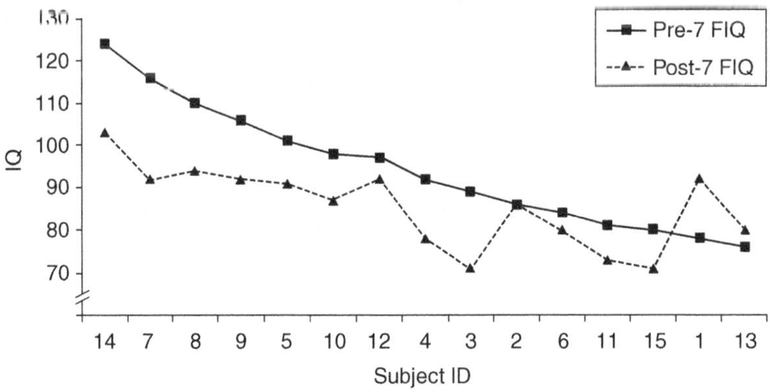

FIGURE 9.3 FIQ scores of individual children with PL assessed before and after age 7 years (from Levine et al., 2005). Note that for most individual children, IQ is higher before age 7 than after age 7.

Several other studies have reported more specific declines in IQ over time in children with PL. For example, in a 2-year longitudinal study in which children with PL were assessed at 3 and 5 years of age, Muter, Taylor, and Vargha-Khadem (1997) report stability in FIQ and VIQ over time. However, whereas PIQ decreased slightly over time in the PL group (by 1.6 points on average) it increased in the control group (by 4.1 points on average), resulting in a significant time-related group difference in PIQ. As noted by these researchers, the short two-year time window coupled with the young age of the participants leaves open the possibility that IQ level may decline with increasing age in children with PL. In a longer term 7-year longitudinal follow-up study of the intellectual development of children with congenital hemiplegia, Gonzalez-Monge et al. (2009) found a significant decrease in PIQ but not VIQ or FIQ over time. Further, these authors reported that PIQ was negatively associated with seizure history in the children with PL. Another longitudinal study carried out by Ballantyne, Spilkin, Hesselink, and Trauner (2008) also found that the IQ decline over time was restricted to those children with PL who had a history of seizures.

Still others have reported stability in the IQ levels of children with PL over time (Aram & Eisele, 1994; Muter, Taylor, & Vargha-Khadem, 1997). However, a re-analysis of the Aram and Eisele (1994) data revealed that the sub-sample of children (N = 11) in their study who had early lesions (dating from prior to age 2) showed a nearly significant main effect of time of assessment, with earlier assessments occurring on average at 6 years 0 months of age and later assessments occurring on average at 10 years 3 months of age (Levine et al., 2005). The remaining children in the Aram and Eisle (1994) study had lesions that were acquired later in childhood, a group that had been previously reported to show stability in IQ over time, unlike the children with PL (Banich et al., 1990). Thus, although the stability of IQ levels of children with PL remains an open question, there is some indication that IQ levels in this population may decline over the course of development. If this is indeed the case, it is important for researchers to examine the question of whether certain kinds of interventions are effective in mitigating this decline.

4. *What Are the Biological Factors that Relate to IQ Levels?*

There is general agreement in the literature about the correlations of various biological factors with the IQ levels of children with PL. The factors that have received the most attention in the literature are lesion laterality, lesion size, and seizure history. The increased use of MRI data is now providing the opportunity to examine the relation of more fine-grained lesion location information to cognitive performance measures, including IQ.

With respect to lesion laterality, existing studies are in general agreement that left and right hemisphere lesions have similar effects on FIQ, VIQ, and PIQ (e.g., Bates et al., 1999; Levine et al., 2005; Muter et al., 1997; Vargha-Khadem, Isaacs, & Muter, 1994). Another point of agreement occurs for lesion size, where there is general agreement that larger lesion size is associated with lower IQ levels (e.g., Cohen & Duffner, 1981; Levine et al., 1987, 2005).

With respect to seizures, some studies report that seizures are a negative predictor of IQ in children with PL (Muter et al., 1997; Vargha-Khadem, Isaacs, van der Werf, Robb, & Wilson, 1992). These studies report that while PIQ is somewhat lower in the PL group compared to typical controls regardless of whether the children have seizures, for VIQ, only the children in the PL group who have seizures score lower than the typical controls (see Bates et al., 1999). Although Levine et al. (2005) and Bates et al. (2007) did not find an effect of seizure history on IQ, this may be because their sample only included children who did not experience seizures and those with mild seizure disorders. Information is lacking concerning the extent to which the seizure disorder *per se*, the underlying pathology associated with the seizure disorder, and/or the anticonvulsant drugs taken to control the seizures may have a negative impact on the IQ level of children with PL (e.g., Bates et al., 1999; Muter et al., 1997).

5. Are the Effects of Input on IQ in Children with PL Similar to Those Observed in Typically Developing Children?

The effects of environmental factors (e.g., the quality of parent input, schools) on IQ and achievement have been documented in numerous studies of typically developing children (e.g., Ceci, 1991; Huttenlocher, Levine, & Vevea, 1998; Nisbett, 2009). Animal studies also indicate that experience is an important factor to consider after early brain injury. For example, Goldman and Mendelson (1977) found that monkeys with neonatal orbitofrontal lesions performed better on a delayed alternation task given when they were 15 months old if they had been assessed earlier on a different task (an object reversal task) than lesioned monkeys who had not received this earlier testing experience. Such findings suggest that early experiences will make a difference in the development of children with early brain injury.

But does input play a differentially important role in the development of children with PL, compared to its role in the development of typically developing children? Despite the importance of this question for theory and intervention efforts, there has been very little research addressing it in children with PL. One possible answer to this question is "no": input may play the *same* role in children with and without early brain injury. Such a finding would indicate that the development of intellectual functions is so buffered that it proceeds in more or less the same manner even when the learner has suffered a significant organic insult. Alternatively, input could play a *less* important role in the development of the intellectual skills of children with brain injury, suggesting that early lesions limit the impact that input has on intellectual development. Finally, environmental input could play a *more* important role for children with focal brain injury than for typically developing children (cf., Wilcox & Shannon, 1996). Such a finding would indicate that augmented environmental input might be needed to ameliorate the impact of brain injury.

A recent study examined the role of input in the language development of children with PL compared to typically developing children. Rowe, Levine, Fisher, and Goldin-Meadow (2009) examined this question with respect to two aspects of language development, vocabulary and syntax. For vocabulary development, findings showed that language input plays a similar role for typically developing children and children with PL. In contrast, for syntactic development, findings showed that language input may play a greater role for children with PL than for typically developing children, possibly because syntactic development is a more challenging aspect of language development than vocabulary development (Fig. 9.4).

With respect to IQ, particularly for the more complex tasks that are given to older children, these findings suggest that input variations may account for considerable variation in children with PL, and possibly more variation than in typically developing children.

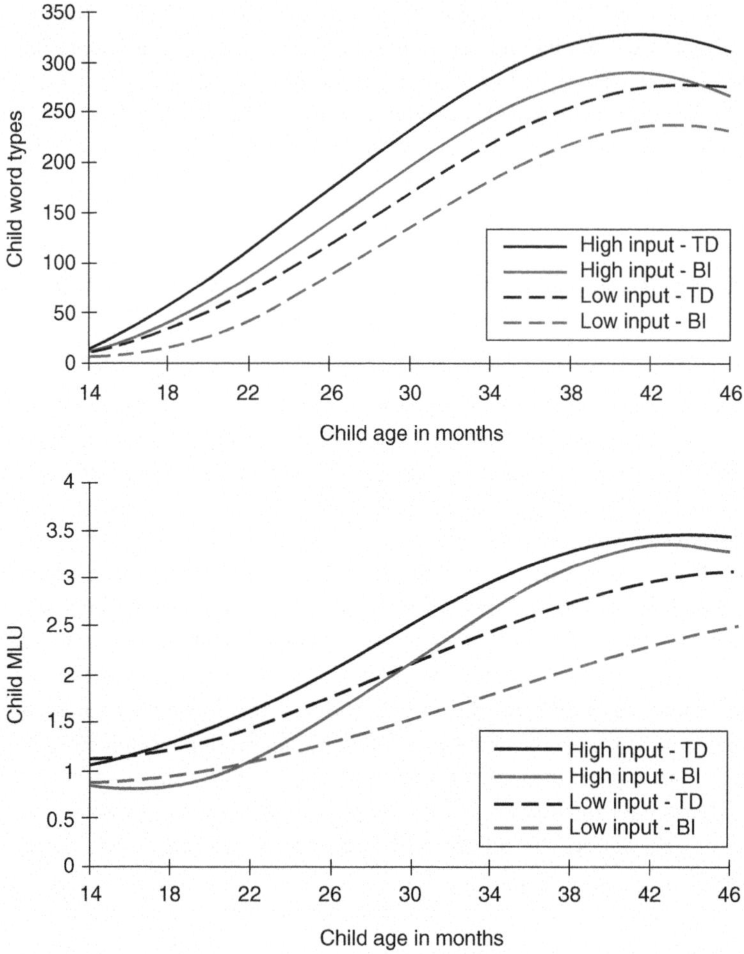

FIGURE 9.4 Model results from hierarchical linear modeling of effects of parent speech on the intercept and growth over time of (1) productive vocabulary measured in word types in the left panel (different words) and (2) mean length of utterance (MLU) in the right panel. Both are plotted for children with PL and typically developing control children. (From Rowe et al., 2009.)

The failure of existing studies of IQ levels in children with PL to consider the impact of input variations may contribute to some of the inconsistencies that have plagued the literature. At the very least, future studies should gather socioeconomic data and measure the quality of the home environment through questionnaires or observation measures such as the H.O.M.E. (Caldwell & Bradley, 2001). Moreover, demonstrating that input plays a particularly important role in the development of children with PL would have important practical implications, suggesting that enhancing the early childhood environments of children with PL would lessen the risks of language and cognitive delays and deficits.

SUMMARY

We organized this chapter by asking five questions. Existing research provides some answers as well as raising important new questions. We briefly review the answers and outstanding issues for each of the questions we asked, beginning with the first, "Is the plasticity of the young brain sufficient to support levels of IQ and school achievement in children with PL that are comparable to typically developing children?" The answer to this question appears to be "almost": the mean IQ level of children with PL is in the low average range. Moreover, there are wide individual variations in levels of performance within the group with PL, and some children with PL have IQs in the fully normal and even above-average range. The disagreements among various studies about the degree of mean IQ deficits in children with PL could be attributable to a variety of factors, including variations in the size of lesions, the presence and nature of seizure disorders, and importantly, whether IQ levels are compared to a well-matched control group or are assessed in relation to test norms. As discussed previously, it is important to consider the demographics and the quality of input of children with PL in assessing and interpreting their IQ levels. Only a few studies have examined the academic achievement levels of children with PL, but there is some indication that children with PL may experience achievement gaps relative to typically developing children in at least some areas. Moreover, for reading comprehension skills in the early elementary school grades, children with PL may lose ground over the summer months compared to typically developing control children. Such findings again implicate the greater importance of input in the growth of language/literacy skills in children with PL than for typically developing children. In this case, our findings suggest that the structured input provided by school may be particularly important (compared to the relatively unstructured input provided in the summer) in promoting the growth of reading comprehension in children with PL.

Moving to our second question, we asked whether the pattern of IQ scores exhibited by children with PL mirrors the pattern seen in adults with similar lesions. Our review shows that unlike adults with unilateral lesions, there is no indication that children with LPL have lower VIQ than PIQ or that children with RPL have lower PIQ than VIQ. Rather, the IQ patterns displayed by children with PL appear to be characterized by somewhat lower VIQ and PIQ levels regardless of their lesion laterality. There is some indication that when unilateral lesions occur after 1 year of age, right hemisphere lesions are associated with lower PIQ than VIQ. However, the age at which left hemisphere lesions are first associated with differential VIQ deficits remains unknown.

The answer to our third question, whether the IQ of children with PL is stable or declines over development, appears to be that there may be a decline in IQ level over the course of development, although there is some disagreement about this in the literature. There is some indication that PIQ may show greater loss over time than VIQ. Moreover, the time interval over which children are assessed, and the age of children at the time of assessment may account for some of the variation in findings with older ages at time of second assessment, and longer time intervals between the assessments more likely to reveal decreases in level of functioning.

Our last two questions concern how the biological characteristics of lesions and input variations, repectively, contribute to the IQ levels of children with PL. Research findings indicate that lesion size and the presence of seizures are negatively associated with IQ levels in children with PL. The role of input has mainly been addressed with respect to language development in typically developing children. Existing findings suggest that high-quality input is even more important to the development of complex language and literacy skills (syntactic skills, narrative skills, and reading comprehension) than it is for typically developing children. These findings are particularly important in terms of formulating educational programs and plans that are likely to support optimal development of cognitive skills in children with PL.

REFERENCES

Aram DM, Eisele JA. (1994). Intellectual stability in children with unilateral brain lesions. *Neuropsychologia* 32:85–95.

Aram DM, Ekelman BL. (1986). Cognitive profiles of children with early onset unilateral lesions. *Dev Neuropsychol* 2:155–172.

Aram DM, Ekelman BL. (1988). Scholastic aptitude and achievement among children with unilateral brain lesions. *Neuropsychologia* 26:903–916.

Ballantyne AO, Scarvie KM, Trauner DA. (1994). Verbal and performance IQ patterns in children after perinatal stroke. *Dev Neuropsychol* 10:39–50.

Ballantyne AO, Spilken AM, Hesselink J, Trauner DA. (2008). Plasticity in the developing brain: intellectual, language and academic functions in children with ischaemic perinatal stroke. *Brain* 131: 2975–2985.

Banich MT, Levine SC, Kim H, Huttenlocher P. (1990). The effects of developmental factors on IQ in hemiplegic children. *Neuropsychologia* 28:35–47.

Bates E, Thal D, Aram D, Eisele J, Nass R, Trauner D. (1997). From first words to grammar in children with focal brain injury. *Dev Neuropsychol (special issue)* 13: 275, 343.

Bates E, Vicari S, Trauner D. (1999). Neural mediation of language development: Perspectives from lesion studies of infants and children. In Tager-Flusberg H (Ed), Neurodevelopmental Disorders: Developmental Cognitive Neuroscience (pp. 533–581). Cambridge, MA: MIT Press.

Bornstein RA, Matarazzo JD. (1982). Wechsler Verbal IQ versus Performance IQ difference in cerebral dysfunction: A literature review with emphasis on sex differences. *J Clin Neuropsychol* 4:319–334.

Brun C, Obiols JE, Cheema A, O'Connor R, Riddle J, Di Maria M, et al. (1995). Longitudinal IQ changes in fragile X females. *Dev Brain Dysfunction* 8:230–241.

Caldwell BM, Bradley RH. (2001). HOME Inventory and Administration Manual (3rd ed). University of Arkansas for Medical Sciences and University of Arkansas, Little Rock.

Carlson, G., Uvebrant, P., Hugdahl, K., Arvidsson, J., Wiklund, L.-M., von Wendt, L. (1994). Verbal and non-verbal function of children with right- versus left-hemiplegic cerebral palsy of pre- and perinatal origin. *Dev Med Child Neurol*, 36:503–512.

Carr J. (1988). Six weeks to twenty-one years old: A longitudinal study of children with Down's syndrome and their families. *J Child Psychol Psychiatry* 29:407–431.

Ceci SJ. (1991). How much does schooling influence general intelligence and its cognitive components: A reassessment of the evidence. *Dev Psychol 27*:702–722.

Cohen ME, Duffner PK. (1981). Prognostic indicators in hemiparetic cerebral palsy. *Ann Neurol* 9:353–357.

Corballis M, Morgan M. (1978). On the biological basis of human laterality: Evidence for a maturational left-right gradient. *Behav Brain Sci* 2:261–336.

Deary IJ, Strand S, Smith P, Fernandes C. (2007). Intelligence and educational achievement. *Intelligence* 35:13–21.

Demir, O.E., Carlson, M., & Levine, S.C. (in preparation). The development of reading skills in children with early brain injury: School year versus summer growth.

Duval J, Dumont M, Braun CMJ, Montour-Proulx I. (2002). Recovery of intellectual function after a brain injury: A comparison of longitudinal and cross-sectional approaches. *Brain and Cognition* 48:337–342.

Feldman HM. (2005). Language learning with an injured brain. *Language Learning and Development* 1:265–288.

Fisch GS, Simensen RJ, Schroer RJ. (2002). Longitudinal changes in cognitive and adaptive behavior scores in children and adolescents with the fragile X mutation or autism. *J Autism Dev Disorders* 32:107–114.

Frith U, Vargha-Khadem F. (2001). Are there sex difference in the brain basis of literacy related skills? Evidence from reading and spelling impairments after early unilateral brain damage. *Neuropsychologia* 39:1485–1488.

Goldman PS. (1971). Functional development of the prefrontal cortex in early life and the problem of neuronal plasticity. *Exp Neurol* 32:366–387.

Goldman PS. (1974). An alternative to developmental plasticity: Heterology of CNS structures in infants and adults. In: Stein DG, Rosen JJ, Butters N (eds), Plasticity and Recovery of Function in the Central Nervous System (pp. 149–174). New York: Academic Press.

Goldman PS, Mendelson MJ. (1977). Salutary effects of early experience on deficits caused by lesions of frontal association cortex in developing rhesus monkeys. *Exp Neurol* 57:588–602.

Gonzalez-Monge S, Boudia B, Ritz A, Abbas-Chorfa F, Rabilloud M, Iwaz J, Barard C. (2009). A 7-year longitudinal follow-up of intellectual development in children with congenital hemiplegia. *Dev Med Child Neurol* 51:959–967.

Goodman R, Yude C. (1996). IQ and its predictors in childhood hemiplegia. *Dev Med Child Neurol* 38:881–890.

Gould SJ. (1981). The Mismeasure of Man. New York: W.W. Norton and Company.

Greenough WT, Black JE, Wallace CS. (1987). Experience and brain development. *Child Dev* 58:539–559.

Hagerman RJ, Schreiner R, Kemper M, Witenberg M, Zahn B, Habitcht K. (1989). Longitudinal changes in IQ among fragile X males: Clinical evidence of more than one mutation? *Am J Med Genetics* 33:513–518.

Hogan AM, Kirkham FJ, Isaacs EB. (2000). Intelligence after stroke in childhood: Review of the literature and suggestions for future research. *J Child Neurol* 15:325–332.

Huttenlocher J, Levine SC, Vevea J. (1998). Environmental effects on cognitive growth: Input from school. *Child Dev* 69:1012–1029.

Irle E. (1990). An analysis of the correlation of lesion size, localization and behavioral effects in 283 published studies of cortical and subcortical lesion in old-world monkey. *Brain Res Rev* 15:181–213.

Kaufman AS. (1990). Assessing Adolescent and Adult Intelligence. Boston: Allyn & Bacon, Inc.

Levine SC, Huttenlocher P, Banich MT, Duda E. (1987). Factors affecting cognitive functioning of hemiplegic children. *Dev Med Child Neurol* 27:27–35.

Levine SC, Kraus R, Alexander E, Suriyakham LW, Huttenlocher P. (2005). IQ decline following early unilateral brain injury: A longitudinal study. *Brain and Cognition* 59:114–123.

McGlone J. (1978). Sex differences in functional brain asymmetry. *Cortex* 14:122–128.

Milner B. (1975). Psychological aspects of focal epilepsy and its neurosurgical management. *Adv Neurol* 8:299–321.

Muter V, Taylor S, Vargha-Khadem F. (1997). A longitudinal study of early intellectual development in hemiplegic children. *Neuropsychologia* 35:289–298.

Nass R, Peterson H, Koch D. (1989). *Differential effects of congenital left and right brain injury on intelligence. Brain and Cognition* 9:258–266.

Nisbett RE. (2009). Intelligence and How to Get It. New York: W.W. Norton and Company, Inc.

Noble KG, McCandliss BD, Farah MJ. (2007). Socioeconomic gradients predict individual differences in neurocognitive abilities. *Dev Sci* 10:464–480.

Perlstein MA, Hood PN. (1955). Infantile spastic hemiplegia. *Am J Phys Med* 34:391–407.

Riva D, Cazzaniga I. (1986). Late effects of unilateral brain lesions sustained before and after age one. *Neuropsychologia* 24:423–428.

Rowe ML, Levine SC, Fisher J, Goldin-Meadow S. (2009). Dow linguistic input play the same role in children with and without early brain injury? *Dev Psychol* 45:90–102.

Schleussner E, Schneider U, Arnscheidt C, Kähler C, Haueisen J, Seewald HJ. (2004). Prenatal evidence of left-right asymmetries in auditory evoked responses using fetal magnetoencephalography. *Early Hum Dev* 78:133–136.

Snow WG, Freedman L, Ford L. (1986). Lateralized brain damage, sex differences and the Wechsler intelligence scales: A reexamination of the literature. *J Clin Exp Neuropsychol* 8: 179–189.

St. James-Roberts, I. (1981). A reinterpretation of hemispherectomy data without functional plasticity of the brain. *Brain and Language* 14:292–306.

Teuber HL. (1975). Why two brains? In Schmitt FO, Worden FG (eds), Neuroscience: Third Study Program. Cambridge: MIT Press.

Tillema JM, Byars AW, Jacola LM, Schapiro MB, Schmithorst VJ, Szaflarski JP, Holland SK. (2008). Cortical reorganization of language functioning following perinatal left MCA stroke. *Brain and Language* 105:99–111.

Todd J, Coolidge F, Satz P. (1977). The Wchsler Adult Intelligence Scale Discrepancy Index: A neuropsychological evaluation. *J Consulting Clin Psychol* 45:450–454.

Trauner DA, Panyar-Davis JL, Ballantyne AO. (1996). Behavioral differences in school age children after perinatal stroke. *Assessment* 3:265–276.

Vargha-Khadem F, Frith U, O'Gorman AM, Watters GV. (June, 1983). Learning Disabilities in Children with Unilateral Brain Damage. Paper presented at the Meeting of the International Neuropsychological Society, Lisbon, Portugal.

Vargha-Khadem F, Isaacs E, Muter V. (1994). A review of cognitive outcome after unilateral lesions sustained during childhood. *J Child Neurol* 9:2S67–2S73.

Vargha-Khadem F, Isaacs E, Van der Werf S, Robb S, Wilson J. (1992). Development of intelligence and memory in children with hemiplegic cerebral palsy: The deleterious consequences of early seizures. *Brain* 115:315–329.

Vargha-Khadem F, O'Gorman A, Watters G. (1985). Aphasia and handedness in relation to hemispheric side, age at injury, and severity of cerebral lesion during childhood. *Brain* 108:677–696.

Warrington EK, James M, Maciejewski C, (1986). The WAIS as a lateralizing and localizing diagnostic instrument: A study of 656 patients with unilateral cerebral lesions. *Neuropsychologia* 24:223–239.

Wechsler, D. (1967). Manual for the Wechsler Preschool and Primary Scale of Intelligence (WPPSI). Cleveland, OH: The Psychological Corporation.

Wechsler, D. (1974). Manual for the Wechsler Intelligence Scale for Children-Revised (WISC-R). San Antonio, TX: The Psychological Corporation.

Wilcox MJ, Shannon M. (1996). Integrated early intervention practices in speech-language pathology: Issues, strategies, and further directions. In: McWilliam R (ed), Proceedings of the 19th Annual Boston University Conference on Language Development.

Wirt RD, Lachar D, Klinedinst JK, Seat PD. (1984). Multidimensional description of child personality: A manual for the Personality Inventory for Children. 1984 edition by David Lachar. Los Angeles: Western Psychological Services.

Woodcock RW, McGrew KS, Mather N. (2001). Woodcock-Johnson III Tests of Achievement. Itasca, IL: Riverside Publishing.

Woods BT. (1980). The restricted effects of right-hemisphere lesions after age one: Wechsler test data. *Neuropsychologia* 18:65–70.

Woods BT, Carey S. (1979). Language deficits after apparent clinical recovery from childhood aphasia. *Ann Neurol* 6:405–409.

Woods BT, Teuber HL. (1973). Early onset of complementary specialization of cerebral hemispheres in man. *Trans Am Neurol Assoc* 98:113–117.

Wulfeck BB, Trauner DA, Tallal PA. (1991). Neurologic, cognitive and linguistic features of infants after early stroke. *Pediatr Neurol* 7:266–269.

Zillmer EA, Waechtler C, Harris B, Khan F, Fowler PC. (1992). The effects of unilateral and multifocal lesions on the WAIS-R: A factor analytic study of stroke patients. *Arch Clin Neuropsychol* 7:29–40.

PART THREE

Clinical and Theoretical Implications

10

Clinical Implications

CLINICIANS FROM MANY specialties will encounter children with early brain damage from numerous causes. These practitioners are expected to provide prognostic information, guidance as to the most effective interventions, and assistance with optimizing the child's potential outcome. To some extent the cause of a particular child's brain insult will affect the outcome. As can be seen from the previous chapters, the recurring themes of adaptability and plasticity that can be observed in the developing brain provide a basis for optimism in the clinical setting. However, the presence of what may be critical, or at least sensitive, periods of brain development that may reflect windows during which specific cognitive processes appear suggests that the clinician may need to take advantage of those windows to maximize cognitive and motor outcomes, regardless of underlying etiology. This chapter will focus on the clinical implications for the perinatal brain injury population, but the discussion provided here may have relevance for children with other neurodevelopmental disorders as well.

CLINICAL PRESENTATIONS OF PERINATAL STROKE

There are two primary ways in which perinatal strokes make their presence known. The first is with seizures in the newborn period. Within the first day or two of life, infants with perinatal stroke may have jerking of one side of the body (or in some cases both sides) recognized as a seizure. This event precipitates a neuroimaging study (preferably an MRI scan of the brain) that demonstrates the stroke. Other forms of neuroimaging, including head ultrasound and a computed tomographic scan of the head, may miss a new-onset lesion. An MRI scan of the brain is the most sensitive means of diagnosing perinatal stroke. Neonatal seizures occur in over 90% of infants diagnosed in the neonatal period (Laugesaar et al., 2007; Mannino & Trauner, 1983; Trauner & Mannino, 1986) and in approximately 30% to 40% of all children with known or presumed perinatal strokes (Ballantyne et al., 2008; Fitzgerald et al., 2007; Trauner et al., 1993). When neonatal seizures occur, they generally resolve within a week or two with anti-epileptic medication (although there is a high risk of later-onset seizures in this population; see below).

Other less common presentations in the neonatal period include poor feeding, lethargy, and low muscle tone. These are nonspecific problems and not all infants with perinatal stroke who have these symptoms will be diagnosed in the newborn period.

The second common mode of presentation of perinatal stroke is with the emergence of a hemiparesis, typically impairment of hand use, around 4 to 5 months of age. This is the time when infants begin to reach for toys, and it becomes quite obvious to the parents when the infant is only using one hand. On closer examination, the parents will usually notice that the infant's other hand is held in a flexed posture most of the time. This observation generally prompts a visit to the pediatrician and subsequently a neuroimaging study that documents a lesion consistent with an old stroke. The lesion then is said to be a "presumed perinatal stroke" (Golomb et al,. 2001). Other less common late presentations of perinatal stroke include later-onset seizures in a previously asymptomatic child, and language or other developmental delay.

The incidence of perinatal stroke is estimated to be approximately 1 in 1,500 to 1 in 5,000 live births (Laugesaar et al., 2007; Lynch, 2009). However, given the subtle and nonspecific nature of some of the presentations, it is likely that the incidence is higher and that some cases are missed entirely.

The remainder of this chapter will discuss clinical implications from the studies of the perinatal stroke population.

FINANCIAL BURDEN OF PERINATAL STROKE

The economic burden of perinatal stroke is high compared to that of healthy infants and children. Five-year direct costs associated with a perinatal stroke diagnosis, adjusted for costs of age-matched controls, was almost $52,000 in a recent study (Gardner et al., 2010). The increased financial cost continued over at least a 5-year period, suggesting that the economic burden of perinatal stroke was not only high but also continued beyond the immediate neonatal period. What has not yet been studied is whether early and intensive intervention can reduce the long-term social and financial burden of this condition.

THE ROLE OF SEIZURES

Studies of clinical outcome following perinatal focal brain damage have shown mixed results, with some showing poor cognitive and/or motor outcomes (Anderson et al., 2010; Kolk et al., 2011; Westmacott et al., 2010, while others suggest more favorable prognoses (Ballantyne et al., 2008; Stiles et al., 2005; Trauner & Mannino, 1986). Some of the variability can be attributed to the differences in the populations studied. For example, many studies have combined children who had a single unilateral perinatal stroke with children who had more global or multifocal brain damage, such as from birth asphyxia, or hypoxic ischemic encephalopathy (Ment et al., 1984). Other studies have used infantile hemiplegia (hemiplegic cerebral palsy) as an indicator of previous stroke without documenting the source or location of the lesion using neuroimaging studies (Banich et al., 1990; Muter et al., 1997). Still others have combined perinatal and later-onset brain damage from infections, trauma, and other mixed etiologies (Aram & Eisele, 1994; Max et al., 2010). The heterogeneity of populations has made it difficult to determine the significance of outcome studies.

Our group has reported on clinical outcomes of a very homogeneous group of children with perinatal stroke. The criteria for the children in the studies have included the presence of a unilateral brain lesion acquired before or around birth, and documented by a neuroimaging study. Children have been excluded if they had prenatal drug exposure or other conditions that might have caused more global or multifocal brain damage, including hypoxic ischemic encephalopathy, meningitis, or trauma. Yet despite the relative homogeneity of the population studied, we have found a great deal of variability in cognitive outcome (Ballantyne et al., 2007, 2008; Bates et al., 1997; Thal et al., 1991). In every study we have conducted, the primary factor in determining outcome appears to be whether the child had a history of seizures beyond the neonatal period. An earlier study documented a high incidence of post-neonatal seizures (greater than 50%) in a group of 29 infants (Trauner et al., 1993). In a recent study, children who had seizures scored over 20 points lower on standardized tests of intelligence and language compared with children who had never had seizures beyond the newborn period (Ballantyne et al., 2008). More importantly, children in the perinatal stroke group who did not have seizures beyond the neonatal period had IQ scores within the normal range (mean IQ 104 ± 18) and standardized language scores that were somewhat below the normal range (total language score 82 ± 10), whereas the children who had post-neonatal seizures were well below the normal range on both IQ (mean 76 ± 10) and standardized language (68 ± 7) measures. Thus, any seizure occurring after 28 days of age may signify a significantly poorer long-term prognosis for the child in terms of intellectual ability, language competence, and future academic success.

Although neonatal seizures have not been found to cause long-term cognitive impairments in our studies to date, a recent report of infants with neonatal stroke treated with hypothermia (Harbert et al., 2011) found that hypothermia reduced the incidence of neonatal seizures in the stroke infants, and the developmental scores of the infants treated with hypothermia were higher than those not treated. However, it is not clear whether the difference in developmental outcome was due to prevention of seizures, or to some other protective effect of hypothermia, such as in reducing metabolic demands on the brain and/or reducing the extent of brain injury. Further studies will be needed in this area to determine whether hypothermia is an effective means of improving long-term outcome in infants with perinatal stroke.

The incidence of seizures that begin after the neonatal period in children with perinatal stroke is 30% to 67% (Ballantyne et al., 2008; Fitzgerald et al., 2007 Trauner et al., 1993; Wanigashinghe et al., 2010; Wusthoff et al., 2011). Thus, this is a common occurrence in the early brain injury population. Many types of seizures have been reported following perinatal stroke, including grand mal or major motor seizures, partial simple seizures, and partial complex seizures. A very ominous form of epilepsy, infantile spasms, has been reported in a small number of children with perinatal stroke (Golomb et al., 2006; Wanigashinghe et al., 2010). This is a severe epileptic encephalopathy that typically begins between 3 and 9 months of age. It is characterized by a specific seizure type, myoclonic seizures, which are brief shock-like episodes that occur in clusters of 10 to 40 at a time, with several clusters occurring every day. The seizures are associated with a classical pattern on the EEG of very disorganized and chaotic electrical activity in the background, as well as very high amplitude multifocal epileptiform discharges that occur almost continuously. Infantile spasms often have a very poor prognosis, with a high incidence of mental retardation and cerebral palsy following the onset of these episodes.

Although the relationship between other types of seizures and cognitive dysfunction in the perinatal stroke population is not clearly defined, there is other evidence that the presence of any seizures may impair cognition, particularly language. This will be discussed below.

Seizures occur as a result of a temporary interruption of normal electrical activity in the brain, in effect "short-circuiting" the brain for a period of time, and thus blocking normal brain function. Seizures can be very obvious and severe, as in the case of grand mal seizures or convulsions, or they may be very subtle, with only brief pauses or staring spells (absence seizures) or even merely brief periods of confusion or unusual motor activity or stereotypies (simple or complex partial seizures). Most seizures last a few seconds to 1 to 2 minutes, but occasionally can be much longer. The abnormal electrical discharges may begin in one area of the brain, such as in the area damaged by a stroke. This is referred to as partial, or focal onset, seizure. This abnormal activity may spread, however, to involve the entire brain, causing secondary generalization of the seizure activity and usually a more severe type of seizure. When a person has two or more unprovoked seizures, this is generally considered to constitute epilepsy. "Unprovoked" refers to the absence of any clear precipitating factor such as fever or head trauma.

The frequency with which seizures occur in someone with epilepsy varies considerably, from multiple daily seizures to an occasional seizure every few months. Even in the absence of clinically visible seizures, however, there may be ongoing epileptiform discharges in the brain that can be identified during an EEG (Fig. 10.1). Normal brain wave activity consists of different frequencies of wave forms depending on whether the person is awake, drowsy, or asleep. Epileptiform discharges are much more sharply contoured and rhythmic than normal brain wave activity, are a sign of brain irritability, and indicate a susceptibility to seizures.

A number of studies have demonstrated cognitive impairments during episodes of epileptiform bursts on the EEG in children with epilepsy (Berman et al., 2010; Kasteleijn-Nolst Trenité et al., 1990; Tromp et al., 2003). In one study, 37 children with childhood absence epilepsy underwent continuous EEG monitoring as well as a functional MRI (fMRI) during a continuous performance task (Berman et al., 2010). The task required the subject to watch a screen on which individual letters were presented for 250 milliseconds, and to push a button when he or she saw an X appear on the screen. During periods of epileptiform (spike wave) discharges on the EEG, in the absence of clinical seizures or loss of consciousness, the patients were impaired in their ability to sustain attention compared to epochs in which epileptiform activity was absent. The error rate (missed targets) was 81% during spike wave discharges, compared with 39% during baseline non-epileptic EEG testing. The simultaneous fMRI showed widespread cortical and subcortical activation during the seizure discharges, particularly in frontal and thalamic regions. The authors suggested that the seizure discharges impair function in two networks necessary for attention, the thalamus and fronto-parietal association cortex, and in this way impair attention and other cognitive functions during the seizure discharge. In an earlier study of 53 children with epilepsy, cognitive tests were performed while recording the EEG (Kasteleijn-Nolst Trenité et al., 1990). The authors found transient cognitive impairments during the time that epileptiform discharges were observed on the EEG in 50% of the test sessions, despite the fact that the patients did not demonstrate any visible signs of seizure activity. Specifically, they found visuospatial

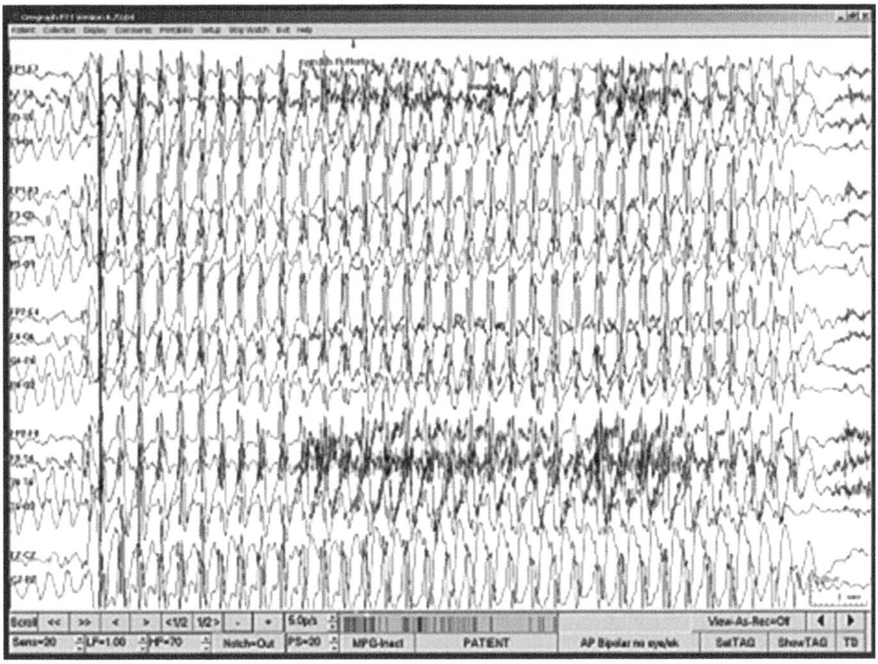

FIGURE 10.1 EEG in a child with petit mal (absence) epilepsy, showing generalized high-amplitude rhythmic spike and wave discharges during a 9-second seizure. During this episode, the patient was staring ahead with slight eyelid fluttering but was totally unaware of surroundings.

errors in association with right-sided epileptiform discharges, and verbal errors associated with left-sided discharges. Although the cognitive changes were transient, repetitive instances of impairment may have serious adverse effects on a child's ability to learn.

Other examples of seizures being associated with long-term cognitive impairments include Lennox-Gastaut syndrome (LGS) and Landau-Kleffner syndrome (LKS). In LGS, an epileptic condition associated with long-term cognitive impairments, there are always clinical seizures of mixed types, with a specific EEG pattern consisting of slow spike and wave discharges. The seizures in LGS are typically very difficult to control. LGS is associated with mental retardation, severe learning disabilities, hyperactivity, and aggressive behaviors, even if the child was developmentally normal prior to the onset of the seizures.

LKS is a severe idiopathic disorder of childhood associated with both epilepsy and severe language impairment (Kleffner & Landau, 2009). The typical presentation of LKS is that of a child who is developing normally and then has a seizure. Following the seizure there is a relatively rapid regression in language. The loss of language may be so complete that the child is unable to comprehend spoken language or to utter words; however, at times the language impairment may be less severe. Although seizures often herald the onset of this condition, it can occur without a prior seizure history. If language recovers, the expressive language of children with LKS is described as sparse, dysfluent, and with poor articulation and syntax (Praline et al., 2003). Children with LKS also display paraphasic errors and neologisms. The only means of diagnosing this condition is from the clinical history of language regression plus the presence on EEG of almost continuous spike or spike wave discharges bilaterally during sleep. These epileptiform discharges may be generalized, bilateral, and independent, or may be focused in perisylvian or frontotemporal-central brain regions.

The most effective treatments for LKS include high-dose corticosteroids, and benzodiazepines. Antiseizure medications may control the seizures but do not improve language function in most cases.

Although there is no current evidence that LKS or a variant of this condition is responsible for the language impairment in children with perinatal stroke, it is important to recognize that seizures can adversely affect cognitive outcome. For children with perinatal stroke, the clinician should be on the alert for evidence of seizure activity and be prepared to treat the child with anticonvulsant medications if there is any indication of seizure activity. Given the information that LKS and absence epilepsy can impair cognition, treating the clinical seizures may not be sufficient to ensure a positive outcome; it may also be necessary to reduce epileptiform activity on the EEG as completely as possible. However, no systematic studies have been conducted to determine whether such treatment would be successful or would make a difference in cognitive outcome.

MOTOR IMPAIRMENT

Motor development is the most obvious feature of an infant's development to most parents. They delight in every new motor milestone, from rolling over to sitting, crawling, walking and waving bye-bye. Parents tend to notice very quickly when motor development is awry. For example, by 4 to 5 months they are aware if their infant is reaching for toys with only one hand, and will bring that to the attention of the pediatrician.

Interestingly, at most only about two thirds of children with perinatal stroke will have a significant hemiparesis (Golomb et al., 2008; Trauner et al., 1993; Wulfeck et al., 1991). When there is weakness on the side opposite the brain lesion, it is generally worse in the arm than in the leg. At its most severe, the child may not be able to use the affected hand at all, making daily living activities such as tying one's shoes or buttoning one's clothes extremely challenging. Virtually all children with a single perinatal stroke will walk independently unless there is some other complicating factor. In fact, many walk at the expected time without significant delay (Trauner et al., 1993), although they may walk with a slight limp or walk on their toes involuntarily on the affected side.

The goal of intervention for motor problems is to allow the child to gain as much use of the affected limb(s) as possible. Physical and occupational therapy, begun early and performed on a regular basis (at least weekly with a home program as well), can help with that goal. For the leg, bracing with a device such as an ankle–foot orthosis (a device to correct alignment and/or provide support) or an orthotic insert in the shoe will help to keep the foot aligned better, prevent toe-walking, and increase stability (Pohl & Mehrholz, 2006). Serial casting of the ankle and lower leg is sometimes used to reduce contractures at the ankles. Contractures involve permanent shortening of the muscles at a joint, usually from spasticity or chronic tightness of those muscles. Once a contracture occurs, the joint cannot be moved. For the upper extremity, occupational therapy is the mainstay of treatment to improve hand and arm function. The use of a hand or thumb splint may help to keep the hand in a more functional position with the thumb abducted (pulled away from the palm) rather than tightly fisted.

Injection of botulinum toxin into a spastic muscle can relieve spasticity for several months and is now commonly used as an adjunct to treatment of cerebral palsy (Wallen et al., 2007). Botulinum toxin works by temporarily blocking neuromuscular transmission. Thus, it alone does not improve function, but merely releases the spasticity to the point that the affected limb can perhaps benefit more from exercise and therapy. There are three limitations to the usefulness of botulinum toxin for hemiplegia. The first is that injection of botulinum toxin relieves spasticity but can also unmask weakness, and this may limit the ability of the individual to use the affected limb. The second is that the effect of botulinum toxin is temporary, and injections typically have to be repeated three or four times per year. Finally, rare and at times serious allergic reactions to botulinum toxin have been reported. However, for many children, the use of this adjunctive therapy can provide additional functional benefit.

The use of constraint-induced movement therapy (CIMT) has been demonstrated in adults and children with hemiparesis to significantly improve hand and arm use on the affected side. This method of treatment has been studied for over 20 years (see Charles & Gordon, 2005, for a review) and its efficacy has been documented in several studies (Wang et al., 2011, in adults; Hoare et al., 2007; Naylor & Bower, 2005; Taub et al., 2011, in children). The technique involves casting or otherwise immobilizing the functional hand and arm while performing intensive therapy with the weak limb. The goal is to make use of the brain's plasticity by forcing the use of the impaired extremity. After 2 to 3 weeks of intensive use of only the affected limb, there is often noticeable improvement in hand use and independent living skills that were absent prior to the CIMT. Casting is generally continued for 2 to 3 weeks, after which the cast is removed but therapy continues to maintain the increased use of the affected extremity.

Because children may not use their impaired hand spontaneously even after CIMT, Hand-Arm Bimanual Intensive Therapy (HABIT) is increasingly being used as a treatment approach (Charles & Gordon, 2006; Gordon et al., 2011; Luft et al., 2004), often in conjunction with CIMT (Gordon et al., 2008). Furthermore, bimanual function is a significant problem for children with hemiplegic cerebral palsy, perhaps even more so than unimanual use where they can rely on their good hand. Structured like CIMT, HABIT, which engages children in play and functional activities that provide structured bimanual practice 6 hours per day for 10 days, has proven effective and improvements persist. Therapies based on bimanual activities should theoretically improve function in the impaired hand (Bleyenheuft & Thonnard, 2011; Carson, 2005; Saposnik et al., 2010). Indeed, a number of studies show that the unaffected hand can enhance the function of the impaired hand. For example, grasping, which requires fingertip force control, can be improved in the affected hand if first performed with the unaffected hand (Steenbergen et al., 2008).

SENSORY IMPAIRMENTS

The incidence of sensory deficits after perinatal stroke is difficult to ascertain because of a paucity of literature on this topic. Most of the reports of sensory abnormalities come from studies of children with cerebral palsy (hemiplegic or diplegic) and report a high incidence (over 50%) of sensory deficits (e.g., Cooper et al., 1995; Wingert et al., 2009). Few studies have documented sensory findings in perinatal stroke patients defined by neuroimaging. We found that almost one third of children with perinatal stroke had evidence of a sensory deficit on follow-up examination (Trauner et al., 1993). The primary type of sensory deficit is a cortical sensory deficit secondary to damage to the parietal lobe. Cortical sensory deficits include agraphesthesia (inability to identify a number written in the palm of the hand); astereognosis (inability to identify familiar objects placed in the palm of the hand by feeling them); proprioceptive deficits (difficulty distinguishing the position of a body part such as a finger when it is moved in one direction or another); and difficulty with separating two stimuli during simultaneous two-point discrimination (see Chapter 4 for more details). In addition to cortical sensory deficits, we and others (Bava et al., 2005; Laurent-Vannier et al., 2006; Trauner, 2003) have described a phenomenon of extrapersonal neglect in children with perinatal stroke. Neglect refers to a situation in which the child ignores the contralateral side of space ("neglect syndrome"). Neglect has been reported for many years in adults primarily after right hemisphere stroke. In children after perinatal brain injury, extrapersonal neglect may be found with either right or left hemisphere lesions, in contrast to the pattern seen in adults. This may reflect a difference in hemispheric dominance for extrapersonal space in the developing brain. When neglect is severe, the person may ignore one entire side of space, and for example write or draw on paper only on the side ipsilateral to the lesion. In less severe cases, neglect may be evident only on formal testing or when constraints such as time limits are placed on the individual. Clock-drawing is a task that has been used by neurologists for many years to check for neglect in a clinical setting. Most children learn to draw clocks in school by second to third grade, so this test can be used in school-age children as well. The child is asked to draw a clock freehand, and to put in the numbers, and then to put in the time (generally 10 minutes past 11 o'clock is the time used). Figure 10.2 shows the results of this task in two teenagers, one with a right hemisphere lesion and the other with a left hemisphere lesion, both of perinatal onset. In Figure 10.2A, drawn by the patient with the left-sided lesion, the numbers are placed correctly but the hands of the clock are both on the left side of the drawing (instructions were to designate the time as 10 minutes after eleven o'clock), suggesting a subtle left-sided spatial neglect. In Figure 10.2B, drawn by the subject with the right brain lesion, all of the numbers are displaced to the right side of the circle, demonstrating a significant left-sided spatial neglect.

Another commonly used test of neglect is a cancellation task. In this test, the person is asked to search a page that contains a large number of letters or symbols, some of which are the target stimuli. The targets are randomly distributed around the page in all four quadrants. The patient is instructed to cancel or strike through all of the target stimuli with a pencil. Adults with spatial neglect will typically be unable to find some or all of the targets on the side of the page contralateral to the lesion. We have unpublished data on the cancellation task in children with perinatal stroke that indicate a much more subtle contralateral neglect in children with right hemisphere lesions, and bilateral inattention and disorganized search strategy in children with left hemisphere lesions. Our findings suggest, as with our other studies, that the adult pattern of neglect is not the same in children.

In a clinical setting, neglect can sometimes be elicited by a test called double simultaneous stimulation. This test consists of having the patient close his or her eyes, and then touching the patient on two different parts of the body at the same time (e.g., left hand and right arm). The examiner then asks the child to tell where he or she was touched. A neurologically intact child will recognize both tactile stimuli. A person with neglect, however, may not recognize being touched on the side contralateral to the lesion, even though he or she can recognize

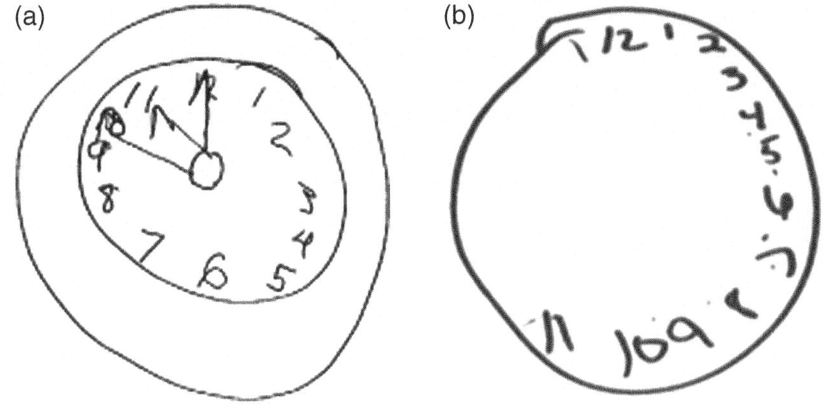

FIGURE 10.2 a) Clock drawn by 17-year-old patient with a left hemisphere lesion of perinatal onset. Note that the numbers are placed correctly, but the hands of the clock are both on the left side of the drawing (instructions were to designate the time as 10 minutes after 11 o'clock), suggesting a subtle left-sided spatial neglect. b) Clock drawn by a 17-year-old subject with a perinatal-onset right hemisphere stroke. Note that all of the numbers are displaced to the right side of the circle, demonstrating a significant left-sided spatial neglect.

being touched in the same location if there is only one stimulus at a time. In our focal lesion population, only children with significant neglect, usually those with large parietal lesions, have difficulty with double simultaneous stimulation (unpublished data).

As can be seen from the way in which neglect manifests, this condition might show up in a school-age child during an arithmetic test, when the child completes the problems on one side of the page only. It is vital to test for and identify neglect if it exists so that measures can be instituted to reduce complications from this condition. Such measures might include reducing the complexity of information placed on a page; training the child to move the page towards the ipsilateral side of the lesion; or increasing awareness of the contralateral side by drawing attention to items on that side prior to testing.

A careful sensory examination should be performed on any child with perinatal stroke, checking for evidence of cortical sensory deficits or neglect. If the child has sensory deficits, therapeutic interventions should be considered. Specific treatment of sensory impairments may improve sensory functioning and secondarily motor function. Standard approaches focus on occupational therapy with brushing and other types of stimulation of the affected side of the body, as well as attempts to improve awareness of the affected side, for example by having the patient look at the hand during functional exercises.

A multisensory approach to the treatment of sensory deficits may be effective in improving deficits in several modalities. For example, tactile acuity may be improved by concurrent visual input (Kennett et al., 2001). In a study of healthy adults, these investigators used a task in which the subjects were told to look at their arm throughout the task. The arm was in a box and the box went dark when a tactile stimulus (one or two points) was applied lightly to the skin. The subjects reliably were able to discriminate two simultaneous stimuli when they were visually attending to (able to see) their arm, even though they could not actually see the stimuli when applied. In contrast, they performed at chance level when they received the tactile stimulation without the visual input. The authors concluded that there are some brain areas that are responsive to both vision and touch, and that if visual input is present, these receptive fields are kept in synchrony or spatial register, and thus are more sensitive to tactile input delivered at the same time as the visual stimulus. Whether this type of intervention will be effective in treating the sensory deficits of children with perinatal stroke has yet to be studied. However, theoretically, given the interaction between different sensory modalities, a multisensory treatment approach might improve the function of individual sensory modalities (Serino et al., 2007).

Sensory integration therapy (SIT) uses multiple sensory and motor modalities to try to improve sensorimotor function and balance. SIT includes techniques such as brushing, deep pressure, swinging, and other activities. No systematic studies have been conducted to demonstrate benefits from this therapy in children with stroke. However, SIT was shown to improve balance and coordination in a small series of adult stroke patients (Smania et al., 2008).

VISUAL FIELD DEFECTS

A small percentage of children with perinatal stroke have a persistent visual field defect. In its most severe form, the child will have a homonymous hemianopsia, meaning that there is essentially blindness in the half of each eye on the side opposite the lesion. This limits the ability to attend to that side of visual space. The incidence of significant and persistent hemi-visual field deficits is difficult to determine, since they may be subtle and require formal ophthalmological testing to identify. Trauner et al. (1993) identified 7 of 29 children who had evidence of a visual field defect on examination at up to 48 months of age. Consistent with that figure is a more recent study by Ballantyne et al. (2008) in which 24% of their subjects with perinatal stroke had visual field defects when tested using confrontation techniques on neurological examination. The few other reports on this topic have shown a relatively low incidence of persistent visual field defects in the perinatal stroke population. At 1 year of age, Mercuri et al. (1996) found 4 of 12 infants post-perinatal stroke to have at least some limitation on visual field testing. However, in a later study of 16 school-age children with perinatal stroke, the same group (Mercuri et al., 2003) found that only 2 of the 16 had a persistent, identifiable visual field defect. Both children had large middle cerebral artery infarcts and contralateral hemiparesis as well. The authors suggested that visual field defects are only likely to be present in children who have a significant hemiparesis because they are related to the size of the brain lesion.

Despite the fact that visual field abnormalities are rare after perinatal stroke, it is important to recognize these as the presence of such a defect may require additional intervention. A child with a right visual field defect, for example, should be seated on the right side of a classroom so that he or she can benefit from the full use of the intact visual field. Similarly, when working with the child one-on-one and even in play situations, it is important that information be presented to the intact visual field to ensure that the child is aware of all visual information being given. There is no definitive evidence that vision therapy improves vision in children with a hemianopsia. Since the condition is quite rare, it would be difficult to conduct such a study with appropriate rigor. In adults, however, two forms of vision therapy, visual exploration training and visual attention training, both appear to improve visual function in post-stroke patients with hemianopsia (**Bergsma & van der Wildt, 2010;** Lane et al., 2010). Certain aspects of vision therapy should be considered for children who have severe and persistent visual field defects as well.

LANGUAGE IMPAIRMENT

As was discussed in detail in Chapters 7 and 8, children with perinatal stroke do not have aphasia, even with large left hemisphere lesions that would cause severe aphasia in adults. However, subtle language deficits may occur and persist in these children, regardless of the side of the lesion. This is particularly true of children with epilepsy, as discussed above. There have been no systematic studies of intervention for speech and language deficits in the perinatal stroke population. There is evidence, however, that parental input may have strong effects on language development after early brain injury. Rowe et al. (2009) studied the amount of talking that parents did with their young children (ages 14–46 months). They studied both typically developing children and a group of children with early brain injury, some of whom had perinatal stroke. They found that the amount of parental interaction in terms of talking with the child directly correlated with both vocabulary development in both groups, and with syntactic development in both groups, but more strongly in the early brain injury group. Thus, parents can play a powerful role in their child's language development by talking and playing actively with the child from early life.

In general terms, there are several approaches to the treatment of any child with a speech or language impairment. These are one-on-one therapy, either with a speech/language pathologist or an assistant who works directly with the child; group speech/language therapy with either a speech/language pathologist or an assistant working with a small group of children; and classroom immersion, in which the child is placed in a special class for children with language disorders, and therapy is incorporated into the classroom setting by teachers and aides as well as speech/language pathologists. A recent study in Scotland (Boyle et al., 2007) evaluated the effectiveness of individual or group therapy approaches with either a speech/language pathologist or an assistant in 152 school-aged children with significant language impairments, using a randomized design with a control group who were receiving standard community-based therapy. Therapy was given three times a week for 30- to 40-minute sessions over 15 weeks. At the end of the study period, the authors found no significant differences in outcome based on a standardized language test between direct and indirect modes of therapy (i.e., therapy given by a speech/language pathologist or an assistant), or between individual and group therapy, on the primary language outcome measures. However, there was a benefit on secondary outcome measures from one-on-one therapy with a speech/language pathologist. Secondary outcome measures included a test of receptive vocabulary, as well as data collected from questionnaires, rating scales, and direct discussion with parents, teachers, and therapists.

All of the language-impaired children, regardless of study intervention, showed significant improvements in expressive but not receptive language scores compared with the control group. Children with expressive language impairment were more likely to show improvement using the study interventions than those with mixed receptive–expressive disorders. Interestingly, nonverbal IQ did not appear to have an impact on outcome.

Although the above study was not specific to children with perinatal stroke, it is likely to have general utility for any child with a language impairment. Individual speech and language therapy, begun early and intensively, may improve ultimate language competence, particularly if seizures can be well controlled to minimize secondary complications from epilepsy.

BEHAVIORAL ISSUES

There is some controversy about the long-term behavioral implications of early focal brain damage. Studies of mixed populations of children (including children with traumatic brain injury, brain tumors, perinatal and childhood-onset strokes) have indicated the potential for significant behavioral problems as children reach adolescence, particularly if the lesion involved the frontal cortex. Max et al. (2010) studied children with early stroke (prenatal to 1 year of age) or later stroke (12 months or older at stroke occurrence) and compared their performance on cognitive and psychiatric tests with those of age-matched orthopedic controls. They found that children with early stroke onset had poorer performance on tests of intelligence, language, memory, academic achievement, and visuospatial skills. The early-stroke group also had a higher incidence and number of psychiatric diagnoses than did the other groups, although specific psychiatric diagnoses were not provided in that study. Interestingly, executive functioning was the one area in which the early-stroke group performed better than the late-stroke children. The authors suggest that there is a period of vulnerability to early insults in the developing brain during the time when myelination and other developmental changes in the brain are occurring, rather than a period of plasticity, to explain their findings of almost uniformly poorer performance in the early-stroke group compared with the later group.

In other studies, children with early right hemisphere damage have been described as having more negative temperaments as infants (Nass & Koch, 1987, 1991; Reilly et al., 1995) and more difficulty reading social cues as they get older (Trauner et al., 1996). Children with left hemiparesis, although not documented to have a right hemisphere lesion, were found to have more social difficulties than children without clinical evidence of such damage (Denkla et al., 1983; Goodman & Yude, 1997; Tranel et al., 1987; Weintraub & Mesulam, 1983).

Children with hemiplegic cerebral palsy and thus presumed to have a unilateral brain insult were found to have a high incidence (around 50%) of psychiatric diagnoses, including hyperactivity, conduct disorders, aggression, and oppositional behavior (Goodman & Graham, 1996; Goodman & Yude, 1997). Such behavioral problems were present in preschoolers and tended to persist into the school-age years.

Most of the above studies assumed a unilateral brain lesion of somewhat early onset based primarily on clinical findings. There has been a paucity of information on behavioral problems associated with documented perinatal unilateral lesions. However, Trauner et al. (1996) studied 17 children with documented unilateral brain damage from perinatal stroke and compared them with 23 typically developing control children using a parent-report questionnaire, the Personality Inventory for Children (Wirt et al., 1984). They reported that children with frontal lobe involvement were thought by their parents to have more cognitive deficits, whereas children with non-frontal (more posterior) lesions had more social deficits, regardless of the side of the lesion. In a later study using the Achenbach Child Behavior Checklist (Trauner et al., 2001), they studied 39 children with unilateral brain damage from perinatal stroke. They found a higher number of children with clinically significant scores on attention and social problems scales compared with controls. These problems did not appear to be related to the side or the size of the lesion.

In terms of clinical utility, this information can be used to heighten awareness among clinicians about the potential behavioral complications of perinatal stroke, particularly as children reach school age. If social problems become apparent, individual psychological counseling or social skills group therapy may be helpful. Problems with attention may be approached with classroom and/or homework modifications, or when appropriate with medication. Given the potential for some medications that treat attention deficit to lower the seizure threshold, one might consider performing an EEG prior to beginning a stimulant medication in children with perinatal stroke.

SUMMARY

The information in this book provides a tremendous resource for clinicians caring for children with perinatal stroke. Parents can be given more accurate information about the likely prognosis for motor, language, and intellectual outcomes, as well as the likelihood of other complications such as epilepsy or behavioral issues. Not all of these are applicable to every child with perinatal stroke, of course, and interventions need to be individualized depending on the particular child's needs. Early intervention with physical and occupational therapy in the first few months of life is advisable until the clinician can determine whether the child has a hemiplegia. Parents can also contribute to their child's developmental progress by providing an enriched environment in which they actively play, read, and talk with their infant. Language development should be followed carefully and speech/language therapy instituted if there is any indication of significant language delay at least by age 2 years. Seizures should be treated promptly and aggressively, with medications that are least likely to cause additional cognitive challenges. Fortunately, a large number of medications are now available to treat various types of seizures, and many of the newer antiepileptic medications have an excellent cognitive profile. As the child reaches school age, consideration will need to be given to classroom modifications if indicated. Early planning for such modifications is important so that the child has a positive school experience. Attention to social issues is also important in the school-age child.

Although the above discussion is focused on children with perinatal stroke, it can apply equally well to children who have other neurodevelopmental disorders, such as genetic and metabolic disorders, traumatic brain injury, and brain tumors, all of which may adversely affect cognition, motor function, and behavior. Awareness, anticipation of needs, and appropriate and timely intervention can make a major difference in the child's social, emotional, cognitive, and academic success.

ACKNOWLEDGMENTS

Much of the author's work described in this chapter was funded by National Institutes of Health grants P50 NS22343, R01 DC06098, R01 NS42584 and the March of Dimes Birth Defects Foundation.

REFERENCES

Anderson V, Jacobs R, Spencer-Smith M, Coleman L, Anderson P, Williams J, Greenham M, Leventer R (2010). Does early age at brain insult predict worse outcome? Neuropsychological implications. *J Pediatr Psychol* 35(7):716–727.

Aram D, Eisele JA (1994). Intellectual stability in children with unilateral brain lesions. *Neuropsychologia* 32:85–95.

Ballantyne A, Spilkin A, Trauner D (2007). Language outcome after perinatal stroke: Does side matter? *Child Neuropsychol* 13:494–509.

Ballantyne AO, Spilkin A, Hesselink J, Trauner DA (2008). Plasticity in the developing brain: intellectual, language and academic functions in children with ischaemic perinatal stroke. *Brain* 131(Pt 11):2975–2985.

Banich MT, Levine SC, Kim H, Huttenlocher P (1990). The effects of developmental factors on IQ in hemiplegic children. *Neuropsychologia* 28:35–47.

Bates E, Thal D, Trauner D, Fenson J, Aram D, Eisele J, Nass R (1997). From first words to grammar in children with focal brain injury. *Dev Neuropsychol* 13:275–343.

Bava S, Ballantyne A, May S, Trauner DA (2005). Perceptual asymmetry for chimeric stimuli in children with early unilateral brain damage. *Brain and Cognition* 59:1–10.

Bergsma DP, van der Wildt G (2010). Visual training of cerebral blindness patients gradually enlarges the visual field. *Br J Ophthalmol* 94(1):88–96.

Berman R, Negishi M, Vestal M, Spann M, Chung MH, Bai X, Purcaro M, Motelow JE, Danielson N, Dix-Cooper L, Enev M, Novotny EJ, Constable RT, Blumenfeld H (2010). Simultaneous EEG, fMRI, and behavior in typical childhood absence seizures. *Epilepsia* 51(10):2011–2012.

Bleyenheuft Y, Thonnard JL (2011). Tactile spatial resolution in unilateral brain lesions and its correlation with digital dexterity. *J Rehabil Med* 43(3):251–26.

Boyle J, McCartney E, Forbes J, O'Hare A (2007). A randomised controlled trial and economic evaluation of direct versus indirect and individual versus group modes of speech and language therapy for children with primary language impairment. *Health Technol Assess* 112(5):iii–iv, xi–xii, 1–139.

Carson RG (2005) Neural pathways mediating bilateral interactions between the upper limbs. *Brain Res Rev* 49(3):641–662.

Charles J, Gordon AM (2005) A critical review of constraint-induced movement therapy and forced use in children with hemiplegia. *Neural Plast* 12(2–3):245–261.

Charles J, Gordon AM (2006). Development of hand-arm bimanual intensive training (HABIT) for improving bimanual coordination in children with hemiplegic cerebral palsy. *Dev Med Child Neurol* 48(11):931–936.

Cooper J, Majnemer A, Rosenblatt B, Birnbaum R (1995). The determination of sensory deficits in children with hemiplegic cerebral palsy. *J Child Neurol* 10:300–309.

Denckla MB (1983). The neuropsychology of social–emotional learning disabilities [editorial]. *Arch Neurol* 40:461–462.

Fitzgerald KC, Williams LS, Garg BP, Golomb MR (2007). Epilepsy in children with delayed presentation of perinatal stroke. *J Child Neurol* 22(11):1274–1280.

Gardner MA, Hills NK, Sidney S, Johnston SC, Fullerton HJ (2010). The 5-year direct medical cost of neonatal and childhood stroke in a population-based cohort. *Neurology* 74(5):372–8.

Golomb MR, Garg BP, Saha C, Azzouz F, Williams LS (2008). Cerebral palsy after perinatal arterial ischemic stroke. *J Child Neurol* 23(3):279–286.

Golomb MR, Garg BP, Williams LS (2006). Outcomes of children with infantile spasms after perinatal stroke. *Pediatr Neurol* 34(4):291–295.

Golomb MR, MacGregor DL, Domi T, Armstrong DC, McCrindle BW, Mayank S, deVeber GA (2001). Presumed pre- or peri-natal arterial ischemic stroke: risk factors and outcomes. *Ann Neurol* 50(2):163–168.

Goodman R, Graham P (1996). Psychiatric problems in children with hemiplegia: cross-sectional epidemiological survey. *BMJ* 312:1065–1069.

Goodman R, Yude C (1997). Do unilateral lesions of the developing brain have side-specific psychiatric consequences in childhood? *Laterality* 2:103–115.

Gordon AM, Chinnan A, Gill S, Petra E, Hung YC, Charles J (2008). Both constraint-induced movement therapy and bimanual training lead to improved performance of upper extremity function in children with hemiplegia. *Dev Med Child Neurol* 50(12):957–958.

Gordon AM, Hung YC, Brandao M, Ferre CL, Kuo HC, Friel K, Petra E, Chinnan A, Charles JR (2011). Bimanual training and constraint-induced movement therapy in children with hemiplegic cerebral palsy: A randomized trial. *Neurorehabil Neural Repair*. June 23 [Epub ahead of print].

Harbert MJ, Tam EW, Glass HC, Bonifacio SL, Haeusslein LA, Barkovich AJ, Jeremy RJ, Rogers EE, Glidden DV, Ferriero DM (2011). Hypothermia is correlated with seizure absence in perinatal stroke. *J Child Neurol* 26(9):1126–1130.

Hoare BJ, Wasiak J, Imms C, Carey L (2007). Constraint-induced movement therapy in the treatment of the upper limb in children with hemiplegic cerebral palsy. *Cochrane Database Syst Rev*.18;2:CD004149.

Trenité et al., 1990Kasteleijn-Nolst Trenité DG, Smit AM, Velis DN, Willemse J, van Emde Boas W (1990). On-line detection of transient neuropsychological disturbances during EEG discharges in children with epilepsy. *Dev Med Child Neurol* 32(1):46–50.

Kennett S, Taylor-Clarke M, Haggard P (2001). Noninformative vision improves the spatial resolution of touch in humans. *Curr Biol* 11(15):1188–1191.

Kleffner FR, Landau WM (2009). The Landau-Kleffner syndrome. *Epilepsia 50(Suppl* 7):3.

Kolk A, Ennok M, Laugesaar R, Kaldoja ML, Talvik T (2011). Long-term cognitive outcomes after pediatric stroke. *Pediatr Neurol* 44(2):101–109.

Lane AR, Smith DT, Ellison A, Schenk T (2010). Visual exploration training is no better than attention training for treating hemianopia. *Brain* 133(Pt 6):1717–1728.

Laugesaar R, Kolk A, Tomberg T, Metsvaht T, Lintrop M, Varendi H, Talvik T (2007). Acutely and retrospectively diagnosed peri-natal stroke: a population-based study. *Stroke* 38(8):2234–2240.

Laurent-Vannier A, Chevignard M, Pradat-Diehl P, Abada G, De Agostini M (2006). Assessment of unilateral spatial neglect in children using the Teddy Bear Cancellation Test. *Dev Med Child Neurol* 48(2):120–125.

Luft AR, McCombe-Waller S, Whitall J, Forrester LW, Macko R, Sorkin JD, Schulz JB, Goldberg AP, Hanley DF (2004). Repetitive bilateral arm training and motor cortex activation in chronic stroke: a randomized controlled trial. *JAMA* 292(15):1853–1861.

Lynch JK (2009). Epidemiology and classification of perinatal stroke. *Semin Fetal Neonatal Med.* 14(5):245–29.

Mannino F, Trauner DA (1983). Stroke in neonates. *J Pediatr* 102(4):605–610.

Max JE, Bruce M, Keatley E, Delis D (2010). Pediatric stroke: plasticity, vulnerability, and age of lesion onset. *J Neuropsychiatry Clin Neurosci* 22(1):30–39.

Ment LR, Duncan CC, Ehrenkranz RA (1984). Perinatal cerebral infarction. *Ann Neurol* 16(5):559–568.

Mercuri E, Anker S, Guzzetta A, Barnett A, Haataja L, Rutherford M, Cowan F, Dubowitz L, Braddick O, Atkinson J (2003). Neonatal cerebral infarction and visual function at school age. *Arch Dis Child Fetal Neonatal Ed* 88(6):F487–491. Erratum in: Arch Dis Child Fetal Neonatal Ed. 2004 Mar;89(2):F187.

Mercuri E, Atkinson J, Braddick O, Anker S, Nokes L, Cowan F, Rutherford M, Pennock J, Dubowitz L (1996). Visual function and perinatal focal cerebral infarction. *Arch Dis Child Fetal Neonatal Ed.* 75(2):F76–81.

Muter V, Taylor S, Vargha-Khadem F (1997). A longitudinal study of early intellectual development in hemiplegic children. *Neuropsychologia* 35:289–298.

Nass R, Koch D (1987). Temperamental differences in toddlers with early unilateral right- and left-brain damage. *Dev Neuropsychol* 3:93–99.

Nass R, Koch D (1991). Specialization for emotion: temperament after congenital unilateral injury. In: Amir N, Rapin I (eds), Pediatric Neurology: Behavior and Cognition of the Child with Brain Dysfunction (pp. 1–17). Basel: Karger.

Naylor CE, Bower E (2005). Modified constraint-induced movement therapy for young children with hemiplegic cerebral palsy: a pilot study. *Dev Med Child Neurol* 47(6):365–369.

Pohl M, Mehrholz J (2006). Immediate effects of an individually designed functional ankle-foot orthosis on stance and gait in hemiparetic patients. *Clin Rehabil* 20:324–330.

Praline J, Hommet C, Barthez M, Brault F, Perrier D, Du Passage G, Lucas B, Bonnard J, Billard C, De Toffol B, Autret A (2003). Outcome at adulthood of the continuous spike-waves during slow sleep and Landau-Kleffner syndromes. *Epilepsia* 44(11):1434–1440.

Reilly JS, Stiles J, Larsen J, Trauner D (1995). Affective facial expression in infants with focal brain damage. *Neuropsychologia* 33:83–99.

Rowe ML, Levine SC, Fisher JA, Goldin-Meadow S (2009). Does linguistic input play the same role in language learning for children with and without early brain injury? *Dev Psychol* 45(1):90–102.

Saposnik G, Teasell R, Mamdani M, Hall J, McIlroy W, Cheung D, Thorpe KE, Cohen LG, Bayley M, Stroke Outcome Research Canada (SORCan) Working Group (2010). Effectiveness of virtual reality using Wii gaming technology in stroke rehabilitation: a pilot randomized clinical trial and proof of principle. *Stroke* 41(7):1477–1484.

Serino A, Bassolino M, Farnè A, Làdavas E (2007). Extended multisensory space in blind cane users. *Psychol Sci* 18(7):642–648.

Smania N, Picelli A, Gandolfi M, Fiaschi A, Tinazzi M (2008). Rehabilitation of sensorimotor integration deficits in balance impairment of patients with stroke hemiparesis: a before/after pilot study. *Neurol Sci* 29(5):313–319.

Steenbergen B, Charles J, Gordon AM (2008). Fingertip force control during bimanual object lifting in hemiplegic cerebral palsy. *Exp Brain Res* 186(2):191–201.

Stiles J, Reilly J, Paul B, Moses P (2005). Cognitive development following early brain injury: evidence for neural adaptation. *Trends Cogn Sci* 93:136–143.

Taub E, Griffin A, Uswatte G, Gammons K, Nick J, Law CR (2011). Treatment of congenital hemiparesis with pediatric constraint-induced movement therapy. *J Child Neurol* 26(9):1163–1173.

Thal DJ, Marchman V, Stiles J, Aram D, Trauner D, Nass R, Bates E (1991). Early lexical development in children with focal brain injury. *Brain & Language* 40:491–527.

Tranel D, Hall LE, Olson S, Tranel NN (1987). Evidence for a right-hemisphere developmental learning disability. *Dev Neuropsychol* 3:114–127.

Trauner DA (2003). Hemispatial neglect in young children after early unilateral brain damage. *Dev Med Child Neurol* 45:160–166.

Trauner DA, Ballantyne A, Chase C (1996). Disorders of affective and linguistic prosody after early unilateral brain damage. *Ann Neurol* 39:361–367.

Trauner DA, Chase C, Walker P, Wulfeck B (1993). Neurologic profiles of infants and children after perinatal stroke. *Pediatr Neurol* 9(5):383–386.

Trauner DA, Mannino FL (1986). Neurodevelopmental outcome after neonatal cerebral vascular accident. *J Pediatr* 108(3):459–461.

Trauner DA, Nass R, Ballantyne AO (2001). Behavioral profiles of children and adolescents after pre- or perinatal stroke. *Brain* 12(4):995–1002.

Trauner DA, Panyard-Davis JL, Ballantyne AO (1996). Behavioral differences in school age children after perinatal stroke. *Assessment* 3:265–276.

Tromp SC, Weber JW, Aldenkamp AP, Arends J, vander Linden I, Diepman L (2003). Relative influence of epileptic seizures and of epilepsy syndrome on cognitive function. *J Child Neurol* 18(6):407–412.

Wallen M, O'Flaherty SJ, Waugh MC (2007). Functional outcomes of intramuscular botulinum toxin type A and occupational therapy in the upper limbs of children with cerebral palsy: a randomized controlled trial. *Arch Phys Med Rehabil* 88(1):1–10.

Wang Q, Zhao JL, Zhu QX, Li J, Meng PP (2011). Comparison of conventional therapy, intensive therapy and modified constraint-induced movement therapy to improve upper extremity function after stroke. *J Rehabil Med* 43(7):619–625.

Wanigasinghe J, Reid SM, Mackay MT, Reddihough DS, Harvey AS, Freeman JL (2010). Epilepsy in hemiplegic cerebral palsy due to perinatal arterial ischaemic stroke. *Dev Med Child Neurol* 52(11):1021–1027.

Weintraub S, Mesulam MM (1983). Developmental learning disabilities of the right hemisphere: emotional, interpersonal, and cognitive components. *Arch Neurol* 40:463–468.

Westmacott R, Askalan R, MacGregor D, Anderson P, Deveber G (2010). Cognitive outcome following unilateral arterial ischaemic stroke in childhood: effects of age at stroke and lesion location. *Dev Med Child Neurol* 52(4):386–393.

Wingert JR, Burton H, Sinclair RJ, Brunstrom JE, Damiano DL (2009). Joint-position sense and kinesthesia in cerebral palsy. *Arch Phys Med Rehab* 90:447–453.

Wirt R, Lachar D, Klinedinst J, Seat P (1984). Multidimensional description of child personality: A manual for the Personality Inventory for Children (revised ed.). Los Angeles: Western Psychological Services.

Wulfeck B, Trauner DA, Tallal P (1991). Neurologic, cognitive and linguistic features of infants after early cerebral infarction. *Pediatr Neurol* 7:266–291.

Wusthoff CJ, Kessler SK, Vossough A, Ichord R, Zelonis S, Halperin A, Gordon D, Vargas G, Licht DJ, Smith SE (2011). Risk of later seizure after perinatal arterial ischemic stroke: a prospective cohort study. *Pediatrics* 127(6):e1550–1557.

11

Towards an Integrative Model of Neurobehavioral Development

NEARLY A HALF-CENTURY ago Hans-Lukas Teuber and Rita Rudel published a paper entitled "Behaviour after cerebral lesions in children and adults" (Teuber & Rudel, 1962). In this seminal study they explored the effects of early versus late brain injury on behavioral functioning. They asked whether and under what conditions the early timing of brain injury can serve to mitigate or promote behavioral disability, thus pitting the notions of equipotentiality and early localization of function against each other. The answer they provided in that paper, though based on very limited data, was essentially that there is no single answer to the question. Rather, the effects of early injury on the developing brain manifest differently depending on the task involved and the developmental level of the child. These findings led them to conclude, "If we admit that the neocortex may be equipotential in some respects, we ought to be able to specify those aspects of performance for which such equipotentiality holds and those other aspects for which it clearly fails" (Teuber & Rudel, 1962, p. 17). With this conclusion, Teuber and Rudel offered both a challenge to the field to better define the interaction of brain injury and behavioral development, and a framework for approaching these deep and important questions.

The ideas set forth in Teuber and Rudel's (1962) paper provided a model for understanding the effects of early brain injury that is still very much a part of thinking in the field of developmental neuropsychology today. This book was intended to provide an overview of the work that has been done in the ensuing years. Following the path set by Teuber and Rudel, it focuses on the behavioral consequences of early injury, and with much greater detail, largely echoes their early findings. But the past half-century has also brought advances in neurobiology and neuroimaging that can provide better insight into not simply the behavioral outcomes of early injury, but also our understanding of why the patterns of outcome emerge as they do. The contributions of work in developmental neurobiology have provided fundamentally different models of typical brain development than those prevalent a half-century ago. These models introduce very different ways of thinking about how an early neural accident might affect the subsequent progression of brain development. Advances in anatomical and functional imaging techniques also hold great promise for actually answering the most basic questions about how the brain develops in the wake of early injury. Why are deficits following early injury often less severe than those following later injury? How has the brain organized to support essential functions that in the typical course of development would have come to rely on injured brain areas? When there is disability, what in the neural circuitry is lacking, or perhaps shared, that prevents full adaptation and development of function?

This last chapter takes up these questions. It begins with an overview and synthesis of the major behavioral findings that were presented in depth in Chapters 5 through 9. The intent of this section is not to recap what has already been presented; rather, the goal is to highlight the major behavioral findings and consider the implications of these data for models of brain development. The second section of the chapter considers models of brain-behavior relationships more generally. Chapter 2 provided an overview of major milestones in typical brain development drawn largely from neurobiological studies of animals. The implications of those data for various models of brain development in typically developing children are the focus of this section. The third section of this chapter will integrate models of typical brain development with data on the effects of early brain injury. This section focuses on dynamic models of brain development and considers what predictions they might make about the effects of early injury on the emerging organization of the neural system. The final section of the chapter looks forward and considers the implications of these new models for both typical and atypical trajectories of neurobehavioral development.

BEHAVIORAL OUTCOMES FOLLOWING PERINATAL BRAIN INJURY

A wide range of factors can affect outcomes following perinatal brain injury. These include such things as timing of lesion, extent of injury, task difficulty, developmental age of the child when assessed, and of course, the behavioral domain under examination. This section will provide a summary of these complex interactions for each of the major behavioral domains reviewed in the earlier chapters of this book. The summaries will include a description of the kinds of deficits observed, the magnitude of impairment, and any evidence of change in the status of deficit with development (i.e., emergence, persistence, or amelioration of deficit). Where the data are available, the patterns of impairment will also be linked to known patterns of deficit or developmental anomaly within the associated neuroanatomical and/or neurofunctional systems.

The section will close with a discussion of the similarities and differences in neurobehavioral outcomes across domains, and a consideration of the kinds of factors that might lead to the more or less effective functioning of neurobehavioral systems. At the heart of this discussion is the central question of neurobehavioral plasticity and its impact on brain development following early injury. As will become clear, the capacity of the developing neural system to adapt to the contingencies imposed by injury may lead to variable outcomes. For some systems the competitive processes that are essential for normal development may also induce compensatory changes that promote the development of highly functional, if atypically organized, neurobehavioral systems. For other systems, these same competitive processes may actually exacerbate the deficit. This discussion will set the stage for the next sections of this chapter, which will consider various models for thinking about the role of neural plasticity in both typical and atypical brain development.

Somatosensory and Motor System Development

The motor and somatosensory systems are evolutionarily older than the neurobehavioral systems mediating higher cognitive function. The basic pathways for both systems form prenatally. The corticospinal tract (CST) efferents originating in the motor cortex begin to innervate both ipsi- and contralateral spinal motor neurons by gestational week 24 (GW24; Eyre, 2007), and thalamocortical tract(TCT) afferent axons reach cortical layer IV by GW26 (Kostovic & Jovanov-Milosevic, 2006; Kostovic & Judas, 2010). Thus, the systems are "early" developing both phylogenetically and ontogenetically, perhaps accounting for their greater vulnerability and more limited resiliency after early injury. The somatosensory and motor cortices are also highly linked, yet the frequently different reorganizational patterns (ipsi- vs. contralateral) of the two systems can interfere with sensorimotor integration.

Motor System

Motor deficits manifest predominantly distally as weakness, spasticity, slowness, impaired dexterity and individuated finger movements, and apraxia. The unaffected hand is sometimes mildly affected. Bimanual activities are often compromised. Although the lesion has been present since the pre-perinatal period, the hemiparesis emerges over time; it is generally apparent by the end of the first year and may even appear to worsen as the distal arm and the leg come "on line" for increasingly complex age-appropriate motor functions. The effects of early damage to the motor system vary by lesion location, type, size, and age at injury even within the context of an 8-week pre-perinatal period; all are interrelated factors. With respect to location, a lesion that compromises the CST anywhere along its path is very likely to cause a hemiparesis; middle cerebral artery territory (MCA) strokes almost invariably do so, while periventricular white matter injury (PVWMI) may not. Lesions associated with PVWMI occur in the early third trimester and tend to be smaller than the late-third-trimester MCA strokes. In most cases of PVWMI, the normal pattern of contralateral CST organization is retained, the hemiparesis is mild, and hand function is only mildly affected. In contrast, after MCA strokes, the most common pattern of reorganization involves the persistence and progressive dominance of the normally transient ipsilateral CST; the contralesional ipsilateral CST controls the affected hand, which would be better served by a contralateral CST from the damaged motor cortex (Eyre, 2007; Staudt, 2010). The persistence and elaboration of ipsilateral CSTs are due to a failure of normal activity-dependent pruning during the first 2 years (Eyre et al., 2007; Martin, 2005). This pattern of reorganization is generally associated with moderate to severe impairment of the affected hand, as well as with mirror movements, which are presumably due to innervation of bilateral spinal motor neurons by efferent axons from the contralesional hemisphere via an ipsilateral CST. Although ipsilateral CSTs are not optimal for motor control, there is a range of residual hand function associated with this reorganization pattern, and good motor function has been reported (Holmstrom et al., 2010). The stabilization of an ipsilateral CST can also have a negative impact on the unaffected hand, presumably because the intact hemisphere is required to support the motor function of both hands; the two hands do not function independently of one another (Utley & Steenbergen, 2006). Furthermore, during complex bimanual tasks that demand planning, the impaired hand can have a negative impact on the intact hand function (Hung et al., 2004, 2010). In addition, mirror movements can interfere with the function of the unaffected hand, particularly on bimanual tasks. While even ipsilateral CSTs allow for better motor function after early injury relative to similar injury in adulthood, an ipsilateral CST may exacerbate or actually create behavioral deficits, and thus may be to some degree maladaptive (Eyre 2007).

Somatosensory System

Somatosensory deficits are very common and can be detected in both the affected hand and relatively frequently in the unaffected hand. Deficits generally affect cortical sensory functions like graphesthesia, stereognosia, as well as two-point discrimination and proprioception. Touch, pain, and temperature perception are less frequently affected. The effects of pre-perinatal injury on the sensory system also vary by lesion type (PVWMI vs. MCA stroke), size, and timing. As noted, lesions associated with PVWMI occur earlier and tend to be smaller than the later-occurring MCA strokes, which are large and more importantly involve the somatosensory cortex itself, as well as thalamocortical afferents. Regional specification of the post-central gyrus as the primary somatosensory cortex occurs early in gestation, even before the development of thalamocortical afferents (Juenger et al., 2011). Unlike the motor cortex, the somatosensory cortex has little capacity for reorganization. Therefore, cortical lesions (like MCA strokes) affect sensory function to a significantly greater degree than even large white matter periventricular lesions (Wilke et al., 2008). However, the somatosensory system does have axonal plasticity (Juenger et al., 2011) and spatial plasticity (Wilke, Staudt, et al. 2009). TCT sensory afferents virtually always retain the typical contralateral distribution, although the pathway from thalamus to cortex can be anatomically unusual. The TCT has the capacity to bypass even large periventricular lesions by traveling through undamaged tissue, presumably into intact somatosensory cortex in the post-central gyrus (Staudt, Grodd et al., 2002, Staudt, Braun, et al. 2006). Although bypass capacity is present after MCA strokes, it may not be as extensive due to the timing of the injury, and because the sensory cortical target is not intact. Thus, sensory deficits occur despite axonal and spatial plasticity. Since sensory afferents remain contralateral, sensory–motor association occurs when CSTs are contralateral in the setting of PVWMI, and sensory–motor dissociation occurs in most cases of MCA strokes with associated ipsilateral CSTs (see Fig. 4.8 in Chapter 4). The former generally results in less clinical deficit than the latter, including intact intrahemispheric sensorimotor integration, and better response to constraint-induced motor therapy (Kuhnke et al., 2008).

Sensory–Motor Interaction

The differences in reorganization patterns of the motor and somatosensory systems place different constraints on the developing nervous system. Unlike the motor system, where activity-dependent reorganization can involve both ipsilateral and contralateral CSTs, somatosensory pathways retain contralateral organization regardless of the time of perinatal injury (Juenger et al., 2011; Staudt, 2010). Despite the reorganizational differences, motor and sensory deficits are both common and persistent and moreover are interrelated. On a behavioral level there is generally a strong correlation between sensibility and motor dexterity (Clayton et al., 2003; Krumlinde-Sundholm & Eliasson, 2002). The negative effect of sensory deficits on motor function reflects the fundamental nature of sensory feedback for the execution of voluntary movement of the hand (Gandevia et al., 1992) and for manual dexterity and precision finger movements (Krumlinde-Sundholm & Eliasson, 2002; Taub & Wolf, 1997). Indeed, recent imaging studies (diffusion tensor imaging [DTI], which tracks axonal pathways) of children born preterm with PVWMI demonstrate that thalamocortical sensory afferent integrity correlates better with motor outcome than does CST integrity (Hoon et al., 2002; Wilke et al., 2009). In contrast to the widely distributed neural circuitry of the cognitive systems, the strong interaction between sensory and motor systems maximizes dysfunction.

Visuospatial Development

The visuospatial processing system has a long evolutionary history and encompasses a wide range of basic skills and abilities. The neural architecture of the visual spatial processing system is complex and includes dozens of posterior brain regions (Van Essen et al., 1992) and a rich array of connections to anterior brain regions. The posterior system is anatomically divided into separate processing streams that subserve distinct higher cognitive functions. The ventral stream mediates information about patterns and objects, while the dorsal stream is involved in processes related to attention, movement, and location, as well as visually guided movement. Much of the early data linking specific functions to the separate processing streams came from adult patients with localized brain injury. Subsequent imaging studies have confirmed the basic divisions and elaborated on their function and organization.

The typical course of development for the two visual systems is quite protracted. Although newborns are capable of very basic dorsal and ventral stream processing, mature levels of functioning are not generally observed until adolescence. The very small number of available neuroimaging studies converge on the profile of neurobehavioral development seen for other higher cognitive functions. Specifically, the neural systems for many spatial functions, including global local processing (Moses, et al. 1997), categorical and coordinate processing (Reese & Stiles, 2005), face processing, and mental rotation (Ark et al., 2003), are initially widely distributed and inefficient; they become gradually more localized with development. Many of the systems display some degree of laterality bias early on (Martinez et al., 1997; Moses, et al. 1997; Holland et al., 2001; Lidzba et al., 2011; Passarotti et al., 2003), but those profiles become refined with development.

Among children with perinatal stroke, the patterns of deficit mirror those observed among adults with comparable extent of brain injury, but the deficits among children with early lesions are much less severe. Across both dorsal and ventral stream processes, development is also observed with age. At each developmental phase, age-appropriate tasks reveal evidence of specific deficit. However, with time, children begin to exhibit some degree of mastery, and their performance on simple spatial tasks becomes indistinguishable from their typical peers. However, in many cases, when more challenging tasks are presented to older children, the same lesion-specific subtle deficits can be detected. This profile suggests that there is evidence of developmental mastery against a backdrop of persistent subtle deficit. These findings suggest that the basic organization of the visuospatial system emerges very early in development, and that early lateralized lesions systematically affect the development of specific functions in ways that generally mirror the organization of the mature system.

Deficits of ventral stream processing manifest as a specific impairment of global/configural or local/featural processing associated with injury to the right or left hemisphere, respectively. Children with right hemisphere injury have greater difficulty reproducing or recognizing the overall configuration of a pattern, while children with left hemisphere injury have difficulty with the local elements (Stiles & Nass, 1991; Stiles et al., 1996, 2006, 2008). Evidence for this pattern of deficit can be found in young preschool-age children, but it is still apparent as the children enter adolescence. For example, teenagers and young adults with perinatal lesions are less accurate on tasks requiring them to say whether two faces presented in sequence are the same. The deficit is more pronounced for adolescents with right hemisphere injury, presumably reflecting the dominance of configural information in face processing, but both groups show evidence for subtle deficits consistent with the idea that featural processing also plays a role. A similar profile of lateralized deficit is also seen for dorsal stream processing. Toddlers with perinatal injury have difficulty compared with typical peers on simple spatial location tasks. Children with right hemisphere injury have particular difficulty coding metric spatial relations. Although improvement is observed with development, more challenging tests of categorical and coordinate processing reveal subtle ongoing deficits in the late school-age and early adolescent periods.

There have been very few neuroimaging studies of visuospatial processing in children with PL. As discussed in Chapter 5, the few studies that exist point to possible reorganization within the normally bilaterally distributed neural system for visuospatial processing (Booth et al., 1999, 2000; Moses, et al. 1997). In the normal course of development, children appear to activate the full functional processing network for a given function, in that sense using all available resources for the task at hand. Thus for global-local processing, children activate both left and right posterior brain regions regardless of task demands; it is only with development that the mature, lateralized patterns of greater left activation for local and greater right activation for global processing emerge. Similarly, for face processing, children appear to activate the entire extended face processing network, even when task demands require only passive viewing; only later do they exhibit the mature pattern of more limited activation within the core face network (Haist et al., submitted). In the wake of early injury, children may also recruit all available resources in their more limited network, which then eventually stabilizes with the nonlesioned hemisphere exhibiting dominance for all of the spatial functions. As is the case with younger typical children, such a neural system may be functional, but not optimal as reflected in the specific patterns of deficit associated with limitations on the plasticity on the visuospatial system.

The Development of Attention, Memory, and Executive Functions

Attention, working memory, and executive functioning are closely interrelated higher-order cognitive domains that to some extent utilize overlapping neural networks. Spatial attention utilizes posterior parietal and inferior frontal cortex, as well as subcortical areas including the thalamus. A fronto-striato-thalamo-cortical network has been described that appears to be integral for spatial attention. Working memory also appears to utilize a distributed network including parietal and both ventral and dorsal lateral prefrontal cortex. While executive function has been thought to require intact prefrontal cortex, in children this does not appear to be the case, and again, a more widely distributed network including posterior parietal lobes has been implicated in early executive functioning.

All of the above skills have a protracted course during development and are not fully operational until late adolescence, particularly certain aspects of executive function. Because of the later emergence of these cognitive skills, there are conflicting theories about the effects of early brain injury on future competence in these areas. Some studies (e.g., Max et al., 2010) find that children with early focal brain damage (prior < 1 yr. of age) have intact executive function skills when tested later in childhood, suggesting that early brain damage may have only limited long-term adverse effects on this aspect of cognition. However, other studies report executive function deficits in children with perinatal lesions, regardless of lesion location, which is consistent with adult studies documenting extended brain networks for these complex functions. Such findings suggest that damage to any part of the extended network may have adverse consequences for this kind of late developing function (Jacobs et al., 2011). Our studies suggest that attention is impaired in older children and adolescents with perinatal damage, suggesting that these late emerging skills are also vulnerable to early brain insults. The developmental constrains on late emerging cognitive functions such as executive function or attention, likely differ from those on earlier developing systems such as language. But because the skills develop over a long time period, there may be means of mitigating adverse consequences (e.g., by early intervention with social skills training). Certainly the long time course of skill development allows the practitioner to identify deficits early on and to address them while the brain is still developing.

Early Communicative Development and the Development of Language

For adults, language is situated in a multimodal communicative system in which language, gesture, and facial expression are temporally integrated within a social context. When we look across the development of communicative systems within the perinatal stroke group, differing degrees of resilience and plasticity are evident.

Emotional expression is a basic signaling system; it is evolutionarily old and highly dependent on subcortical structures (e.g., the amygdala). The findings with respect to the perinatal stroke group show distinctive profiles as a function of lesion site. Children with left hemisphere injury behave like typically developing children: in a free play situation, they smile easily and produce predominantly positive vocalizations. In contrast, infants with right hemisphere injury show flattened affective expression both facially and vocally and increased negativity compared to both the left hemisphere injury group and to controls. It is of note that these hemisphere-specific profiles are not tied to a particular modality (face or voice) but rather reflect a broader system of emotional expression. Moreover, these results map onto those from adult lesion patients in comparable situations. Specifically, adults with left hemisphere stroke look comparable to neurologically healthy adults, whereas those with right hemisphere stroke show flattened affect and increased negativity in spontaneous conversation. Thus affective expression appears to be functionally organized from early infancy and shows little plasticity as it emerges as a communicative system.

Another early-emerging communicative system is that of gesture, and gestures (e.g., pointing) have been found to precede and predict subsequent lexical acquisition in toddlers. The few studies on early gesture in the PL group suggest that these early precursors to language have the same relation to early words as in typically developing children. Although there are some data to suggest that infants with right hemisphere injury may have smaller repertoires of gesture than those with left hemisphere injury, the relation of early gesture to children's later lexical production shows no laterality differences. Such results suggest that although delayed overall, early gesture and language are linked in the PL group, irrespective of lesion site.

For language, the most extensively researched communicative system, the studies show delay in the emergence of all linguistic milestones beginning with babbling. Importantly, the side and site of lesion do not appear to be influential. That is, regardless of lesion side (right hemisphere or left), children with PL are delayed at each linguistic milestone: babbling, early comprehension, first words, and first sentences. Within this broad context of overall delay, a number of studies of toddlers and preschool-age children have observed an increased deficit in productive language (vocabulary and syntax) in the left hemisphere injury group. As the children enter school, side-specific profiles have resolved such that after about age 6 to 7 years, there are no appreciable differences in language measures between children with right or left hemisphere injury. Although they score below their typically developing peers on standardized language measures, and subtle deficits are apparent, in spontaneous speech and narratives the PL group as a whole is within the low normal range for productive language. Such findings suggest that language acquisition and language functions draw on a distributed neural network from the outset. Further, this wide distribution may in large part be responsible for its resilience as a behavioral system. Recent imaging studies from both typically developing children as well as those with left hemisphere lesions are beginning to confirm this notion. Using the verb generation task, which reliably activates the left inferior frontal gyrus in healthy adults, a number of large-scale studies of typically developing school-age children have shown bilateral activation in the younger children, which progressively lateralizes to the left hemisphere in adolescence (Holland et al., 2001, 2007; Ressel et al., 2008). Using this same design, studies of children with left hemisphere injury show either right hemisphere activation, or bilateral activation with perilesional areas in the left hemisphere participating as well (Jacola et al., 2006; Raja Beharelle et al., 2010). Thus the resilience of language in the PL children appears to be due to the initially bilateral and dispersed nature of the neural network underlying language acquisition. The children with left hemisphere injury are then able to exploit this widely distributed network such that the right hemisphere (and what remains active of the left hemisphere) can support language functions.

Finally, with respect to co-speech gesture, more than 20 years ago David McNeill proposed that gesture and speech in adults form an integrated system. The data from the PL group by and large support this position in that gestures from 5- and 6-year-old PL children follow their language profiles. School-age children with right or left hemisphere injury are in the low normal range for productive language, and the quantity and quality of their gestures also follow this pattern. Such findings suggest that similar to language, co-speech gesture is a distributed and relatively resilient system.

In sum, across communicative systems the behavioral data demonstrate gradients of neural plasticity from the more vulnerable evolutionary old and subcortically mediated emotional expression to the more resilient, more recent, and widely distributed system for language.

MODELS OF TYPICAL BRAIN DEVELOPMENT

The profiles of behavioral outcome following perinatal brain injury present a complex, multifaceted puzzle. Outcomes vary by behavioral domain, age at lesion, lesion location and size, and experience. For most but not all domains, the effects of early injury on behavior are less severe than those observed among adults with comparable extent of injury. But in nearly every case and for all domains there is some measurable level of deficit, indicating that there is a neurobehavioral cost to early brain injury. The challenge is to provide an account of the effects of early brain injury that captures the complexity of the neurological and behavioral events that begin at a discrete moment in the perinatal period but then unfold gradually over many months and years. The story is ultimately one about development, and how and to what extent a complex developing system can adapt to a serious, early perturbation. But there are many models of development, ranging from those proposing strong predeterminism to those stressing equipotentiality. The question is: What kind of model of typical development best accounts for the patterns of data observed in children with perinatal brain injury? The remainder of this section will consider a variety of accounts that have been offered to explain the complex events of typical brain development, and how well they fit the observed data.

Three Models of Functional Brain Development in the Postnatal Period

Perinatal brain injury represents an anomaly of normal brain development. It is an interruption of an ongoing developmental process that happens at a discrete moment in time but then affects the subsequent developmental trajectory. To understand the effects of early injury on the developing brain, it is necessary to first understand the mechanisms that underlie typical brain development—that is, to understand the processes that are being interrupted by injury to the emerging neural system. However, different models make very different assumptions about the processes that underlie normal brain development. Thus the model of development one brings to the study of early injury will influence both the questions that are asked and the interpretation of the observed data. In a recent series of papers, Johnson (Johnson, 2001, 2005, 2011) summarized three major viewpoints concerning the functional development of the brain: the Maturational view, the Skilled Learning view, and the Interactive Specialization view. Each makes very different assumptions about how neural systems develop and about the relationship between brain and behavioral development.

The Maturational viewpoint focuses on linking the emergence of individual sensory, motor, and cognitive behaviors to the maturation of specific brain areas, usually within the cerebral cortex. The functionality of a cortical region is presumed to emerge discretely as the region matures and comes online. By this model, neural maturation enables the emergence of behavioral function in a unidirectional causal fashion, such that biological development precedes and permits behavioral development. This model of functional development is closely allied with genetic models that postulate a unidirectional line of influence from genes to cells to networks to function (Gottlieb, 1992, 2007). Nativist models of behavioral development, which assume innate specification of core knowledge (Carey, 2011; Carey & Xu, 2001; Kinzler & Spelke, 2007; Spelke, 2003; Spelke & Kinzler, 2009), are compatible with the Maturational view. The Maturational view presumes evolutionarily derived, genetic predetermination of the basic features of brain organization. Nativist models of behavioral development suggest that the human capacity for conceptual understanding is anchored to innate, domain-specific evolutionarily derived conceptual primitives (Carey, 2011) that serve as the basis for later learning. Thus, as Johnson (Johnson, 2005) notes, the maturational model of brain development is consistent with strongly localizationist views from adult neuropsychology. In development, discrete, domain-specific functional modules successively come online as brain areas mature, while injury to the adult brain discretely produces lesions in those modules, resulting in functional loss.

The second viewpoint described by Johnson (Johnson, 2001, 2005, 2011) is what he has termed the Skill Learning view. The Skill Learning view suggests that the brain regions that are active in infants and young children during very early learning of basic perceptual and motor skills are the same as those engaged by adults during complex skill acquisition. Thus, while the nature or complexity of the task within the domain may change with development, neural mediation of skill acquisition remains constant. To illustrate the point Johnson (Johnson, 2001) cites data from early- and late-acquired motor skill learning tasks. Specifically, over the course of learning a new, complex visuomotor skill, adults show a decline in activation in dorsolateral prefrontal cortex accompanied by increases in posterior parietal regions. Similarly, young infants show greater activation in frontal than posterior regions when learning a simple visuomotor task, and with development, activation on these tasks shifts posteriorly. The Skill Learning view suggests that there is early specification of brain regions for certain types of functions, but the content of the to-be-learned skills can vary in complexity. Thus, the Skill Learning view implies early specification of neural systems for broad classes of domain-general functions, without necessarily positing prespecification (Johnson, 2011).

The Interactive Specialization view emphasizes the role of interactions among brain regions in shaping emerging brain organization. It posits that changes in the response properties of cortical regions arise as the product of their competitive interactions with other cortical regions. These interactions occur in the process of acquiring new skills and abilities in what is described as a domain-relevant fashion. By this view, cortical regions do not begin as domain-specific or even domain-general neural modules. Rather, different regions have neuronal and neurochemical properties that make them more suitable for processing some kinds of inputs rather than others, but they are initially poorly defined and broadly functional, and active in a wide range of networks. Activity-dependent interactions sharpen and narrow functions within a cortical region as skills are acquired. Because response properties of a cortical region reflect connectivity to multiple brain regions, the acquisition of new behavioral competencies will be associated with changes in several networks. This model of functional development is closely allied with dynamic, multilevel models of development, and most specifically with Neuroconstructivism (Karmiloff-Smith, 1998a, 2009; Mareschal et al., 2007; Westermann et al., 2007; Westermann et al., 2011). Neuroconstructivism characterizes development as a trajectory that is shaped by multiple, interacting biological and environmental influences (Mareschal et al., 2007). Brain and behavior are linked within the theory by characterizing mental representations as neural activation patterns. Across development the activation patterns associated with a given behavior change, becoming more finely tuned and efficient. The refinement of neural networks derives from the mutual influence of factors arising from many different levels, ranging from genes to cells to brain networks to the active body and the physical and social environment. Interactive Specialization focuses on emerging cortical specialization in the postnatal period and is thus a component within the larger Neuroconstructivist model.

The Fit of the Models to the Data

Each of the models outlined in the last section provides a different perspective on the mechanisms that support brain development. A principal way in which the models diverge is in the postulated sources of constraint on development. The Maturational view emphasizes the priority of neural maturation and genetic specification as the principal factors directing and constraining the developmental process. The Skill Learning view posits early neural specification and functional continuity across the lifespan but leaves open the mechanism for initial neural specification. The Interactive Specialization highlights the role of multiple interacting levels of organization and input in the gradual shaping of functional brain organization, suggesting that the multiple levels of interaction impose dynamic constraints on the development process. The question addressed in this section is which of the three models is best aligned with the available data on brain development, and thus the optimal model for considering the effects of early brain injury. The discussion draws upon data presented in Chapter 2 but is organized around the question of constraints and how they operate to support the orderly development of the neurobehavioral system. It is of note that in his review of the models, Johnson focused primarily on the development of brain–behavior relations, and thus focused on development in the postnatal period. But the arguments from any of the models should apply to the earlier-occurring events of the prenatal period as well. This section considers how data taken from major events in both the pre- and postnatal period align with the various models.

Constraints on Neurological Development

Chapter 2 provided an overview of the major milestones of brain development beginning in the embryonic period and extending into the postnatal period. Studies elucidating the neurobiology of brain development span the levels of neural organization from the macroanatomical, to the cellular, to the molecular. Together this large body of work provides a picture of brain development as the product of a complex series of dynamic and adaptive processes. But for the outcome of these processes to be successful, they must also operate within highly constrained and genetically organized but constantly changing contexts (Morange, 2001; Stiles, 2008; Waddington, 1939). The question addressed in this section concerns the sources of constraint on neurobehavioral development. There are three principal types of constraint on neurobehavioral development: genetic, environmental, and temporal. Each will be considered.

Genetic Constraints

Genes provide the templates for creating particular proteins that are essential for the development and functioning of the organism. Many genes, particularly developmental genes, have a long evolutionary history that shaped their functional roles both phylogenetically and ontogenetically. Abnormalities in gene expression affect development by altering the critical signaling pathways. There were many examples provided in Chapter 2 of a modification in the level of expression of a particular gene altering the developmental trajectory of, for example, cell differentiation, cell migration, or pathway formation. Gene products must be available at the right time and in the right quantities for development to proceed normally. In that way genes provide powerful constraints on the course of brain development.

Environmental Constraints

The environment also provides essential input that influences the development of the emerging neural networks. Here the notion of what constitutes the "environment" is broadly construed and includes many different levels ranging from the cell, to cell assemblies, to neural systems, to the world outside the organism (Gottlieb, 2007). Thus, for example, environmental influences on a single neuron can derive from gene expression within the cell, molecular signaling produced by other cells, nutrients or toxins in the surrounding cellular environment, or input from the external environment that propagates to the cell via the activation of neural networks. Interactions are also bi- or multi-directional. Thus, for example, a cell can be the recipient of a molecular or electrical signal from an external source, and it can also produce a signal that influences other cells and cell networks. Further, interactions at one level often have cascading effects that propagate and produce effects on other levels. For example, severing the major input pathway to primary auditory cortex (PAC) in 1-day-old ferrets alters the balance of competition for resources in PAC. The normally transient inputs to PAC from the retina stabilize and the input from the eye changes the function of PAC from auditory to visual (Sur et al., 1999; Sur & Leamey, 2001; Sur & Rubenstein, 2005).

Some aspects of the environment are the product of the neurodevelopmental process itself. For example, the subplate cells of the neocortex are an early-produced but transient population of neurons whose function is to guide the thalamocortical and corticothalamic axons to their appropriate locations in the somatosensory system (Kostovic et al., 2011). Thus, a subplate cell is the product of complex developmental processes that then goes on to serve a particular function in the subsequent development of neural networks.

Many environmental factors are external to the organism. Nutrients provided by the maternal system, infection of the mother or fetus, teratogens introduced to the fetus via ingestion, gravity, light, temperature, and sensory input are all examples of factors that affect and constrain the development of the organism. As is the case with gene products, environmental factors, whether intrinsic to the organism or from the outside world, must be present at the right time and in the right quantities for normal development to proceed. Indeed, one way to think about the effects of early brain injury is as a very serious perturbation of the developmental environment that affects all levels of the developing system from the molecular, to the cellular, to the neural systems levels.

Time-based Constraints

A third essential constraint on neural development arises from the fact that developmental processes unfold over time. The integrity of the developmental process depends absolutely upon the availability of the right neural elements appearing at the appropriate moment in developmental time. Often the emergence of a new element depends upon developmental events that immediately precede its appearance. The earlier-discussed example of subplate cell production preceding the formation of the thalamocortical pathway is one such instance of this kind of developmental scaffolding. What this type of event illustrates is that the process of development itself introduces levels of structure and function that constrain the range of possible developmental trajectories for the organism. In that sense, development can be construed as a self-organizing process.

Two important aspects of the temporal constraints on neurodevelopment are manifest in the complementary principles of progressive differentiation and progressive commitment of neural elements (Stiles, 2008). While each is an ongoing process across the course of development, snapshots of the organism at successive moments in time can illustrate the ways in which these temporally based constraints support the neurodevelopmental process.

Progressive Differentiation

Progressive differentiation refers to and reflects the ongoing increases in the complexity of the organism. There were many examples of this phenomenon given in Chapter 2, but the major events of gastrulation, which includes the very first step in brain development, provide one clear example of the ongoing differentiation of the embryo. Specifically, during gastrulation the embryo goes from a two-layered to a three-layered structure as new cell lines differentiate and become organized and integrated. Migrating cells that will by the end of gastrulation form the mesodermal germ layer of the embryo also establish signaling pathways that promote the differentiation of the neural progenitor cell population in the epiblast layer. This progressive differentiation of neural progenitors also has a spatial component that is critical for establishing the basic functional organization of the embryo. Concurrent with the signaling that promotes the differentiation of the neural progenitor cell lines, more specific signaling establishes subpopulations of neural progenitors along the emerging neuraxis of the embryo. Cells in rostral regions differentiate to become forebrain progenitors, while more caudally positioned cells differentiate to become spinal and hindbrain progenitors. A few weeks later, the gradient expression of multiple transcription factor proteins in the rostral progenitor cell population will promote further differentiation within cells destined to form the major sensory and motor areas of the emerging neocortex. Thus, one hallmark of development is the progressive differentiation of neural elements that is observed in the increasing diversity of cell types, cell assemblies, and cell networks.

Progressive Commitment

The complement of progressive differentiation is the progressive commitment of resources that serves to stabilize the developing neural systems. Developing systems exhibit considerable plasticity and capacity to adapt to varying signals and contingencies. But that plasticity is progressively constrained and declines with development as different neural populations become committed to particular systems. For example, at the onset of gastrulation the embryonic cells are totipotent; that is, they are capable of differentiating into any cell type in the body (Stiles, 2008). But with development there is progressive restriction of potential. The epiblast cells that receive molecular signals from migrating mesodermal cells differentiate to become neural progenitor cells. The subset of those cells that also receive anteriorizing signals are further restricted to producing neurons for the forebrain. Later, during the formation of the neocortex, those same progenitor cells become progressively more restricted in the specific types of neurons they can produce (McConnell, 1992). Thus the potential of progenitor cells becomes more and more restricted as a consequence of emerging constraints on progenitor cell plasticity. This kind of waning plasticity is also observed much later in development. For example, in the early postnatal period, connectivity in the brain is exuberant, with most regions making transient connections with multiple brain regions that are not observed in the mature brain (Innocenti & Price, 2005). In the normal course of development exuberant connections are retracted and mature patterns of connectivity stabilize and are retained. It is assumed that competitive forces act to shape the final patterns of connectivity, such that optimally efficient networks are retained and stabilized and less optimal patterns of connectivity are eliminated.

State and History of the Organism

At all levels of the neural system, progressive differentiation of specific elements and structures and progressive commitment of those elements to functional systems serve to constrain and shape the developmental trajectory of the neural system. The degree of differentiation and commitment of neural elements defines the developmental state of the organism at any given moment in time; the series of events leading up to a given state defines the developmental history of the organism. The state of the organism constrains which factors can influence its development. Many developmental events can happen only in certain contexts. For example, visual and auditory signals have little effect on the gastrulating embryo, but both are essential for the typical development of vision and audition in the newborn. Thus the state of the organism represents both the current structure and functional capacity of the organism, as well as its potential for further change. In short, development does not happen all at once. Rather it builds upon itself, often creating as it goes the tools necessary for each successive step in the developmental process.

Reconsidering Models of Neurobehavioral Development

At the beginning of this section, three very different models of neurobehavioral development were presented, the Maturational model, the Skill Learning model, and the Interactive Specialization model. The question posed in this section is: Which model best fits the available data on the basic processes and progress of brain development? As outlined in detail in Chapter 2 and summarized in this section, the hallmark of pre- and postnatal brain develop is dynamic, interactive, and progressive change. The processes that underlie and support brain development involve the ongoing interplay of genetic and environmental factors. Brains do not develop normally in the absence of critical genetic signaling *and* they do not develop normally in the absence of essential environmental input. Rather, at each point in development, organism-intrinsic and environmental factors interact to support the increasingly complex and elaborate structures and functions of the brain. Constraints that arise from genetic, environmental, and temporal sources account for the orderly progression of brain development. Considering the various models outlined at the beginning of this section, the data presented here are most consistent with the Neuroconstructivist view of development and least compatible with a strongly Maturational account. Skill Learning represents an interesting intermediate position involving early stabilization of neural systems that may well be important for learning in some domains.

THE EFFECTS OF PERINATAL BRAIN INJURY

The dynamic and interactive nature of the process of brain development as posited by the Neuroconstructivist model has important implications for the study of children with perinatal brain injury. On one hand, it provides an instructive model for considering the implications of the profiles of data observed in this population and may provide a model for explaining the documented profiles of behavioral strength and weakness. On the other hand, the variable outcomes across domains in this population may also serve to inform the Neuroconstructivist model. Why are some systems better preserved than others, and what are the implications of the documented weaknesses for the model? Do the limits on plasticity suggest that some combination of elements from different models might best accommodate the data on the effects of early brain injury? The next section will focus on linking models of behavioral development to the outcome data from the perinatal lesion population. It begins with a discussion of the most prominent historical account of behavioral functioning after perinatal lesions, the so-called crowding effect, and considers the limits of this account. It then turns to a discussion of how a Neuroconstructivist perspective, or some mix of that model with elements of other models, might provide a different view of the observed data and what the implications of that view are for our understanding of brain development following early injury.

The Right Hemisphere "Crowding Effect" for Language

In 1974 Teuber (Teuber, 1974) published an influential chapter in which he discussed a possible account of the patterns of functional deficit and sparing in children with early brain injury. In that chapter he suggested that the preferential sparing of language over other functions such as visuospatial processing might be accounted for by what he termed the right hemisphere "crowding effect" for language. He argued that because language is an essential human function, in the aftermath of injury to left hemisphere language areas, linguistic functioning is preferentially supported by homologous regions of the right hemisphere. Thus, he suggested that language would "crowd out" the spatial or other functions that would have been mediated by these regions. He further argued that data supporting a crowding effect for language would suggest very early hemispheric specialization for language.

Subsequent behavioral studies have generally confirmed the greater resiliency of language functions, and that has been taken as support for the crowding hypothesis (Aram & Eisele, 1994; Carlsson et al., 1994; Gonzalez-Monge et al., 2009; Rasmussen & Milner, 1977; Vargha-Khadem et al., 1994). However, studies that have actually measured brain laterality for language following early left hemisphere injury have reported considerable variability in the extent of right hemisphere involvement (Everts et al., 2010; Jacola et al., 2006; b et al., 2006a, 2006b; Liegeois et al., 2004; Strauss al., 1990; Tillema et al., 2008). Indeed, recent fMRI studies have suggested that right lateralization of language function does not predict the best outcomes in children with early left hemisphere injury. Rather, the combination of left frontal activation and bilateral activation in posterior brain regions is associated with optimal language outcomes following early left hemisphere injury (Raja Beharelle et al., 2010). Further, one study explicitly examined the association between extent of right hemisphere involvement and visuospatial outcomes, and reported that right hemisphere lateralization, but not bilateral organization, for language is associated with greater levels of impairment of visuospatial functions (Lidzba et al., 2006b).

At the neural level, the construct of a "crowding effect" derives directly from the fact that early injury compromises significant regions of neural tissue, leaving a smaller brain substrate to accommodate the full range of important behavioral functions. However, while the facts of the reduced neural space do make some kind of "crowding" notion likely, there are few data to support the specific assumptions of the most prominent version of the crowding effect hypothesis. Teuber's original conceptualization of the crowding effect began with the observation that language tends to show greater resiliency following early injury than other behaviors. That resiliency was thought to reflect the importance and thus priority of language over other cognitive functions. The assumption of linguistic priority was then used to draw inferences about the effects of the presumed behavioral priorities on emerging neural organization. Thus the logic of the "crowding effect" as it was originally formulated and as it is commonly applied today is that because language is the most important behavioral function, it will be given priority, effectively crowding out other functions, at the level of neural structure during development.

This very top-down approach to the question of neurobehavioral development has very little grounding in the neurobiological or even within the neurobehavioral literature. The mechanism for the crowding event is not specified; the strongest available neural data come from consistent reports of a rightward shift in laterality of language function. But an account of what induces the lateralized shift is lacking, as is the evidence of how a change in the neural substrate for language could affect other functions.

The traditional crowding argument postulates a trade-off between preservation of language and impairment in other, particularly visuospatial, processes. The presumption is that because spatial functions are strongly right lateralized from very early in development, injury to the left hemisphere should not directly affect those processes. Thus any decrement in spatial processing following left hemisphere injury should be attributed to the effects of crowding. However, while some spatial functions such as spatial attention, spatial localization, and face processing are right dominant, they are bilaterally represented in typical brains (Fink et al., 2001; Kanwisher & Yovel, 2006; Siman-Tov et al., 2007). Further, other spatial functions, such as object processing, categorical and coordinate processing, and global–local processing, are strongly bilateral in their representations (Keita & Bedoin, 2011; Meadmore et al., 2009; Ng et al., 2000; van der Ham et al., 2009). There is also evidence for left hemisphere dominance for some spatial functions such as shift attention (Asari et al., 2005). Thus an injury to the left hemisphere might well affect the development of spatial functions quite apart from a loss of neural territory to language functions in the unlesioned hemisphere. Indeed, as reported in Chapter 5, left *and* right perinatal brain injury have quite specific and differential effects on spatial processing that are consistent with injury to the brain systems that mediate lateralized components of those functions in typically developing children and adults.

Sources of Functional Vulnerability and Resilience

The data that prompted the initial formulation of the classical crowding effect hypotheses have not changed a great deal in the past 50 years. There are substantially more data, but the basic, broad strokes of evidence remain. This leads to an important question: If the strongly top-down, "linguistic priority" version of the crowding hypothesis does not account for the patterns of observed neurobehavioral data, are there other possible factors that might? It is likely that the basic construct of "crowding" plays some kind of role in the emergence of the neural organization aftermath of early brain injury. Injury compromises neural tissue, leaving a reduced brain substrate, and there is evidence for at least mild neurobehavioral deficits across domains. However, it is also clear that not all functions are affected equally. Somatosensory and motor deficits are more pronounced than deficits of higher cognitive functioning. Among higher cognitive functions, language appears to exhibit somewhat greater resilience than other functions. A similar continuum of impact is evident at the neural level. The somatosensory system exhibits the lowest level of plastic adaptation, maintaining the same basic pattern of organization following injury. The motor system can develop anomalous ipsilateral connections through preservation of a pathway that is usually largely transient. However, the recruitment of that pathway is often associated with worse motor outcome (Staudt et al., 2002). For higher cognitive functions, bilaterality of function, or in some cases recruitment of the nondominant hemisphere, is often reported following early injury, with variable but largely preserved function associated (Jacola et al., 2006; Liegeois et al., 2004; Staudt, 2007; Tillema et al., 2008). The key questions are: How and why do these particular patterns of organization arise? Why are some functions more impaired than others? Why is there such variability in adaptation at the neural level?

Two factors could contribute to the profiles of observed neurobehavioral outcome. The first concerns the dependency of a particular function on basic sensorimotor systems. The second is the evolutionary "age" of the function involved. It is very likely that these two factors are related. Rather than representing two alternative accounts of the observed patterns of data, they may represent two different levels of analysis of a common factor.

Dependence on Sensorimotor Functions

Rank ordering of the behavioral functions by severity of deficit on the one hand, and plasticity evidenced by the emergence of alternative pathways on the other, yields similar lists. Though there are exceptions, level of functional outcome roughly parallels degree of plastic reorganization. Somatosensory and motor functions show the greatest and most persistent deficits and the most limited or dysfunctional patterns of neural reorganization. Among higher cognitive functions, visuospatial processes show less resilience than other functions, and the pattern of lesion site to deficit mapping preserves the patterns observed among adults most veridically. Although imaging data are very limited, neural organization appears to exploit the same neural regions typically associated with visuospatial processes, but consolidates the normally bilaterally distributed spatial functions into the nonlesioned component of the system, perhaps reflecting a kind of within-domain crowding effect. Language, by contrast, shows the least functional decrement and perhaps the greatest neural resourcefulness.

One possible account of these findings is that the more reliant a function is on the primary somatosensory and motor input/output systems, the less resilience both behaviorally and neurologically will be observed. Both the somatosensory and motor systems develop early, forming their basic connections prenatally. The thalamocortical pathway is in place by GW26 (Kostovic & Judas, 2010) and the corticospinal tract by GW24 (Eyre, 2007). The greater vulnerability of the two functions in cases of early injury may be accounted for by the fact that both are typically very early-developing systems. The two systems comprise critical input/output pathways for the entire nervous system. They underpin and provide essential information for all other behaviors. Thus, in the normal course of development, their early emergence, stability, and limited capacity for plastic adaptation may be optimal. The most basic information entering or exiting the neural system needs to be stable and reliable in order to support the development of other functions.

Higher cognitive functions also show differing degrees of resiliency, and it is possible that this could be in part related to their specific dependency on associated sensorimotor systems. Visuospatial processing arguably relies on a more specific and narrower set of basic sensory inputs (visual, vestibular, and in the case of vision for action, motor) than a function like language, which is amodal. Higher-level visuospatial processes rely, obviously, on an intact, functioning visual system. Even brief periods of selective visual deprivation can have long-term negative effects on higher-level visuospatial functions. For example, the studies by Maurer et al. (Le Grand et al., 2003, 2004; Lewis & Maurer, 2005) of the effects of congenital cataracts have shown that a few months of monocular visual deprivation in the first year of life can permanently impair configural processing. But visuospatial processing also involves other basic sensorimotor processes. Vision for action is tied to movements of the body and body position in space. In that sense, basic sensorimotor deficits would limit the component of visuospatial learning that relies on what has been termed embodiment. Embodiment refers to the fact that the body is the principal conduit for interactions with the world (Clark 1999; Mareschal et al., 2007; Smith & Gasser, 2005). Thus neural activations associated with sensorimotor processing introduce powerful filters that shape and constrain mental representations. Actions in the world generate and/or modify new representations. Thus, impairment of the basic sensory and motor systems can have downstream effects on the development of the higher-level visuospatial cognitive functions.

In the normal course of development, language also relies on both sensory and motor input and output. But that reliance may be broader and less rigidly tuned. Language is demonstrably more flexible than other functions in that it can rely on a wider range of input and output systems. Work on the major sign languages of the world has demonstrated that fully articulated language can develop in the absence of auditory input and oral–motor output. Studies of brain organization for language in congenitally deaf individuals suggests that even though sign languages operate in a manual/spatial medium, they nonetheless activate the major brain areas observed in oral/auditory language processing (Emmorey, Allen, et al., 2003; Emmorey, Grabowski, et al. 2003; McCullough et al., 2005), suggesting that these brain areas code linguistic representations rather than modality-specific input and output systems. Thus linguistic functioning may be able to rely on a broader and more varied set of inputs and outputs, such that in the face of early sensorimotor impairment it can exhibit stronger—though not complete—resilience.

Phylogenetic Constraints on Neural Representation

The continuum of neurobehavioral resiliency also maps onto the phylogenetic age of the behavioral functions. Somatosensory and motor systems show the least resiliency and are among the oldest behavioral functions. Language is the most recent acquisition and is arguably unique to humans, at least in its most fully elaborated form, and it shows the greatest resiliency at both the neurological and behavior levels. This pattern raises the possibility that factors related to differences in the phylogenesis of behavioral functions may contribute to the varying levels of resilience among behavioral functions. Evolutionary theories vary greatly in their account of the emergence of higher cognitive functions. On one hand, modular accounts from evolutionary biology suggest that the mind can be decomposed into specialized, separately modifiable functions (Cosmides & Tooby, 1994; Duchaine et al., 2001). Each specialized module is postulated to have arisen over the course of evolution to serve a specific and independent function. It is difficult to reconcile this kind of model with the pattern of data observed in the perinatal lesion population. However, a number of recent models, falling generally under the category of "neural reuse" models, make interesting claims about the evolution of neural systems for cognitive functions that are consistent with the PL data.

Two evolutionary models that are closely aligned with theories of situated and embodied cognition suggest that sensorimotor functions may have anchor the emergence of higher cognitive functions. Gallese and Lakoff's (Gallese, 2008; Gallese & Lakoff, 2005) Neural Exploitation Hypothesis (NEH) begins with the well-documented findings from the neuroimaging literature that imagining an action and executing an action (e.g., grasping an object) activate the same neural system. Based upon these widespread reports, NEH proposes that as new cognitive functions emerge, they exploit, or reuse, the same neural circuitry as the more basic actions. However, because cognition is complex and multimodal, the evolutionary processes that give rise to higher cognitive functions also link circuitry from different modalities to form higher-order functional systems. Thus the emergence of higher cognitive functions is achieved by exploitation of existing neural systems and clustering of systems across modalities to form higher-level units. The "exploited" neural networks come to serve the new higher cognitive function while retaining their original functions. Hurley's (Hurley, 2008) Shared Circuits (SC) model also posits neural reuse that is anchored by the sensorimotor system. She proposes a five-layered network ranging from very basic sensorimotor processes to conceptual representation, in which interactions between levels link processing across levels. Because of this linkage, all levels of the system reuse the basic information derived from the lowest level. Thus, by both of these accounts, the effects of injury to the sensorimotor system could cascade through the cognitive system.

Anderson's (Anderson, 2010) Massive Redeployment Hypothesis (MRH) offers a somewhat different take on the construct of neural reuse. As an alternative to neural architectures organized around functional modules (or even particular domains such as vision, audition, or language) MRH postulates an organization in which, across the course of evolution, low-level neural circuits are used, and reused, for a variety of purposes across a range of task domains. The model is related to the NEH and SC models but does not limit adaptation to the sensorimotor circuits. Recruitment (reuse) of a particular neural circuit is constrained by the functional properties and biases of local circuitry, thus promoting efficient functioning. Further, the model predicts that there should be a strong correlation between the phylogenic age of a neural system and both its degree of anatomical localization and the frequency with which is it redeployed for other functions. Specifically, an older system should be more highly localized because the neural system was more primitive when it emerged; and it should be more widely integrated with later-emerging functions, because its circuits have been available for reuse for a longer time. By contrast, newer functions should be both more adaptable and exhibit more widely distributed neural circuitry. This account of the emergence of higher cognitive functions is reminiscent of our colleague Elizabeth Bates' description of language as "a new machine built out of old parts" (Bates et al., 1991). Anderson (2010) conducted a large meta-analysis of nearly 1,500 neuroimaging studies that supported the predictions of his model. The objective of the study was to determine the frequency with which brain regions were activated by very different types of tasks. The results showed that more than 90% of the brain regions were activated by tasks from multiple domains, suggesting widespread reuse of neural circuitry. Further, areas that activated during a perceptual or motor task exhibited greater levels of reuse, lending support to the idea that brain areas associated with somatosensory functions exhibit greater reuse.

While all of the neural reuse models are broadly compatible with the data from the perinatal lesion population, Anderson's MRH makes a set of specific predictions that are closely aligned with the observed findings. His model predicts that the older sensorimotor systems will be less flexible and more highly localized, which would make them more vulnerable in the wake of early injury. That is what is observed in the data from the perinatal lesion population. It also predicts that because later functions reuse a wide variety of existing neural circuits and integrate across several neural systems to execute complex functions, they will be more highly distributed and more flexible. Again, this is consistent with the profile observed in the data from the perinatal lesions group. Language functions are more highly distributed than the visuospatial processing systems, and they exhibit greater resilience in the wake of early injury.

An Alternative Account of the Crowding Effect

The sensorimotor dependency and the neural reuse hypotheses both argue for developmental grounding of higher cognitive functions within sensorimotor processes. Sensorimotor dependency takes an ontogenetic perspective suggesting that the early development of the basic input and output systems anchors the subsequent development of other higher cognitive functions. It draws from ideas in theories of embodied cognition (Clark, 1999; Mareschal et al., 2007; Smith & Gasser, 2005) in suggesting that sensorimotor processing shapes and constrains the development of higher-order representations. In the wake of perinatal injury, the early-developing sensorimotor systems are more vulnerable and less resilient than later-developing higher cognitive systems. Further, the higher cognitive systems exhibit different degrees of vulnerability, depending on how broadly or narrowly dependent they are on the basic systems. Neural reuse theories also argue for a link between sensorimotor and higher cognitive functions, suggesting that the emergence of new functions makes use of existing neural circuitry. The more recent the function, the more widespread the array of neural circuits that are incorporated into the new system. That makes new systems both more distributed and more flexible.

These two ideas offer a different perspective of the effects of early brain injury than the older ideas associated with the classical crowding effect. Rather than positing the functional priority of language as the basis for neural crowding effects, these accounts are anchored in developmental and/or evolutionary processes. The vulnerability or resiliency of a function is not related to its hypothesized value or merit, but instead it is based on the temporal and functional dynamics of developmental processes. When injury to the developing neural system occurs, the most vulnerable systems are those that emerge and stabilize earliest, specifically the somatosensory system. Impairment of those systems likely impacts the development of other systems in ways that we have yet to specifically define. It is also the case that the impact of early sensorimotor impairment may vary across cognitive functions. The more narrow and specifically reliant a cognitive function on the sensorimotor system, the greater the impact. The more widely distributed the neural system, and the wider the array of sensorimotor inputs that the network exploits, the more resilient the function. Thus, this is a specifically developmental account of crowding effects that is anchored in basic developmental processes of both ontogenesis and phylogenesis.

PERINATAL BRAIN INJURY AND THE DEVELOPMENTAL PROCESS

In this section, we return to the questions that inspired this book, indeed inspired the work of all of the authors decades ago: How does perinatal brain injury affect neurobehavioral development? Our knowledge of outcomes has expanded greatly over the years. We know what kinds of functions seem to be more vulnerable or more resilient. We understand more, though not enough, about patterns of neural organization after early injury. We have new ideas about clinical intervention. But another thing that has changed considerably over the years is our models of why the observed outcomes emerge. Thirty years ago the model of neural development was strongly maturational, reflecting the dominant models in developmental neurobiology at the time. Tremendous progress has been made in our understanding of the basic mechanisms of brain development, and that progress has fundamentally changed the way we think about the effects of injury. In the next sections we consider how our thinking has changed and what contemporary models of brain and cognitive development can tell us about the effects of perinatal brain injury.

Organization or Reorganization

An interesting small issue has arisen in the literature on the effects of early brain injury that might at first glance appear to be a trifling over words. Several years ago Martin Staudt introduced a seemingly odd orthographic variation in his use of the term "reorganization": he began spelling it (re-)organization. The note that accompanied this new form said, "Note: Whether lesions to a developing CNS induce actual "reorganization" (i.e., changes of an already existing organization), or whether they primarily cause abnormalities of organization can often not be decided. Therefore, the term "reorganization" might often be inappropriate in patients with developmental lesions. In order to express this uncertainty, the term (re-)organization is used" (Staudt, 2007, p. 1151). It is an interesting point and one that is worth considering further, both for what is implied by the distinction and how it fits within models of neurobehavioral development.

Staudt's definition of (re-)organization distinguishes between the possibilities that early injury changes an existing organization or that it creates abnormalities in an existing organization. However, both options seem to imply some kind of change or reorganization of the neural systems. Thus, one possible interpretation of the distinction is that neural "reorganization" results in a less impaired and more functional behavioral system, while neural change that creates abnormalities leads to behavioral impairment. Thus, for example, the neural changes that result in bilateral mediation of language function would constitute a "reorganization" of the language system because the changes largely preserve linguistic function. By contrast, the changes involving the ipsilateral mediation of the motor system would be considered to have created abnormalities of organization because function is poor. The distinction between types of neurobehavioral outcome is an important observation, but tying it to a notion of (re-)organization is somewhat more difficult to reconcile. Both developmental outcomes involve a change in the typical patterns of organization, and both were induced by an early pathological event. Thus both could be considered to constitute reorganization of the typical neural system; it is just that some kinds of reorganization ameliorate deficit and others exacerbate it.

However, there is the more basic question as to whether it is ever appropriate to apply the term "reorganization" to the events that unfold after perinatal brain injury. This question is important because how one describes the differences in brain organization following early injury reflects an underlying model of neurobehavioral development that affects the interpretation of how the changes came about and what they mean. The (re)organization interpretation takes the somewhat static view that there is a single typical form of neural organization that is changed by the lesion event. It is a kind of snapshot approach that actually focuses on typical and atypical neurobehavioral *outcomes*, or more accurately on status reports taken later in development that reflect a comparatively stable and mature organizational state. But both the typical and atypical "outcomes" are the products of developmental processes that extend over many years. Lesions happen at a discrete moment in time and they have a destructive immediate effect. Neural tissue is lost, cascades of molecular signaling are triggered that have widespread effects throughout the brain, and established patterns of neural organization are disrupted. Thus, at that particular moment in time, both the state and the developmental history of the organism are altered. But the other thing that is changed by the lesion events is the trajectory of development. Neurobehavioral outcomes are snapshots, summary statements of functionality at a particular moment in time late in development. But these "outcome states" are the consequence of developmental processes that extend over years. In the wake of early injury, the brain continues to develop, and that development is supported by the same processes that operate in typical development. Lesions introduce a new and important factor in the developmental process, but the basic processes are the same. Genes are expressed, cells die off, synapses are exuberantly produced and pruned away, and environmental factors influence neural changes at all levels. Lesions do not change those basic processes; rather, they change the specific ways in which the basic processes of development are implemented. They change the developmental trajectory. Thus, when the neurobehavioral outcomes for typical children and children with early brain lesions are compared, what is observed is not the "reorganization" of the injured brain, but rather the effects of an altered developmental trajectory that is induced by the lesion event and results in the development of alternative patterns of brain organization. They are not "reorganized" mature states; they are alternative organizations that are the product of development. To understand neurodevelopmental outcomes, typical or atypical, it is necessary to understand development. Because of that, the models of typical development that one brings to the study of neurodevelopmental disorders are of critical importance.

Neuroconstructivist Views of Neurodevelopmental Disorders

In a long series of papers published over many years Annette Karmiloff-Smith has argued for what, in recent years, has coalesced into a Neuroconstructivist view of neurodevelopmental disorders (Karmiloff-Smith, 1998ab, 2002, 2007, 2010; Karmiloff-Smith & Thomas, 2003; Paterson et al., 1999; Thomas & Karmiloff-Smith, 2002, 2005; Westermann et al., 2011). According to this view, the key to understanding a disorder lies in its developmental trajectory and how the pathology of the disorder, whether a gene mutation or an early lesion, interacts with and affects that trajectory. It stands in contrast to the dominant view from adult neuropsychology, in which behavioral deficits are attributed to the disruption of independent neural modules. When the adult model is applied to the study of developmental disorders, as it frequently is, this leads to an approach in which the brains of children with disorders are "viewed as normal brains with parts intact and parts impaired…[rather than as]…brains that have developed differently throughout embriogenesis and postnatal development" (Karmiloff-Smith, 2007). The Neuroconstructivist approach to the study of developmental disorders provides a different and dynamic framework for understanding the effects of perinatal brain injury and for explaining the patterns of observed data. It also offers very different strategies for exploring the nature of deficit and development in this population. But before considering the potential contributions of Neuroconstructivism to the study of disordered populations, a brief summary of the general framework of the theory will be considered.

Neuroconstructivism

The Neuroconstructivist approach views development as a trajectory that is shaped by multiple, interacting biological and environmental constraints (Mareschal et al., 2007; Westermann et al., 2007). In this model, the key to understanding cognitive development lies in understanding how constraints on neural development affect the emergence of neural networks, so they can in turn give rise to more and more complex mental representations. Central to this approach is the idea that brain and cognitive development are linked by characterizing mental representations as activation states within the neural networks. Neuroconstructivism postulates five levels of constraint on the developing neural system. Note that the constraints proposed by this neuro*behavioral* model of development are very similar to those described earlier for models of neuro*biological* development, thus providing an alignment of perspectives on brain and behavioral development.

1. *Genes*. Genes provide the material code for the development and functioning of all biological structures and processes. Molecular signaling plays a central role in all aspects of development and thus serves as a powerful constraint on development. However, genes are not prescriptive. Gene expression is a process that requires the interaction of multiple factors within the environment of the cell.
2. *Encellment (neural constructivism)*. Neuronal development is also a process. Cells differentiate and take on changing roles in response to cues from the local environment, and via signaling from more distant cells, and from the environment. Neural activity can affect nerve growth factor production and synapse formation or elimination, and can trigger cell death cascades.
3. *Enbrainment (interactive specialization)*. Cortical regions arise as the product of their competitive interactions with other cortical regions. These interactions occur in the process of acquiring new skills and abilities. Activity-dependent interactions sharpen and narrow functions within a cortical region as skills are acquired.

4. *Embodiment.* The fact that the brain is embedded in a body introduces powerful constraints on cognitive development. The body develops in parallel with cognitive abilities and serves to change the information available to the child. It also serves to constrain the mental computations necessary to solve a problem. Exploration of the environment is an essential component of cognitive development.
5. *Ensocialment.* The social world in which the child lives provides the last level of constraints on development. The amount and quality of social interaction has profound effects on the development of neurobehavioral processes.

Within the Neuroconstructivist model, a number of common principles apply to all levels of developmental constraint. The first is the idea of context dependency, which states that the complex of constraints arising from all levels of the system establishes a context that shapes both the trajectory of development and eventual outcome. Context is realized through competition among neural elements, cooperation among elements and systems, time constraints that limit what kinds of factors can affect the system at a given moment, and the proactivity of the organism in selecting inputs from the environment. The constraints all lead to progressive specialization, or commitment, of systems and resources. Thus the trajectory of development is determined across time by ongoing interactions across the multiple levels of the neurobehavioral system. The processes of progressive differentiation and commitment continuously modify the existing state of the organism, such that the system is reorganized not once, but many times across the course of development. In that sense, development can be construed as process of continuous, successive reorganization. The product of these developmental processes is a relatively stable (though still plastic) end-state organization that is characteristic of the mature individual.

Neuroconstructivism and the Effects of Perinatal Lesions

Because of its emphasis on developmental trajectories, the Neuroconstructive approach leads to very different ways of thinking about the effects of early brain lesions than more static approaches that are focused on interpreting outcome. It also leads to different sets of questions and research strategies. Rather than focusing on intact or impaired neurobehavioral modules, the emphasis shifts to understanding developmental trajectories, and what in the course of neural development might lead to the constellation of neurobehavioral systems observed at the end state of development. An example from language acquisition data in the perinatal lesion populations illustrates this point.

The neuroimaging studies of brain laterality for linguistic functioning following early brain injury all report a rightward shift in brain activation during language tasks, relative to the more highly left-lateralized activation patterns typical of older children and adults. Further, the best functional outcomes for language are associated with bilateral patterns of organization (Raja Beharelle et al., 2010). Indeed, there are very few cases of complete right lateralization, and those are associated with poorer linguistic functioning. This shift in lateralization certainly reflects the effect of loss of optimal brain regions due to injury, but it is also important to consider the effects of the developmental trajectory on the emergence of these altered patterns of organization. As Teuber (Teuber & Rudel, 1962) stressed many years ago, to evaluate the effects of early injury it is important to have appropriate normative control data.

But in the case of early injury the optimal control data may not be those obtained from outcome measures, but rather from developmental studies. In the case of the language data from the perinatal lesion population, the developmental imaging data from normal controls is revealing. Specifically, the profile of bilateral mediation in the perinatal lesion population is also consistent with the growing body of evidence for neural mediation of language in young typically developing children. Those data suggest that in the course of typical development activation patterns for language tasks are initially strongly bilateral and only gradually become left-lateralized (Everts et al., 2009; Holland et al., 2001; Plante et al. 2000; Ressel et al., 2008; Szaflarski et al., 2006). It is of note that most of the perinatal lesion imaging studies are done when the children reach the late school-age or adolescent period. Thus, what is known about their brain organization for language, at least for the cases of bilateral organization, is that it is similar to that of younger normal children. Given these findings, an alternative interpretation of the laterality data is that the injury interrupts the typical developmental process in which more efficient and more highly lateralized neural systems would have emerged over time and with the experience of the child. The observed alterations in neurobehavioral outcomes could be interpreted as an injury-induced divergence from the normal developmental trajectory to an alternative trajectory that produces, over time, the profiles of neurological and behavioral organization that are characteristic of this population of children.

The Neuroconstructivist approach encourages a very different way of thinking about the effects of neurodevelopmental disorders. The injury introduces a set of "bad actors" into the developmental context. These abnormal events do not just affect local areas of neural tissue, they change the course of development throughout the neural system by affecting local processes across a range of levels and altering constraints throughout the system. A large cortical and subcortical lesion not only disrupts major pathways but also alters early-emerging patterns of cortical organization, changes the balance of competition among systems, disrupts local processes of differentiation and commitment, and affects the ability of the child to interact with the world. Thus the effects of early injury cascade through the developing neurobehavioral system for month and years, inducing not one instance of reorganization, but rather altering the entire trajectory of development.

Despite these large-scale alterations in the developmental trajectory, the effects of perinatal injury on neurobehavioral functioning are for most, but not all, functions attenuated relative to the effects of injury in adults. One way to think of development is as a dynamic and interactive process, but also as an adaptive process. Over the course of evolution new systems have emerged to serve the demands of new functions. Neural reuse theories propose that their emergence is very much an adaptation, a reuse, of existing functions. The data from the perinatal lesion populations provide an interesting parallel to this notion of adaptation and reuse. Rather than introducing demands for new skills that must be accommodated by the neural architecture, lesions compromise regions of the available neural substrate, requiring functional adaptation to conditions of reduced neural resources. But unlike the evolutionary case, these adaptations must unfold across the course of development.

DEVELOPMENTAL PLASTICITY

The title of this book, *Neural Plasticity and Cognitive Development: Insights from Children with Perinatal Brain Injury*, emphasizes the central role of plasticity in neurobehavioral development. But the definition of plasticity that emerges from the perspective and models discussed here is somewhat different and in some ways more specific than the usual, often vague, usage of the term as generally applied to studies of neurobehavioral development. Here plasticity is construed as an adaptive process that is very much a part of the dynamic interactions that underpin all of brain and behavioral development. It is the capacity of the system to adjust to changing circumstances (i.e., changing constraints) and to alter the developmental trajectory to maintain optimal functionality at each moment in developmental time. Note that this dynamic temporally bound account of plasticity may not always result in optimal outcomes. Thus, while the adaptive stabilization of an ipsilateral motor pathway in response to injury may temporarily solve a local optimization problem, it does so within a developmental context that is ultimately detrimental to the organism. By contrast, the pattern of adaptive plasticity for the language system optimizes both the immediate state of the organism and the eventual outcome. As discussed earlier, two very different profiles of development likely reflect the operation of adaptive processes within two very different contexts. The motor system is more localized and more constrained, while language is more distributed and can exploit a wider range of resources; it is thus more flexible in its organization.

This is a very different way to think about the construct of plasticity, but it is one that links plastic change to the fundamental processes of typical development. Thus, in the case of early brain damage the mechanism of plastic adaptation does not reflect the workings of an ancillary system that is triggered by pathology. Rather, it is a fundamental process and an essential aspect of both typical and atypical brain development. The events of early injury may make the processes of plastic adaptation more apparent because the pathological event necessitates adaptation to an altered set of conditions that requires an alternate developmental trajectory. Thus the plasticity, the capacity for adaptation, is brought into high relief by virtue of the divergence of the developmental trajectory. But the processes that underlie plastic change following early injury exploit the same basic adaptive mechanisms that are a central feature of typical development; and those processes are well described by dynamic and interactive models of neurobehavioral development.

FUTURE DIRECTIONS

Much of this book is a progress report on the effects of early brain injury that incorporates the findings from the past 30 years. The organization of the book reflects the predominant approach to these questions during much of this time. First, the neurobiological questions are considered separately from behavioral questions. Further, there is a tendency for studies of behavior to balkanize along domain-specific lines. Reflecting this state of the field, this book is divided into two main parts, one focused on the neurobiology of brain development and the other on outcomes from individual behavioral systems. But the development of a child is not compartmentalized into the biological and the behavioral, or even the linguistic and the spatial. A major objective of future work will be to understand the relationships between the development of neurobiological and behavioral systems. This will require an integration of models of neurobiological and neurobehavioral development. But it will also require an understanding of how the development of one behavioral system affects another, and how those complex interactions are related to neural development.

This final chapter has attempted to propose a way of integrating models of biological and behavioral development, but it provides only the barest framework of an approach. As discussed earlier in this chapter, over the past two decades, the separate models of brain and behavioral development have each proposed new and productive approaches to understanding how complex structures emerge. Neurobiological models construe brain development as the product of a complex series of dynamic and adaptive processes. Neuroconstructivist models view behavioral development as a trajectory that is shaped by multiple, interacting constraints. Importantly, although the models were developed independently, they converge on a common set of principles that are each anchored in basic developmental processes. This convergence of ideas permits the alignment of disciplines, and thus the opportunity and the challenge of creating an integrated model of neurobehavioral development. This integrated model has critical implications for our understanding both typical and atypical neurobehavioral development.

Many of the tools necessary for addressing this challenge already exist and have begun to produce exciting data. Probably the largest body of data for the school-age and adolescent periods comes from various types of magnetic resonance imaging (MRI) studies, including functional magnetic resonance imaging (fMRI), anatomical MRI, and diffusion-weighted and diffusion tensor imaging (DWI and DTI, respectively). FMRI studies have provided important insights into the changes in patterns of neural activation across development for both typical and atypical populations. Very recently this work has begun to focus on defining patterns of functional connectivity that will provide a more precise and refined perspective on change in neural systems (Fairet al., 2008, 2009; Lopez-Larson et al., 2011). To date there are only a handful of functional imaging studies focused on children with early injury, but this in part reflects the state of progress in the field. As Teuber stressed many years ago, developmental disorders can only be understand in the context of substantive data from typical controls. As those data become more and more available, functional imaging will become a powerful tool for understanding the effects of early injury on neurobehavioral development. In addition, recent improvements in structural imaging and refinements in protocols for tissue segmentation also have great potential for informing our understanding of the effects of early injury on brain structure (Dale et al., 1999; Destrieux et al., 2010; Fischl et al., 2004). These more refined methods will not only make lesion description more precise, but they also offer the potential for examining secondary changes in brain anatomy. For example, a number of studies have identified cortical thinning as a marker of functional brain maturation and have reported systematic regional differences in the progress of cortical thinning across the period of childhood and adolescence (Gogtay et al., 2004; Sowell et al., 2004; Thompson et al., 2005; Westlye et al., 2010). Divergence from typical development trajectories within specific cortical regions may provide an important index of the effects of early injury on brain regions remote from the actual site of lesion. Finally, DWI and DTI can provide important information on the development of brain pathways. Recent work mapping the developmental trajectories for the major projection, callosal, and association pathways have revealed substantial diversity in the time course of development for the pathways (Lebel et al., 2008; Lebel & Beaulieu, 2011). These changes are very likely related to the changes in patterns of functional activation and connectivity seen in the fMRI studies, to the anatomical changes in cortex seen in the structural imaging studies, and to cognitive changes observed in behavioral measures. Thus an important future direction for research on neurobehavioral development will be the integration of data from these very different levels of analysis. This kind of data convergence will prove essential to our understanding of the trajectories of neurobehavioral change in both typically and atypically developing children.

While MRI technologies have already proven to be effective tools for exploring developmental changes from the late preschool period through adolescence, the application of these technologies to younger children has proved challenging. Yet, the trajectories of change, both typical and atypical, find their origins in this early period of development. Thus, finding the means to document early changes is critical. Anatomical imaging of brains in the first year of life is challenging. Movement can degrade the quality of images, requiring the use of sleep or sedation protocols for image acquisition. Further, the MRI analyses rely to a large extent on the contrast of gray and white matter structures, but the process of myelin deposition is gradual, making tissue segmentation challenging with data from infants and young children. However, very recent advances in anatomical image acquisition protocols have introduced dynamic motion correction that may largely solve the movement problems at least for anatomical MRI data (Keating et al., 2010; White et al., 2010). Further, improvements in tissue segmentation protocols may help improve resolution of infant data. Importantly, the introduction of DTI and DWI protocols with very young children has provided important data on early changes in major pathways in both typical and atypical populations (Huppi & Dubois, 2006). Nonetheless, fMRI continues to present technical problems for use with young children. In addition to movement problems, which within the fMRI protocols cannot as yet be compensated for by dynamic motion correction during acquisition, the task demands of fMRI are challenging. A small number of studies have used passive protocols with sleeping or sedated children (Dehaene-Lambertz et al., 2006) with promising results, but passive protocols can address only a subset of behavioral questions. Thus, the limitations on the fMRI methodology make it a less promising approach for many research questions in the first years of life. However, both magnetoencephalographic (MEG) and near-infrared spectroscopy (NIS) offer possible ways of circumventing the problems associated with fMRI (Lloyd-Fox et al., 2010; Travis et al., 2011). Both are less sensitive to movement artifact and both can be used with awake and alert children, thus greatly extending the range of neurobehavioral questions that can be addressed.

Another approach that has already produced important and informative data is neuromodeling. Connectionism, in particular, provides a powerful and compatible tool for exploring the kinds of issues raised by dynamic and interactive models of neurobehavioral development (Elman et al, 1996; Mareschal et al., 2007; Raz et al., 1995; Spencer et al., 2009). Connectionist models typically consist of a large number of interconnected units, which are conceptualized as simplified neuron-like elements. These units are connected to other units, forming a multilayered network. Units receive input and produce outputs. The sum of the inputs to a unit determines its level of activation. Patterns of activity throughout the neural network represent activation states that change over time, and the record of change in activity state over time represents the network's history. Connectionist models typically study learning within a network. Networks can be designed to incorporate various constraints on learning. Constraints can include things such as network structure, environmental complexity, noise in the input or representations, or output parameters. Constraints can be systematically manipulated, thus providing the opportunity to examine how the effects of a change in one level of the neurocomputation system propagate and affect the trajectory of learning for the network (Thomas & Karmiloff-Smith, 2002). The organization and functioning of connectionist models mirror, in a very simplified way, neurobehavioral structure and function in biological systems. They are excellent tools for studying the effects of alterations in constraints on the trajectory of learning, and thus can inform our understanding of the effects of constraint variation on the development of neurobehavioral systems.

While all of these tools have enormous potential to inform our understanding of specific aspects of neurobehavioral development, ultimately the threads of data from different techniques, modalities, and developmental epochs will need to be integrated. A unified model of neurobehavioral development will need to describe the trajectory of development, not for a single domain or neurological system, but for the complete complex of behaviors and neural systems. It is a very large task, but if the ultimate goal is to provide an account of neurobehavioral development, the approach cannot be fragmentary. The task of building a unified model also places additional burden on researchers because informed discussions across disciplines require not only expertise in one's own discipline but also understanding of the basic issues and core vocabulary of the sister disciplines. The goal is to build a comprehensive and integrated model of neurobehavioral development that can capture and explain both typical and atypical trajectories and outcomes; and that requires a multidisciplinary effort. This is an exciting and challenging enterprise with enormous potential rewards for both advancing the basic science disciplines and for the impact such knowledge may have on the everyday lives of children whose development we seek to understand.

REFERENCES

Anderson ML. (2010). Neural reuse: a fundamental organizational principle of the brain. *Behav Brain Sci* 33(4):245–266; discussion 266–313.

Aram DM, Eisele JA. (1994). Intellectual stability in children with unilateral brain lesions. *Neuropsychologia* 32(1):85–95.

Ark W, Stiles J, et al. (2003). *Ventral temporal processing further distinguishes mental rotation and feature matching*. Paper presented at the Human Brain Mapping meeting.

Asari T, Konishi S, et al. (2005). Multiple components of lateral posterior parietal activation associated with cognitive set shifting. *NeuroImage* 26(3):694–702.

Bates E, Thal D, et al. (1991). Symbols and syntax: A Darwinian approach to language development. In Krasnegor NA, Rumbaugh DM, et al. (eds), Biological and behavioral determinants of language development. Hillsdale, NJ: Erlbaum, pp. 29–65.

Booth JR, MacWhinney B, et al. (1999). Functional organization of activation patterns in children: whole brain fMRI imaging during three different cognitive tasks. *Progress Neuropsychopharmacol Biol Psychiatry* 23(4):669–682.

Booth JR, MacWhinney B, et al. (2000). Developmental and lesion effects in brain activation during sentence comprehension and mental rotation. *Dev Neuropsychol* 18(2):139–169.

Carey S. (2011). Precis of "The Origin of Concepts." *Behav Brain Sci* 34(3):113–124; discussion 124–162.

Carey S, Xu F. (2001). Infants' knowledge of objects: Beyond object files and object tracking. *Cognition* 80(1–2):179–213.

Carlsson G, Uvebrant P, et al. (1994). Verbal and non-verbal function of children with right-versus left-hemiplegic cerebral palsy of pre- and perinatal origin. *Dev Med Child Neurol* 36:503–512.

Clark A. (1999). An embodied cognitive science? *Trends Cogn Sci* 3(9):345–351.

Clayton, K., Fleming, J. M., & Copley, J. (2003). Behavioral responses to tactile stimuli in children with cerebral palsy. *Physical & occupational therapy in pediatrics*, 23(1), 43–62.

Cosmides L, Tooby J. (1994). Beyond intuition and instinct blindness: toward an evolutionarily rigorous cognitive science. *Cognition* 50(1–3):41–77.

Dale AM, Fischl B, et al. (1999). Cortical surface-based analysis. I. Segmentation and surface reconstruction. *NeuroImage* 9(2):179–194.

Dehaene-Lambertz G, Hertz-Pannier L, et al. (2006). Nature and nurture in language acquisition: anatomical and functional brain-imaging studies in infants. *Trends Neurosci* 29(7): 367–373.

Destrieux C, Fischl B, et al. (2010). Automatic parcellation of human cortical gyri and sulci using standard anatomical nomenclature. *NeuroImage* 53(1):1–15.

Duchaine B, Cosmides L, et al. (2001). Evolutionary psychology and the brain. *Curr Opinion Neurobiol* 11: 225–230.

Elman JL, Bates EA, et al. (1996). Rethinking Innateness: A Connectionist Perspective on Development. Cambridge, MA: MIT Press.

Emmorey K, Allen JS, et al. (2003). A morphometric analysis of auditory brain regions in congenitally deaf adults. *Proc Natl Acad Sci U S A* 100(17):10049–10054.

Emmorey K, Grabowski T, et al. (2003). Neural systems underlying lexical retrieval for sign language. *Neuropsychologia* 41(1):85–95.

Everts R, Lidzba K, et al. (2009). Strengthening of laterality of verbal and visuospatial functions during childhood and adolescence. *Hum Brain Mapp* 30(2):473–483.

Everts R, Lidzba K, et al. (2010). Lateralization of cognitive functions after stroke in childhood. *Brain Injury* 24(6):859–870.

Eyre JA. (2007). Corticospinal tract development and its plasticity after perinatal injury. *Neurosci Biobehav Rev* 31(8):1136–1149.

Fair DA, Cohen AL, et al. (2008). The maturing architecture of the brain's default network. *Proc Natl Acad Sci U S A* 105(10):4028–4032.

Fair DA, Cohen AL, et al. (2009). Functional brain networks develop from a local to distributed organization. *PLoS Computational Biology* 5(5):e1000381.

Fink GR, Marshall JC, et al. (2001). The neural basis of vertical and horizontal line bisection judgments: an fMRI study of normal volunteers. *NeuroImage* 14(1 Pt 2):S59–67.

Fischl B, van der Kouwe A, et al. (2004). Automatically parcellating the human cerebral cortex. *Cerebral Cortex* 14(1):11–22.

Gallese V. (2008). Mirror neurons and the social nature of language: the neural exploitation hypothesis. *Social Neurosci* 3(3–4):317–333.

Gallese V, Lakoff G. (2005). The brain's concepts: the role of the sensory-motor system in conceptual knowledge. *Cognitive Neuropsychol* 22(3):455–479.

Gandevia SC, McCloskey DI, Burke D (1992). Kinaesthetic signals and muscle contraction. *Trends Neurosci* 15: 62–65.

Gogtay N, Giedd JN, et al. (2004). Dynamic mapping of human cortical development during childhood through early adulthood. *Proc Natl Acad Sci U S A* 101(21):8174–8179.

Gonzalez-Monge S, Boudia B, et al. (2009). A 7-year longitudinal follow-up of intellectual development in children with congenital hemiplegia. *Dev Med Child Neurol* 51(12):959–967.

Gottlieb G. (1992). Individual Development and Evolution: The Genesis of Novel Behavior. New York: Oxford University Press.

Gottlieb G. (2007). Probabilistic epigenesis. *Dev Sci* 10(1):1–11.

Haist F, Adamo M, et al. (submitted). On the development of visual processing for faces.

Holland SK, Plante E, et al. (2001). Normal fMRI brain activation patterns in children performing a verb generation task. *NeuroImage* 14(4):837–843.

Holland SK, Vannest J, et al. (2007). Functional MRI of language lateralization during development in children. *Intl J Audiol* 46(9):533–551.

Holmstrom, L., Vollmer, B., Tedroff, K., Islam, M., Persson, J. K., Kits, A., . . . Eliasson, A. C. (2010). Hand function in relation to brain lesions and corticomotor-projection pattern in children with unilateral cerebral palsy. *Developmental medicine and child neurology*, 52(2), 145–152.

Hung, Y. C., Charles, J., & Gordon, A. M. (2004). Bimanual coordination during a goal-directed task in children with hemiplegic cerebral palsy. *Developmental medicine and child neurology*, 46(11), 746–753.

Hung, Y. C., Charles, J., & Gordon, A. M. (2010). Influence of accuracy constraints on bimanual coordination during a goal-directed task in children with hemiplegic cerebral palsy. *Experimental brain research*, 201(3), 421–428.

Hoon AH Jr, Lawrie WT, Jr, et al. (2002). Diffusion tensor imaging of periventricular leukomalacia shows affected sensory cortex white matter pathways. *Neurology* 59(5):752–756.

Huppi PS, Dubois J. (2006). Diffusion tensor imaging of brain development. *Semin Fetal Neonatal Med* 11(6).489–497.

Hurley S. (2008). The shared circuits model (SCM):how control, mirroring, and simulation can enable imitation, deliberation, and mindreading. *Behav Brain Sci* 31(1):1–22; discussion 22–58.

Innocenti GM, Price DJ. (2005). Exuberance in the development of cortical networks. *Nat Rev Neurosci* 6(12):955–965.

Jacola LM, Schapiro MB, et al. (2006). Functional magnetic resonance imaging reveals atypical language organization in children following perinatal left middle cerebral artery stroke. *Neuropediatrics* 37(1):46–52.

Johnson MH. (2001). Functional brain development in humans. *Nat Rev Neurosci* 2(7): 475–483.

Johnson MH. (2005). Sensitive periods in functional brain development: problems and prospects. *Dev Psychobiol* 46(3):287–292.

Johnson MH. (2011). Interactive Specialization: A domain-general framework for human functional brain development? *Dev Cogn Neurosci* 1(1):7–21.

Juenger, H., de Haan, B., Krageloh-Mann, I., Staudt, M., & Karnath, H. O. (2011). Early determination of somatosensory cortex in the human brain. *Cerebral cortex*, 21(8), 1827–1831.

Kanwisher N, Yovel G. (2006). The fusiform face area: a cortical region specialized for the perception of faces. *Philos Trans R Soc Lond B Biol Sci* 361(1476):2109–2128.

Karmiloff-Smith A. (1998a). Development itself is the key to understanding developmental disorders. *Trends Cogn Sci* 2(10):389–398.

Karmiloff-Smith A. (1998b). Is atypical development necessarily a window on the normal mind/brain? The case of Williams syndrome. *Dev Sci* 1(2):273–277.

Karmiloff-Smith A. (2002). Development itself is the key to understanding developmental disorders. In Johnson MH, Munakata Y, Gilmore RO (eds), Brain Development and Cognition: A Reader. Malden, MA, Blackwell Publishers, pp. 375–391.

Karmiloff-Smith A. (2007). Atypical epigenesis. *Dev Sci* 10(1):84–88.

Karmiloff-Smith A. (2009). Nativism versus neuroconstructivism: rethinking the study of developmental disorders. *Dev Psychol* 45(1):56–63.

Karmiloff-Smith A. (2010). Multiple trajectories to human language acquisition: domain-specific or domain-general? *Hum Dev* 53(5):239–244.

Karmiloff-Smith A, Thomas M (2003). What can developmental disorders tell us about the neurocomputational constraints that shape development? The case of Williams syndrome. *Dev Psychopathol* 15(4):969–990.

Keating B, Deng W, et al. (2010). Prospective motion correction for single-voxel 1H MR spectroscopy. *Magnetic Resonance in Medicine* 64(3):672–679.

Keita L, Bedoin N (2011). Hemispheric asymmetries in hierarchical stimulus processing are modulated by stimulus categories and their predictability. *Laterality* 16(3):333–355.

Kinzler KD, Spelke ES (2007). Core systems in human cognition. *Prog Brain Res* 164:257–264.

Kostovic I, Jovanov-Milosevic N (2006). The development of cerebral connections during the first 20-45 weeks gestation. *Semin Fetal Neonatal Med* 11(6):415–422.

Kostovic I, Judas M (2010). The development of the subplate and thalamocortical connections in the human foetal brain. *Acta Paediatr* 99(8):1119–1127.

Kostovic I, Judas M, et al. (2011). Developmental history of the subplate zone, subplate neurons and interstitial white matter neurons: relevance for schizophrenia. *Intl J Dev Neurosci* 29(3):193–205.

Krumlinde-Sundholm L, Eliasson AC (2002). Comparing tests of tactile sensibility: aspects relevant to testing children with spastic hemiplegia. *Dev Med Child Neurol* 44(9):604–612.

Kuhnke, N., Juenger, H., Walther, M., Berweck, S., Mall, V., & Staudt, M. (2008). Do patients with congenital hemiparesis and ipsilateral corticospinal projections respond differently to constraint-induced movement therapy? *Developmental Medicine and Child Neurology*, 50(12), 898–903.

Lebel C, Walker L, et al. (2008). Microstructural maturation of the human brain from childhood to adulthood. *NeuroImage* 40(3):1044–1055.

Lebel C, Beaulieu C (2011). Longitudinal development of human brain wiring continues from childhood into adulthood. *J Neurosci* 31(30):10937–10947.

Le Grand R, Mondloch CJ, et al. (2003). Expert face processing requires visual input to the right hemisphere during infancy. *Nat Neurosci* 6(10):1108–1112.

Le Grand R, Mondloch CJ, et al. (2004). Impairment in holistic face processing following early visual deprivation. *Psychol Sci* 15(11):762–768.

Lewis TL, Maurer D (2005). Multiple sensitive periods in human visual development: evidence from visually deprived children. *Dev Psychobiol* 46(3):163–183.

Lidzba K, Schwilling E, et al. (2011). Language comprehension vs. language production: Age effects on fMRI activation. *Brain and Language [e-pub March 29]*.

Lidzba K, Staudt M, et al. (2006a). Lesion-induced right-hemispheric language and organization of nonverbal functions. *NeuroReport* 17(9):929–933.

Lidzba K, Staudt M, et al. (2006b). Visuospatial deficits in patients with early left-hemispheric lesions and functional reorganization of language: Consequence of lesion or reorganization? *Neuropsychologia* 44(7):1088–1094.

Liegeois F, Connelly A, et al. (2004). Language reorganization in children with early-onset lesions of the left hemisphere: an fMRI study. *Brain* 127(Pt 6):1229–1236.

Lloyd-Fox S, Blasi A, et al. (2010). Illuminating the developing brain: the past, present and future of functional near infrared spectroscopy. *Neurosci Biobehav Rev* 34(3):269–284.

Lopez-Larson MP, Anderson HS, et al. (2011). Local brain connectivity and associations with gender and age. *Dev Cogn Neurosci* 1(2):187–197.

Mareschal D, Johnson MH, et al. (2007). Neuroconstructivism: How the Brain Constructs Cognition. Oxford: Oxford University Press.

Martin JH (2005). The corticospinal system: From development to motor control. *Neuroscientist* 11:161–173.

Martinez A, Moses P, et al. (1997). Hemispheric asymmetries in global and local processing: evidence from fMRI. *Neuroreport* 8(7):1685–1689.

Max, J. E., Bruce, M., Keatley, E., & Delis, D. (2010). Pediatric stroke: plasticity, vulnerability, and age of lesion onset. *The Journal of neuropsychiatry and clinical neurosciences*, 22(1), 30–39.

McConnell SK. (1992). The control of neuronal identity in the developing cerebral cortex. *Curr Opin Neurobiol* 2(1):23–27.

McCullough S, Emmorey K, et al. (2005). Neural organization for recognition of grammatical and emotional facial expressions in deaf ASL signers and hearing nonsigners. *Brain Res Cogn Brain Res* 22(2):193–203.

Meadmore KL, Dror IE, et al. (2009). Lateralisation of spatial processing and age. *Laterality* 14(1):17–29.

Morange M. (2001). The Misunderstood Gene. Cambridge, MA: Harvard University Press.

Moses P, Martinez A, Roe K, Frank L, Buxton R, Wong E, Stiles J. (1997). Functional magnetic resonance imaging of children's spatial analysis of hierarchical forms.

Ng VWK, Eslinger PJ, et al. (2000). Hemispheric preference in visuospatial processing: a complementary approach with fMRI and lesion studies. *Hum Brain Mapp* 10:80–86.

Passarotti AM, Paul BM, et al. (2003). The development of face and location processing: An fMRI study. *Dev Sci* 6(1):100–117.

Paterson SJ, Brown JH, et al. (1999). Cognitive modularity and genetic disorders. *Science* 286(5448):2355–2358.

Plante E, Holland S, et al. (2000). Functional MRI in normal language development. Presented at the Symposium on Research in Child Language Disorders, Madison, WI.

Raja Beharelle A, Dick AS, et al. (2010). Left hemisphere regions are critical for language in the face of early left focal brain injury. *Brain* 133(Pt 6):1707–1716.

Rasmussen T, Milner B (1977). The role of early left-brain injury in determining lateralization of cerebral speech functions. *Ann NY Acad Sci* 299:355–369.

Raz N, Torres IJ, et al. (1995). Selective neuroanatomic abnormalities in Down's syndrome and their cognitive correlates: evidence from MRI morphometry. *Neurology* 45(2):356–366.

Reese CJ, Stiles J (2005). Hemispheric specialization for categorical and coordinate spatial relations during an image generation task: Evidence from children and adults. *Neuropsychologia* 43(4):517–529.

Ressel V, Wilke M, et al. (2008). Increases in language lateralization in normal children as observed using magnetoencephalography. *Brain and Language* 106(3):167–176.

Siman-Tov T, Mendelsohn A, et al. (2007). Bihemispheric leftward bias in a visuospatial attention-related network. *J Neurosci* 27(42):11271–11278.

Smith L, Gasser M (2005). The development of embodied cognition: six lessons from babies. *Artificial Life* 11:13–29.

Sowell ER, Thompson PM, et al. (2004). Longitudinal mapping of cortical thickness and brain growth in normal children. *J Neurosci* 24(38):8223–8231.

Spelke E. (2003). Core knowledge. In Kanwisher N, Duncan J (eds), Attention and Performance: Functional Neuroimaging of Visual Cognition. Oxford: Oxford University Press, pp. 29–55.

Spelke E, Kinzler KD (2009). Innateness, learning, and rationality. *Child Dev Perspectives* 3(2):96–98.

Spencer J, Thomas MSC, et al. (2009). Toward a Unified Theory of Development: Connectionism and Dynamic Systems Theory Re-Considered. Oxford, UK: Oxford University Press.

Staudt M. (2007). (Re-)organization of the developing human brain following periventricular white matter lesions. *Neurosci Biobehav Rev* 31(8):1150–1156.

Staudt, M. (2010). Reorganization after pre- and perinatal brain lesions. *Journal of anatomy, 217*(4), 469–474

Staudt, M., Braun, C., Gerloff, C., Erb, M., Grodd, W., & Krageloh-Mann, I. (2006). Developing somatosensory projections bypass periventricular brain lesions. *Neurology*, 67(3), 522–525.

Staudt M, Grodd W, et al. (2002). Two types of ipsilateral reorganization in congenital hemiparesis: a TMS and fMRI study. *Brain* 125(Pt 10):2222–2237.

Staudt M, Ticini LF, et al. (2008). Functional topography of early periventricular brain lesions in relation to cytoarchitectonic probabilistic maps. *Brain and Language* 106(3):177–183.

Stiles J. (2008). The Fundamentals of Brain Development: Integrating Nature and Nurture. Cambridge, MA: Harvard University Press.

Stiles J, Nass R. (1991). Spatial grouping activity in young children with congenital right or left hemisphere brain injury. *Brain & Cognition* 15(2):201–222.

Stiles J, Paul B, et al. (2006). Spatial cognitive development following early focal brain injury: evidence for adaptive change in brain and cognition. In Munakata Y, Johnson MH (eds), Process of Change in Brain and Cognitive Development. Attention and Performance XXI. Oxford: Oxford University Press, pp. 535–561.

Stiles J, Stern C, et al. (1996). Developmental change in spatial grouping activity among children with early focal brain injury: Evidence from a modeling task. *Brain & Cognition* 31(1):46–62.

Stiles J, Stern C, et al. (2008). Effects of early focal brain injury on memory for visuospatial patterns: Selective deficits of global-local processing. *Neuropsychology* 22(1):61–73.

Strauss E, Satz P, et al. (1990). An examination of the crowding hypothesis in epileptic patients who have undergone the carotid amytal test. *Neuropsychologia* 28(11):1221–1227.

Sur M, Angelucci A, et al. (1999). Rewiring cortex: the role of patterned activity in development and plasticity of neocortical circuits. *J Neurobiol* 41(1):33–43.

Sur M, Leamey CA. (2001). Development and plasticity of cortical areas and networks. *Nat Rev Neurosci* 2(4):251–262.

Sur M, Rubenstein JL. (2005). Patterning and plasticity of the cerebral cortex. *Science* 310(5749):805–810.

Szaflarski JP, Holland SK, et al. (2006). fMRI study of language lateralization in children and adults. *Hum Brain Mapp* 27(3):202–212.

Taub E, Wolf SL (1997). Constraint-induced (CI) movement techniques to facilitate upper extremity use in stroke patients. *Topics Stroke Rehab* 3:38–61.

Teuber HL. (1974). Why two brains? In Schmitt FO, Worden F (eds), The Neurosciences: Third Study Program. Cambridge, MA: MIT Press, pp. 71–74.

Teuber HL, Rudel RG (1962). Behaviour after cerebral lesions in children and adults. *Dev Med Child Neurol* 4: 3–20.

Thomas M, Karmiloff-Smith A. (2002). Are developmental disorders like cases of adult brain damage? Implications from connectionist modelling. *Behav Brain Sci* 25(6):727–750; discussion 750–787.

Thomas M, Karmiloff-Smith A. (2005). Can developmental disorders reveal the component parts of the human language faculty? *Language Learning and Development* 1(1):65–92.

Thompson PM, Sowell ER, et al. (2005). Structural MRI and brain development. *Int Rev Neurobiol* 67:285–323.

Tillema J, Byars A, et al. (2008). Cortical reorganization of language functioning following perinatal left MCA stroke. *Brain and Language* 105(2):99–111.

Travis KE, Leonard MK, et al. (2011). Spatiotemporal neural dynamics of word understanding in 12- to 18-month-old-infants. *Cerebral Cortex* 21(8):1832–1839.

Utley, A., Steenbergen, B., & Sugden, D. A. (2004). The influence of object size on discrete bimanual co-ordination in children with hemiplegic cerebral palsy. *Disabil Rehabil, 26*(10), 603–613.

van der Ham IJ, Raemaekers M, et al. (2009). Categorical and coordinate spatial relations in working memory: an fMRI study. *Brain Res* 1297:70–79.

Van Essen DC, Anderson C, et al. (1992). Information processing in the primate visual system: An integrated systems perspective. *Science* 255(5043):419–423.

Vargha-Khadem F, Isaacs E, et al. (1994). A review of cognitive outcome after unilateral lesions sustained during childhood. *J Child Neurol* 9 Suppl 2: 67–73.

Waddington CH. (1939). An Introduction to Modern Genetics. New York: Macmillan.

Westermann G, Mareschal D, et al. (2007). Neuroconstructivism. *Dev Sci* 10(1):75–83.

Westermann G, Thomas MSC, et al. (2011). Neuroconstructivism. In Goswami U (ed), The Wiley-Blackwell Handbook of Childhood Cognitive Development. Chichester, West Sussex: Blackwell Publishing Ltd.

Westlye LT, Walhovd KB, et al. (2010). Life-span changes of the human brain white matter: diffusion tensor imaging (DTI) and volumetry. *Cerebral Cortex* 20(9):2055–2068.

White N, Roddey C, et al. (2010). PROMO: Real-time prospective motion correction in MRI using image-based tracking. *Magnetic Resonance in Medicine* 63(1):91–105.

Wilke M, Staudt M, et al. (2009). Somatosensory system in two types of motor reorganization in congenital hemiparesis: topography and function. *Hum Brain Mapp* 30(3):776–788.

INDEX

Note: Page numbers followed by *f* or *t* indicate figures or tables, respectively.

The manufacturer's authorised representative in the EU for product safety is Oxford University Press España S.A. of El Parque Empresarial San Fernando de Henares, Avenida de Castilla, 2 - 28830 Madrid (www.oup.es/en or product.safety@oup.com). OUP España S.A. also acts as importer into Spain of products made by the manufacturer.
Printed and bound by CPI Group (UK) Ltd, Croydon, CR0 4YY
14/09/2026
02216286-0014